Digital Imaging and Communications in Medicine (DICOM)

Oleg S. Pianykh

Digital Imaging and Communications in Medicine (DICOM)

A Practical Introduction and Survival Guide

Second Edition

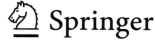

Oleg S. Pianykh, Ph.D.
Harvard Medical School
Beth Israel Deaconess Medical Center
Department of Radiology
Brookline Ave. 330
02215, Boston Massachusetts
USA

ISBN 978-3-642-10849-5   e-ISBN 978-3-642-10850-1
DOI 10.1007/978-3-642-10850-1
Springer Heidelberg Dordrecht London New York
Library of Congress Control Number: 2011939482

© Springer-Verlag Berlin Heidelberg 2012

This work is subject to copyright. All rights are reserved, whether the whole or part of the material is concerned, specifically the rights of translation, reprinting, reuse of illustrations, recitation, broadcasting, reproduction on microfilm or in any other way, and storage in data banks. Duplication of this publication or parts thereof is permitted only under the provisions of the German Copyright Law of September 9, 1965, in its current version, and permission for use must always be obtained from Springer. Violations are liable to prosecution under the German Copyright Law.

The use of general descriptive names, registered names, trademarks, etc. in this publication does not imply, even in the absence of a specific statement, that such names are exempt from the relevant protective laws and regulations and therefore free for general use.

Product liability: The publishers cannot guarantee the accuracy of any information about dosage and application contained in this book. In every individual case the user must check such information by consulting the relevant literature.

Printed on acid-free paper

Springer is part of Springer Science+Business Media (www.springer.com)

To my parents

Preface: DICOM in Radiology

Digital Imaging and Communications in Medicine (DICOM) standard is the backbone of modern image display, equivalent only to film in the pre-digital era. Since the inception of this standard some 20 years ago, it has become the driving force behind the entire imaging workflow. DICOM truly controls all parts of digital image acquisition, transfer, and interpretation, and many radiologists and other imaging specialists and users may not realize to what extent their work relies on DICOM capabilities.

We depend on DICOM extensively. We use DICOM to collect the original medical images. This process is much more complex compared to X-ray film but is also more accurate and complete. We use DICOM to send, distribute, and store images, irrespective of machine, manufacturer, or modality. DICOM controls proper image display, and without DICOM we would not have any image post-processing – whether it is simple multiplanar reconstruction, or more advanced perfusion analysis, virtual colonoscopy, volume segmentation, or computer-aided diagnosis. We owe to DICOM much of the ease and flexibility that we enjoy in our work.

As digital medicine becomes increasingly complex and imaging projects globalize, knowledge of DICOM basics for any healthcare professional becomes crucial. Whether you are thinking about your next PACS upgrade, or a new teleradiology project, or simply about installing a new digital modality, DICOM should be the crucial reference. Standard, DICOM-based workflow is the only way to build a robust and efficient radiology practice. It is also the only way to integrate your medical imaging into a complete enterprise-wide electronic patient record solution.

This book, written from a hands-on angle, gives the healthcare professional a comprehensive introduction to the evolving and multifaceted standard that is DICOM. It may become your daily reference, a teaching guide, or a tool to prepare you for dealing with the intricacies of original DICOM volumes and supplements. Take full advantage of it, and take full advantage of DICOM.

Vassilios Raptopoulos, M.D.
Vice Chair of Clinical Services
Beth Israel Deaconess Medical Center
Professor of Radiology, Harvard Medical School

Preface: DICOM in Healthcare IT

Unlike healthcare standards such as HL7, the DICOM standard is not as well known or understood by IT professionals. On one hand, DICOM stands and delivers on the promise of interoperability and cost effectiveness. On the other hand, it requires some tweaking to work. DICOM planning and implementation errors are common, often resulting in operational nightmares. Given that digital medicine and PACS require a substantial investment and are critical, getting the DICOM part right up front is essential.

Frequently overlooked is the impact of DICOM and PACS on the actual patient. DICOM drives clinical workflow from the moment a patient enters Radiology, collecting important imaging data from the digital modality and delivering it to the radiologist in the most accurate and diagnostically complete form within minutes. Comparing previous studies with the current study is effortless with DICOM, resulting in more skillful diagnosis and treatment. No film to lose, misplace, under- or overexpose, and fewer repeated studies – all add up to faster and vastly improved healthcare. DICOM is beneficial to the patient, provider, and the facility; and IT professionals owe it to them to get it right. The importance of DICOM as a working, integral part of the IT infrastructure will continue to expand. The number of present and available DICOM and PACS applications is staggering. Selecting the PACS right for you becomes more challenging with each passing year and a good understanding of DICOM is now essential.

Without a basic and practical understanding of DICOM you risk making embarrassing mistakes in such areas as security, equipment specification, capacity planning, network configuration, and disaster recovery/continuity of operations.

The built-in security of DICOM is not going to be adequate to address HIPAA requirements and will need to be augmented. The various modalities have different image resolutions, which affect choice of viewing monitors. DICOM supports several image compression technologies. The tradeoff between image sizing and quality will affect equipment sizing and network bandwidth requirements. The DICOM connectivity model is still very much static IP centric. Remote access through VPN needs to be carefully planned. The complexity and interactions of all of the above are interrelated and can make upgrades difficult. The aspect of disaster recovery and continuity of operations emerge as so technically challenging that they are frequently ignored. The practical way of dealing with these issues begins with an understanding of DICOM.

In the following pages you will not have to wade and sift through volumes of technical specifications to get the knowledge you need. Consider it your one-stop-shopping experience for a good understanding of DICOM.

New Orleans, LA

David Troendle
Assistant Vice Chancellor
for Information Technology
LSU Health Sciences Center

Who Needs This Book?

If you are involved in any form of medical work, decision making, image analysis, or research and development, this book is for you. As "digital" spreads even into the most veiled areas of contemporary medicine, understanding DICOM becomes increasingly imperative for ensuring accuracy, efficiency, and reliability of any medical application or process. DICOM is an extremely powerful tool when you can harness its power. But it could just as easily be the doom of an ill-planned project. Helping you learn DICOM was the principal reason for writing this book.

A lesser, but no less important, reason was the sheer repetitiveness of DICOM problems that I learned to deal with personally as a medical IT administrator, researcher, and developer. To a great extent this book has evolved from my personal "DICOM diary," which I started writing to record the problems and the solutions of my countless experiences. A seemingly inexhaustible list of DICOM-related questions is inevitably asked wherever digital medicine is practiced; and many practitioners continue to fall into numerous DICOM traps as they attempt to bring new equipment and applications online. Although it would be too ambitious on my part to protect you from all possible DICOM traps, together we will try to identify and avoid the most common ones.

Finally, DICOM – being a very complex and evolving standard – is not exactly fun to read. On the other hand, many popular overviews tend to be sketchy and introductory. In this book, I try to help you navigate between the Scylla and Charybdis of *simple to understand* and *important to know*. Do not expect the journey to be easy, but rest assured that it will be rewarding. You will become familiar with the principal DICOM concepts and terminology; you will see how they fit together; and you will gain sufficient knowledge to start dealing with DICOM in all its complexity. Your next best resource after reading this book is the DICOM standard itself – then you will be prepared for the rest of your own DICOM Odyssey.

I hope that this educational foray will be entertaining, informative, and will change the way you look at your work. So let's go!

Acknowledgments

Knowledge is always shared, and many things I described in this book I learned with the help of others. It was my pleasure to work with many radiologists, researchers, computer scientists, technicians, engineers, and students – listing all of their names would be virtually impossible. I would like to thank all of them for their time and patience. I would also like to thank:
- My dear, wonderful family.
- The faculty and students of Harvard Medical School, BIDMC Radiology, and LSUHSC Radiology, from whom I learned so much.
- The countless clients I worked with.
- David Troendle, for his very valuable comments and discussions on this book; Oliver Lenhart, for his helpful suggestions; John Tyler, for his lessons.
- Roger Cote for turning this book into something that not only the author can understand.
- You, my dear readers, for taking the time. Your feedback will be very helpful, and you can always reach me at opiany@gmail.com.

  I hope this book will make your work easier and your goals higher.

New Orleans, USA–
Moscow, Russia–
Boston, USA

Best regards
Oleg Pianykh

Contents

Part I Introduction to DICOM

1. What Is DICOM? 3
2. How Does DICOM Work? 7
3. Where Do You Get DICOM from? 11
   3.1 DICOM Versus Digital 11
   3.2 DICOM, DICOM-Compatible, DICOM-Ready? 13
   3.3 In the Middle of Nowhere 14

Part II DICOM and Clinical Data

4. Brief History of DICOM 19
   4.1 How Did This All Get Started? 21
5. Parlez-vous DICOM? 27
   5.1 IT Boot Camp 27
   5.2 Text Versus Binary 29
   5.3 DICOM Grammar: VRs 31
        5.3.1   VR Length 36
        5.3.2   Characters: Foreign and Wild 37
        5.3.3   Text VRs: CS, SH, LO, ST, LT, UT 38
        5.3.4   Dates and Times: DA, TM, DT, AS 38
        5.3.5   Numbers in Text Format: IS, DS 39
        5.3.6   Numbers in Binary Format: SS, US,
                SL, UL, FL, FD, OB, OW, OF, AT 39
        5.3.7   PN – Storing Person's Names 40
        5.3.8   AE – Naming Application Entities 41
        5.3.9   UI – Unique Identifiers 41
        5.3.10 SQ – Sequencing Data Sets 41
        5.3.11 UN – Representing Unknown Values 43
   5.4 DICOM Data Dictionary 43
        5.4.1   Standard DICOM Data Dictionary 43

		5.4.2 Private DICOM Data Dictionaries.......................... 47
		5.4.3 Standard DICOM Command Dictionary................... 47
	5.5 DICOM Objects.. 48
		5.5.1 Encoding Data Elements...................................... 49
		5.5.2 Encoding Data Groups... 53
		5.5.3 Example: Element and Group Lengths 55
		5.5.4 Encoding DICOM Data Objects 56
		5.5.5 SQ: Encoding DICOM Object Sequences................. 57
		5.5.6 Required and Optional Data Elements 62
		5.5.7 Storing Image Data 62
		5.5.8 Unique Identifiers 64
	5.6 DICOM Information Hierarchy................................... 66
		5.6.1 Problems with Patient ID..................................... 68
		5.6.2 Problems with Study, Series, and Image UIDs 70
		5.6.3 Hierarchical and Relational Data........................... 71
	5.7 Modules, IODs and IEs 71
		5.7.1 Attribute Macros: Making It Easier........................ 72
		5.7.2 Information Modules: Basic Data Blocks 73
		5.7.3 Information Entities... 77
		5.7.4 DICOM Information Objects................................ 77
		5.7.5 IODS and Their Instances 77
		5.7.6 Learning More... 80

6   **Medical Images in DICOM** 81
	6.1 DICOM Bitmaps 82
	6.2 Image Compression... 86
		6.2.1 Lossless Compression 88
		6.2.2 Lossy Compression 88
		6.2.3 Streaming Compression...................................... 91
		6.2.4 Choosing the Right Compression Technique.................. 93
	6.3 Working with Digital Medical Images.......................... 97
		6.3.1 Image Interpolation 97
		6.3.2 Image Reconstructions.. 100
		6.3.3 Grayscale Depth.. 102
		6.3.4 Waveforms... 107
		6.3.5 Overlays.. 108
		6.3.6 Supporting True Video in DICOM 111

Part III   DICOM Communications

7   **DICOM SOPs: Basic**... 117
	7.1 Identifying Units on the DICOM Network 118
	7.2 Services and Data 121
		7.2.1 DIMSE Services 122
		7.2.2 Simple DIMSE Example: C-Echo........................... 124

    19.2.10 Do You Have Full-Fidelity DICOM? 389
    19.2.11 Do You Have Free DICOM? 389

Appendix 391

References 411

Index 413

Part I
Introduction to DICOM

What Is DICOM? 1

> *When working toward the solution of a problem,*
> *it always helps if you know the answer*
>
> – *Murphy's Law*

You can walk with this question into most modern, digital, state-of-the-art hospitals and spend hours looking for someone who could answer it correctly. We all get used to buzz words and acronyms, and rarely think about their meanings. Unfortunately, nothing distances you more from success than not knowing what you are dealing with!

DICOM stands for *Digital Imaging and COmmunications in Medicine* and represents years of effort to create the most universal and fundamental standard in digital medical imaging. As such, it provides all the necessary tools for diagnostically accurate representation and processing of medical imaging data. Moreover, contrary to popular belief, DICOM *is not just an image or file format*. It is an all-encompassing data transfer, storage and display protocol built and designed to cover all functional aspects of contemporary medicine (which is why many view DICOM as a *set* of standards, rather than a single standard). Without a doubt, DICOM truly governs practical digital medicine.

Another important acronym that seemingly all DICOM vendors plug into their names is PACS (*Picture Archiving and Communication Systems*). PACS are medical systems (consisting of necessary hardware and software) built to run digital medical imaging. They comprise:
1. *Modalities*: Digital image acquisition devices, such as CT scanners or ultrasound.
2. *Digital image archives*: Where the acquired images are stored.
3. *Workstations*: Where radiologists view ("read") the images.

When you play with your digital camera (modality), store the images on your computer (archive), and send them to your friends (reviewers), you use the exact same model (Fig. 1.1).

PACS are directly related to DICOM: they are the standard incarnate. Their functionality is DICOM-driven, which guarantees their interoperability. However, each DICOM unit has its own purpose, implementing only a subset of DICOM required for the task. For that reason, any PACS device or software comes with its own

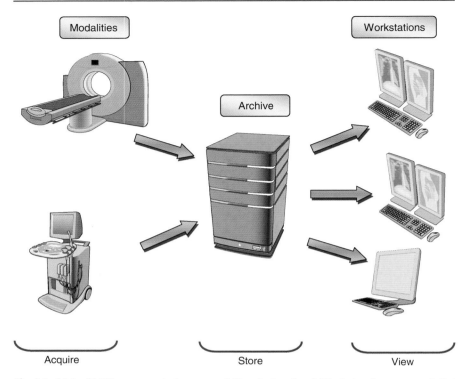

Fig. 1.1 Major PACS components: image acquisition devices (modalities) store images on a digital archive. From there images are accessed by radiologists at the viewing workstations

DICOM Conformance Statement – a very important document explaining the extent to which the device supports the DICOM standard.[1] In this way, a digital CT scanner uses DICOM to acquire and distribute computed tomography images; a DICOM printer to print; a DICOM archive to store and query DICOM data; and so on.

One can hardly imagine modern digital medicine without DICOM and PACS. The DICOM standard – conceived over 20 years ago – plays an integral role in the digital medicine evolution, ensuring the highest diagnostic standards and the best performance. DICOM truly shaped the landscape of contemporary medicine by providing:
1. *Universal standard of digital medicine*. All current digital image acquisition devices produce DICOM images and communicate through DICOM networks. Modern medical workflow is implicitly controlled by a multitude of DICOM rules, which we will review in this book.

---

[1]PS3.2 part of DICOM standard covers conformance statements, and provides a detailed conformance statement template (Appendix) with samples.

2. *Excellent image quality.* Just to give you an example, DICOM supports up to 65,536 (16 bits) shades of gray for monochrome image display, thus capturing the slightest nuances in medical imaging. In comparison, converting DICOM images into JPEGs or bitmaps (limited to 256 shades of gray) often renders the images unacceptable for diagnostic reading. DICOM takes advantage of the most current and advanced digital image representation techniques to provide the utmost diagnostic image quality.
3. *Full support for numerous image-acquisition parameters and different data types.* Not only does DICOM store the images, it also records a legion of other image-related parameters such as patient 3D position, sizes and orientations, slice thickness, radiation doses and exposures, image processing filters, and so on. This data immensely enriches the informational content of DICOM images, and facilitates processing and interpreting the image data in various ways (for example, creating 3D images from several sequences of 2D CT slices).
4. *Complete encoding of medical data.* DICOM files and messages use more than 2000 standardized attributes (defined in the *DICOM Data Dictionary*) to convey various medical data from patient name to image color depth to current patient diagnosis. Often essential for accurate diagnostics, the data captures all aspects of the current radiology.
5. *Clarity in describing digital imaging devices and their functionality – the backbone of any medical imaging project.* DICOM defines medical device functionality in very precise and device-independent terms. Working with medical devices through their DICOM interfaces becomes a straightforward, predictable process leaving little room for errors.

At the time this book was written, the DICOM standard consisted of 16 volumes (from 1 to 18, volumes 9 and 13 being retired) known as parts, and traditionally numbered from PS3.1 to PS3.18.[2] We used the last publicly available revision of the standard, performed in 2009.[3]

---

[2] Number 3 representing DICOM 3.0, the current version of the standard.
[3] See DICOM home page at NEMA's web site, http://medical.nema.org.

How Does DICOM Work?

2

> *Everything in life is important, important things are simple,*
> *simple things are never easy*
>
> *– Murphy's Law*

To introduce order into the complex medical environment, DICOM uses its own lingo, based on its model of the real world (*DICOM information model*). Here is that model in a nutshell.

All real-world data – patients, studies, medical devices, and so on – are viewed by DICOM as objects with respective properties or *attributes*.[1] The definitions of these objects and attributes are standardized according to DICOM *Information Object Definitions* (IODs). Think about IODs as collections of attributes, describing IOD properties. A *Patient IOD*, for example, can be described by patient name, ID, sex, age, weight, smoking status, and so on – as many attributes as needed to capture all clinically relevant patient information. As the famous "philosopher" Popeye was fond of saying: "I ams what I ams and that's all that I ams." Bearing that wisdom in mind, a patient (just like any other DICOM object) *is* the set of attributes of which he consists, as you can see in Fig. 2.1. DICOM maintains a list of all standard attributes (more than 2,000 of them), known as the *DICOM Data Dictionary*, to ensure consistency in attribute naming, formatting, and processing. For example, our patient attributes – name, date of birth, sex, and so on – are included in the DICOM Data Dictionary as well. All DICOM attributes are formatted according to 27 *Value Representation (VR)* types which include dates, times, names, identifiers, and so on.

As soon as the data is captured as DICOM data attributes, it can be transmitted and processed between various DICOM devices and software – known as *Application Entities (AEs)* in DICOM. DICOM represents this processing with a service-rendering model: Application Entities *provide services* to each other (Fig. 2.2).

Because each service usually involves some data exchange (typically performed over a computer network) it becomes natural to associate particular

---

[1] If you have an IT background, you will certainly recognize object-oriented design.

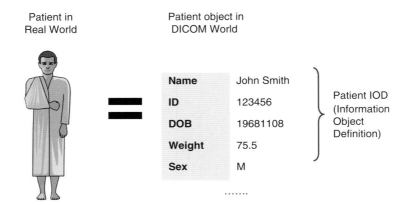

Fig. 2.1 From real data to DICOM IODs. Each IOD is a collection of attributes

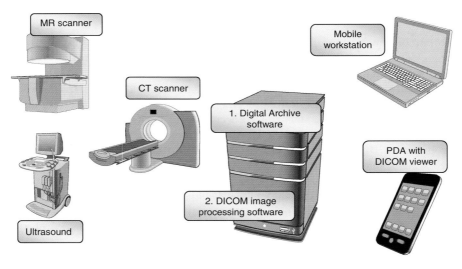

Fig. 2.2 DICOM Application Entities. Note that Application Entities can be programs, so multiple AEs can be running on the same device, as shown for the archive server

service types with the data (IODs) that they process. DICOM calls these associations *Service-Object Pairs* (SOPs), and groups them into *SOP Classes*. For example, storing a computed tomography (CT) image from a digital CT scanner to a digital PACS archive corresponds to the CT Storage Service-Object Pair (SOP), as shown in Fig. 2.3.

In this particular example, the CT image represents the DICOM Information Object Definition (Computer Tomography IOD). The CT scanner *requests the CT*

2 How Does DICOM Work?

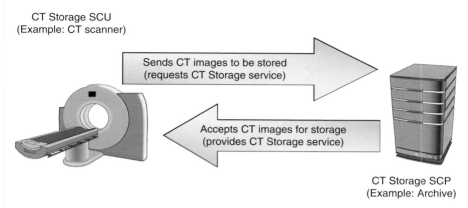

Fig. 2.3 DICOM services

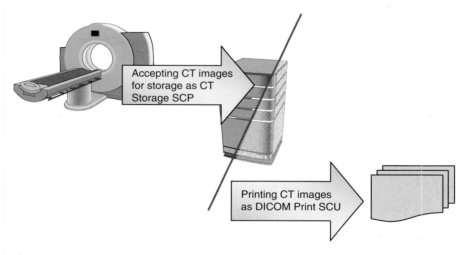

Fig. 2.4 Different SCP and SCU processing on the same AE

storage service from the archive, and the archive *provides the CT storage service* to the scanner. Therefore, DICOM calls the service requestors *Service Class Users* (SCUs) and the service providers *Service Class Providers* (SCPs). In the same CT example, the CT scanner acts as the CT Storage Service Class User (SCU), and the digital archive as the CT Storage Service Class Provider (SCP). Everything is relative, and SCU/SCP roles may change depending on the processing logic. Imagine that the same digital archive needs some of its images to be printed on a DICOM printer. In this case, the archive acts as an SCU and the printer as an SCP (Fig. 2.4).

Each data exchange between SCU and SCP peers is called *association*. Consequently, each network transfer begins with *Association Establishment* – the DICOM handshake-used when the two connecting applications exchange information about each other. This information is called *Presentation Contexts*. If the two applications can match their contexts, they can connect and start SCU-SCP processing. In our example in Fig. 2.3, the CT scanner will open association to the Archive with CT image storage presentation context. The Archive will check its current settings – which may include storing different types of images such as MR or X-rays – and if CTs are among them, it will accept the scanner association.

Because hundreds of DICOM devices and applications are produced by hundreds of DICOM manufacturers, each DICOM unit will be accompanied by its own *DICOM Conformance Statement*. This statement explains which SOPs (services) the unit supports, and to what extent (SCU, SCP, or both) it supports them. The DICOM Conformance Statement is your most essential planning guide for any DICOM-related project. Obtain it from the manufacturer ahead of time and read it carefully. For example, if you buy a digital archive that supports CT Storage SCU only (does *not* support CT Storage SCP), you won't be able to store CT images in it. The archive won't be able to *provide* the CT storage *service*.

This brief summary reflects the core DICOM functionality, and as you can see, it is quite straightforward. In fact, understanding the theory of DICOM is easy; dealing with DICOM in real life is often the challenge. Most of this book is committed to helping you meet that challenge.

Where Do You Get DICOM from? 3

If anything can go wrong, it will

– Murphy's Law

The DICOM standard is free and can be found on the official DICOM website (http://medical.nema.org) maintained by the National Electrical Manufacturers Association (NEMA). However, from a practical perspective, you usually deal with DICOM implementations in *devices and software*. Currently, hundreds of these products are on the market constantly transforming and vying for your attention. This natural selection, however, only adds another layer of commonly misunderstood and confusing concepts to the original complexity of the DICOM standard.

Moreover, the question "Are you completely DICOM-compatible?" can never be answered with a simple Yes or No. In fact, this question is simply inaccurate. All DICOM devices and software support *only specific parts* of the DICOM standard required for their functionality. As a result of this selectiveness, implementing a DICOM workflow that is *completely* DICOM-compatible is tricky business, making it one of the most critical and treacherous phases in organizing any medical imaging practice. So, just how do you introduce DICOM into your practice and what should you avoid? Well, let's start with the basics.

3.1 DICOM Versus Digital

Like all human beings, we perceive the world around us in *analog mode* – that is, as continuous shapes and shades. Computers on the other hand function in *digital mode* – they store and process images pixel-by-pixel, number-by-number. DICOM, as its very name suggests, also deals only with digital images. Digital images can be acquired in this manner (computed tomography being an example), or digitized from analog (consider scanned patient reports). In any case, acquiring or converting images into digital format is the very first step required for any DICOM implementation.

All contemporary image-acquisition modalities provide digital image output. Such modalities include computed tomography (CT), magnetic resonance (MR), ultrasound (US), nuclear medicine (NM), and more. By their nature, some of these devices have always acquired images digitally; others were complemented with digitizing circuits as technology progressed.

The problem, however, is that *while DICOM implies digital, digital does not guarantee DICOM*. You could very well purchase a digital medical imaging device that has no DICOM support whatsoever. You are not making DICOM images with your point-and-shoot camera, are you?

How would you know if you can use DICOM with your medical imaging device?

It is easy: as I already mentioned, any DICOM device should come with a DICOM Conformance Statement.[1] The Conformance Statement, in many cases, is more important than the device's user manual and should be supplied by the device manufacturer to outline the DICOM functions supported by the device. For this very reason, the statement should leave no room for errors or false assumptions about the device's functionality.

You should be conjuring the guardian spirits of DICOM Conformance Statements any time you plan or perform any DICOM-related installation. *Always ask for it, and always make sure that you have the correct version for your model.* Even the same device or software can come in a variety of revisions, and your Conformance Statement should correspond to the version that you are using. Upgrade wisely!

Blame It on the New Guys?

Keeping up with DICOM upgrades can be an expensive and workflow-critical proposition. I know of a hospital that used to have a nice DICOM printer from a well-known company – I'll call them A – that was set up to print CT images from a DICOM-compatible scanner, produced by another well-known company – I'll refer to as B. When the scanner aged enough to go up in smoke (literally), B replaced it with a brand new model; only to discover that it could not print to A's printer. Did I forget to mention that *all* devices were *DICOM-compliant*?

So the hospital IT staff contacted A and the printer company recognized that the printer software version was old (circa Windows NT) and had eminent bugs. They said that it was no longer supported and beyond repair; the only solution was an upgrade – for a *reasonable* fee of course.

What did the hospital IT do? Complained to B for breaking their DICOM network, and got a new DICOM printer from them – *for free*. The moral of the story? When you run out of money, just learn to be more ... um ... *creative*.

---

[1] Sorry for beating you over the head with countless references to these documents; you will see them again and again as we continue. But because they are so important in any DICOM project, I implore you to forgive me for the browbeating.

3.2 DICOM, DICOM-Compatible, DICOM-Ready?

Let's say that you have identified your imaging needs and you are ready to purchase a DICOM unit. Is there anything you need to know *before* writing that check? Definitely.

Buying a DICOM-compatible device or software application is like having dinner in an expensive restaurant. Your device manufacturer presents you with a wonderful entrée (the device), and the option to add a fancy decadent dessert (the entire DICOM functionality). Perhaps, to save on your budgetary diet, you think about passing on dessert. Many clinical practitioners have committed this very mistake: skipping what is presented as optional to save a little and not ordering what they really should have – and found themselves eating crow in the end.

You might ask: "Why should we pay for DICOM functionality as an additional DICOM device option when having a DICOM device without DICOM is nearly meaningless?"

Well, it might be meaningless *to you*, but it surely is not meaningless to the device manufacturers. To better comprehend this paradox, let's recall what we learned in the previous section.

All current, medical image-acquisition devices are digital, which does not necessarily mean that they inherently provide DICOM functionality.

Device manufacturers can implement their own *proprietary* protocols for digital image acquisition, storage, and display. Those manufacturer-dependent protocols will suffice to allow the device to operate as a standalone unit, or possibly connected to other units *from the same manufacturer*. In other words, the device will work as expected, but only inside its little proprietary shell. When manufacturers use proprietary protocols, it results in convenience and clever marketing – for them. Convenience, because the manufacturers can do anything they want to implement the device functionality internally – they are not limited by any standard or any particular requirement. Marketing, because proprietary standards make you dependent on your manufacturer – you simply cannot connect to another vendor's equipment or software.

This might sound like just another conspiracy theory, but pragmatically any proprietary format inevitably segments the medical device market. We will discuss this in more detail toward the end of the book (see Chap. 12). The bottom line is that in many cases, *you must explicitly purchase device DICOM functionality as an option* (in addition to the DICOM device purchase itself). If you do not purchase the DICOM functionality option, you end up with what some manufacturers label as a "DICOM-Ready" device – a device that *could have been* running DICOM, if you *had paid* for it.

Another way of looking at this problem is to realize that, in its very essence, DICOM is a device-interfacing standard. It connects the devices externally, but it is not meant to drive them internally. DICOM provides a standard for device output (which also ensures that various devices can be connected to each other). When you purchase a DICOM option, you pay for this conversion, you pay for uniformity, and you pay for the ability to export and process device data in the standard format.

If you are serious about your medical imaging workflow, all DICOM *options* on your manufacturer's price list should be treated as mandatory.

What should you do if any of these options are missing? Heed these words of wisdom: despite the urgency and possible sense of guilt, *never attempt to fix this problem yourself*. If you have a *DICOM-Ready* device that is lacking DICOM options, the only way to remedy the problem is to contact the device manufacturer. Resolving all DICOM issues with the manufacturer should become your standard approach under any circumstance. Not only does it deliver the best functional solution (even if you have to pay for it), but it also preserves the device warranty and ensures that no harm will be done to the unit.

A similar DICOM-compatibility problem can arise with an old imaging unit. As you will see in Chap. 4, the DICOM standard has been around for a long time and has evolved considerably. As DICOM devices age, they need to be updated with current DICOM software from their manufacturers. In general, this is the same approach I just described with one new catch: the original device manufacturers might not exist anymore. If this is the situation, you will more than likely have one of the following choices:

1. Your original DICOM unit manufacturer was purchased by another, which will help you with the unit support.
2. Your original DICOM unit manufacturer went out of business. In this case, the unit support may have been transferred to another DICOM provider. Many discontinued DICOM units from out-of-business companies are still sold refurbished and supported by other manufacturers.

Rule of thumb: digital medical devices that are more than 10 years old should be replaced. In addition to advances in the DICOM standard, the entire digital medicine technology has made great strides. After a certain age, older units not only start looking primitive, they also lack many features and functions – some of which are standard with current technology. When this becomes the case, do not keep patching these dinosaurs; you will do much better replacing them with contemporary models.

3.3 In the Middle of Nowhere

There remains one more common case of providing DICOM functionality: medical devices that were never meant to support the DICOM standard. Despite the rapid progress in digital medicine technology, and the growing *DICOMization* of the medical imaging workflow, *DICOM-free* units are still numerous and can come from several sources:

1. Digital medical devices manufactured with no DICOM interface: film scanners, digital microscopes.
2. Generic nonmedical devices (digital or analog).
3. Analog medical devices with no digital output: analog X-rays and more.
4. Old, pre-DICOM medical devices: old CTs, MRs, etc.

3.3 In the Middle of Nowhere

The last case of pre-DICOM units is the least interesting and will be discussed in the following chapter on DICOM history. In general, if your device is older than DICOM (which is quite old in itself) you have a no-brainer: replace the device.

The first case on our list is much more typical: contemporary digital medical imaging devices (such as many popular film digitizers) that were never meant to have a DICOM interface. This usually happens when device manufacturers want to keep their distance from the medical imaging domain; either because the manufacturer works in other areas/markets, or because it considers medical imaging too complex and troublesome for a stronger commitment. For example, if a CT scanner must be DICOM-compliant, a simple flatbed scanner used elsewhere might not.

The problem with digital non-DICOM devices is bigger than their lack of DICOM output. They simply do not fit well into the clinical workflow. For example, each DICOM image must contain patient name and ID tags – indispensably important for accurate image routing and identification. If you have a film digitizer that scans films into plain, non-DICOM digital image formats (such as bitmaps), tagging them with patient or study information is simply impossible. Non-DICOM image formats cannot support DICOM tags. Diagnostic image quality (excellent in DICOM and greatly varying in conventional image formats) is another issue. While DICOM modalities store all clinical data automatically in DICOM image tags, their less-advanced and more generic non-DICOM counterparts require human assistance, which inevitably leads to data entry errors and lost time.

> **Creative Thinking**
> One high-profile hospital, where I was making rare consulting appearances, was particularly famous for two things: a lack of PACS and an abundance of clinical IT personnel. The latter kept claiming that one day they will develop their own digital system. After many years of flowcharts and spreadsheets, they indeed came up with their own "PACS solution" – a $100 scanner.
> The scanner – a bold answer to the overcharging PACS industry – was plugged into the hospital network, and contained the following set of instructions:
> 1. Keep printing on film
> 2. Scan film into the system using the scanner
> 3. Saved scanned files on the computer
> 4. Name scanned files with patient name and IDs – something like JohnSmith_ID12345.bmp
>
> Please do not do this. Just do not. Please.

With all this in mind, if you still want to buy a digital medical device with no DICOM interface, at least take the following precautions:
1. Try to buy from a DICOM manufacturer, which might resell the device with its own DICOM interface.
2. Do not make a non-DICOM device a centerpiece of your clinical workflow.

The same logic applies to using generic, nonmedical devices (digital or not). For example, many dermatologists would like to use off-the-shelf digital cameras to record images of their patients' skin patterns, infections, and other conditions (which makes perfect sense clinically). Clearly, off-the-shelf digital cameras have no DICOM functionality whatsoever, and likely never will. Therefore, if you want to incorporate those images into your PACS or medical imaging workflow in general, you face the same problem of DICOM conversion and image identification. Because those devices were never meant to be medical, your chances of getting any DICOM assistance from their manufacturers are beyond slim. Instead, look for image importing options in your existing DICOM/PACS software. Many current DICOM workstations and file viewers offer various options for DICOM import, enabling you to convert a plain, conventional digital image (bitmap, JPEG, and such) into a standard DICOM file. Once again, you will have to manually enter the missing information (patient name, ID, study date, and so on), but you will be rewarded with the ability to include this image into your clinical all-digital cycle. In a more general sense, the same approach works for any non-DICOM data, wherever it might come from.

Finally, many medical devices are still analog and could stay analog for some time (for example, nonimaging units such as ECG, or even certain modalities such as ultrasound are sometimes not equipped with digital interfaces.) As we know, a device must be digital to be DICOM. Therefore, analog images must be digitized: still images can be converted into digital format and video can be broken into digital image frames. The task of digitization and DICOM conversion is commonly performed with *DICOM converters* – small box-like devices capable of converting analog images, video, and cine loops into digital, DICOM-compliant images. Moreover, DICOM converters can often interface with standard hospital information systems (to obtain patient data instead of relying on error-prone manual entry) and can send converted images to PACS and other DICOM devices, thus supporting DICOM networking in addition to plain image conversion. DICOM converters are primarily marketed for legacy analog imaging systems, but will do the job with any analog imaging device in general. Another good thing about them, some DICOM converters are actually smart enough to work with certain proprietary imaging formats from the main medical producers and can convert those formats to work with DICOM as well. In addition to DICOM converters, more and more current DICOM/PACS products offer advanced image export options, accommodating at least digital (but non-DICOM-compliant) images.

To conclude, it is still very possible to create a DICOM workflow from generic, somewhat crude, and non-DICOM-compliant imaging devices. Nevertheless, as I have mentioned, image quality and bookkeeping can be problematic. And the need for human interaction makes such solutions slower and more error-prone. Therefore, making DICOM out of nothing is more appropriate for low-volume, marginal imaging solutions, or as a temporary solution in the midst of your transition from a legacy system to a contemporary PACS. However, steady, *industrial* medical imaging workflow definitely needs to be based on 100% DICOM-compliant devices.

Part II
DICOM and Clinical Data

Whatever you need to accomplish in a medical workflow, you will face one of two principal tasks: *collecting* clinical data or *processing* clinical data. DICOM was designed to assist you with both in a consistent, clinically-sound manner. To eliminate ambiguity in data interpretation, the standard uses a formal set of rules for representing and encoding data. This part of the book introduces you to these rules.

In many ways, this might sound like an introduction to a foreign language spoken by bulb-eyed robots from planet DICOM. This language might not sound pretty to the human ear, but it definitely serves the purpose of making many DICOM conversations easier. Its longevity has become the best proof of its value: despite all the *Sturm und Drang* changes that the medical and computer industries have experienced since the inception of DICOM in the mid-1980s, it is still spoken and – with occasional updates to the vocabulary – will be spoken for many years to come.

Knowing the basics of DICOM lingo is indispensable for any human venturing into the DICOM world – the bulb-eyed robots may get moody. As with any language, DICOM learning begins with an introduction to its dictionary and its grammar.

Brief History of DICOM

4

Every solution breeds new problems

– Murphy's Law

Because the DICOM standard is some 30 years old, its history has become an integral part of its being; and knowing DICOM's past can help answer many current questions. Moreover, despite having undergone frequent revisions, the standard has never truly been revolutionized. It has continually evolved, adjusting itself to current practices, yet preserving many original historical features.

The natural process of DICOM device manufacturing, selling, upgrading, and using spans many years[1]; modalities are expensive, and hospital administrators are typically conservative and budget-conscious, trying to get the most out of equipment – sometimes even to the point of keeping things until they fall apart. Should I also mention all discontinued, refurbished, and simply old units that many practices still purchase as the most affordable alternatives? This creates an environment in which drastic updates are not really welcome, and compatibility with older equipment (and, consequently, older DICOM) becomes a must.

How Old Is *Your* Computer?
If you still believe in quick technology upgrades, consider Table 4.1. It shows web site attendance statistics, collected for a private DICOM vendor in 2011 – thus representing a fairly objective sample of users interested in DICOM products. Who would expect Windows XP (released in 2001) to be on top? And in this age of mobile gadgets, who would imagine Windows NT 4.0 (released in 1996) would make a stunningly triumphant run over Android and Mobile?

---

[1]According to the 2011 CapSite report on PACS replacement (www.capsite.com), 52% of PACS in US hospitals are more than 5 years old – quite an age in this fast-changing field.

While manufacturers take time improving their products, users take even longer to embrace these improvements. The result: manufacturers forcing their users to upgrade. Let's look at a good example in the common world: the Microsoft Internet Explorer 6 countdown project (ie6countdown.com), proactively suggesting that its users abandon the old IE6 browser for much newer versions. Looking at a better example from my own experience: when we informed one PACS company that we were still running an old version of their software, their hilarious response about their own product was: "Are you still using this old crap?"

We laughed: only a year before the same guys sold us the "crap" as "a new revolutionary product." Viva la revolution!

Table 4.1 DICOM web site users by their operating system

Operating system	Percentage
Windows XP	49.04
Windows Vista	17.17
OS X	15.79
Windows 7	12.67
Linux	2.66
Windows NT 4.0	0.73
Windows 2000	0.64
Windows 98	0.64
Mobile	0.28
Windows 2003	0.18
Android	0.09
Windows 32	0.09

The standard itself adds another layer of complexity – even the pure task of DICOM maintenance requires Herculean efforts, due to many tiny, crisscrossed details and plain subjectivities involved in resolving most of them. It is not easy to keep all DICOM vendors, users, and workgroups equally happy – in fact, it is just impossible. As David Clunie pointed out in his DICOM blog (www.dclunie.com), "If we ever had the chance to start DICOM all over again and 'do it right,' I am sure that despite our best intentions we would still manage to screw it up in equally egregious ways." So despite the best intentions, do not be surprised to trip over DICOM's "egregious ways" in your own practice.

In brief, if you work in the current, multifaceted clinical environment you will have to work with multi-generation equipment (DICOM-compliant and not), and you are bound to make occasional *archeological* discoveries, and find yourself dealing with many layers of DICOM history.

4.1 How Did This All Get Started?

> **Data** = [data element 1] + [data element 2] + ... + [data element N]
>
> *Example:*
>
> **Patient** = [Name] + [Age] + [Weight] +...+ [Sex]

Fig. 4.1 Breaking data into data elements

4.1 How Did This All Get Started?

The standard was conceived in 1983 by a joint committee formed by the American College of Radiology (ACR), and the National Electrical Manufacturers Association (NEMA).[2] The primary goal was to develop a standard that would make digital medical imaging independent of particular device manufacturers, thus facilitating the expansion of digital imaging and PACS. If we look at a number of other industries currently struggling with compliance issues, we should admire the foresight of those who reflected upon the structure of digital medical applications long before the spread of contemporary computers and networks.

The joint committee – named ACR-NEMA Digital Imaging and Communications Standards Committee – began its work by reviewing many other standards established at that time. Although the committee found nothing specifically fitting for its needs (Horill), it did glean a few valuable hints from the study. The American Association of Physicists in Medicine (AAPM) had recently adopted a standard for recording images on magnetic tape. AAPM took the approach of encoding all information as sequences of *data elements;* each element could have a variable length (size) and was identified by its unique name (tag). The idea of representing the data as a sequence of tagged data elements was adopted by the ACR-NEMA group. If you have any experience with HTML, or better yet XML, you should immediately recognize the same approach in those very current and popular standards. The concept of using data elements as small building blocks to represent data of any complexity has proven to be extremely useful and robust (Fig. 4.1).

The first version of the standard – called ACR-NEMA 300-1985 or ACR-NEMA 1.0 – was published in 1985 and distributed at the Radiological Society of North America (RSNA) annual meeting. Officially, the original ACR-NEMA standard was proposed as a guideline and NEMA did not assume any responsibility for its

---

[2] Part PS3.1 of DICOM standard includes a brief historical overview of DICOM.

enforcement or interpretation.[3] But the objectives for standardization were well set and well needed. Compliance with the standard has become the de facto imperative for the medical community.

As with any first version, ACR-NEMA 1.0 contained errors and imperfections. It was soon realized that the standard required further work with continuous effort and better structure. For these reasons, ACR-NEMA embraced the idea of Working Groups (WG), which are separate subcommittees dedicated to improving specific parts of the growing standard. The first WG VI (currently known as WG-06, Base Standard) was created to work on improving ACR-NEMA 1.0. The result of this work was the second revised version – ACR-NEMA 2.0 (or ACR-NEMA 300-1988) – released in 1988. The revised version was sturdy enough to be adopted by the medical device manufacturers, and slowly but surely it started to work its way into medical device interfaces. Even today, you can still find an old CT scanner or digital archive running ACR-NEMA 2.0. The basic compatibility with the current DICOM standard still keeps ACR-NEMA 2.0 afloat, no matter how obsolete it has become.

ACR-NEMA 2.0 could have ruled the medical world for much longer had it not been for computer networks. ACR-NEMA 2.0's ability to communicate medical data between devices was extremely limited. For example, a user could send an image to a remote device, but the standard did not specify what the device should do with the image. Such functional gaps, along with the emergence and rapid spread of networking technology in the late 1980s, demanded more than a simple standard patchwork; they called for another major revision.

Another issue mandating a major revision was the need to accommodate the increasing variety of digital devices and their communications protocols. Not only did these devices need a new and more abstract way of looking at the digital information workflow, they also required a solid information model for digital medicine.

In response to these changing needs, a third version of the ACR-NEMA standard was created and showcased at RSNA in 1992 in its most basic, prototypical form. The following year was spent in monthly Working Group meetings. The first nine parts of the new ACR-NEMA standard were completed by September 1993 and presented at RSNA 1993 in a much more functional form. The revamped standard was called ACR-NEMA DICOM (*Digital Imaging in COmmunications and Medicine*) or, because it followed the first two ACR-NEMA editions, DICOM **3.0**. Thus the standard became **DICOM 3.0** (even though it had no DICOM 2.0 or DICOM 1.0 predecessors). For this same reason the number 3.0 is often omitted and the standard is commonly referred to as DICOM.

---

[3] As noted in the current edition of the standard: "NEMA has no power, nor does it undertake to police or enforce compliance with the contents of this document. NEMA does not certify, test, or inspect products, designs, or installations for safety or health purposes."

Parlez-vous DICOM? 5

> *Each profession talks to itself in its own language, apparently there is no Rosetta Stone*
>
> – Murphy's Law

In Chap. 2, we briefly touched on the subject of DICOM data representation. DICOM segments all real-world data into standardized attributes (listed in the DICOM Data Dictionary) and describes any real object as a collection of these attributes known as the *Information Object Definition*. In this chapter, we look at this process more carefully.

5.1 IT Boot Camp

Because DICOM is all about *digital*, we should brush up on our computer basics.

In our daily lives, we deal with the *decimal* system: we count by tens, and we have ten digits representing numbers 0–9. Computer data is stored and processed in *binary* format. Binary, or base-2 system, means that any value will be represented by only two digits: 0 or 1. A *bit* is a digit in the binary system. Consequently, any bit can take only one of two possible values: you guessed it, 0 or 1.

A *byte* is simply eight bits (8-digit binary number). If you write all possible combinations of eight 0s and 1s, you would get $2^8 = 256$ binary numbers: 00000000, 00000001, 00000010, 00000011, 00000100... 11111110, 11111111. In other words, one byte can store values from 0 to 255. All computer hardware (hard drives, RAM memory, flash drives, and so on) stores, reads, and writes binary data in bytes.[1] For example, to store 13 bits of data, a computer must allocate a full two bytes (16 bits) of memory. Conventional monitors (and graphics cards) use one byte for each

---

[1] According to Wikipedia, the term "byte" comes from "bite," as in the smallest amount of data a computer could "bite" at once. Clever, n'est pas?

Table 5.1 Multiples of bytes

Prefix	Name	Binary meaning	Metric meaning	Size difference: binary vs. metric (%)
K	Kilo (KB)	$2^{10} = 1024^1$	$10^3 = 1000^1$	2.40
M	Mega (MB)	$2^{20} = 1024^2$	$10^6 = 1000^2$	4.86
G	Giga (GB)	$2^{30} = 1024^3$	$10^9 = 1000^3$	7.37
T	Tera (TB)	$2^{40} = 1024^4$	$10^{12} = 1000^4$	9.95
P	Peta (PB)	$2^{50} = 1024^5$	$10^{15} = 1000^5$	12.59

primary color (red, green, or blue) to represent its 256 shades. Consequently, only one byte is available to represent grayscale shades used in radiology. This means that you will get 256 shades of gray on any conventional monitor – you simply cannot squeeze more options into a single available byte. Special radiological monitors and hardware overcome this limitation by allocating more bytes to grayscale shades.

One byte also provides enough choices to store all Latin characters (lowercase, uppercase, punctuation signs), so a byte is often viewed as a single-character unit. For example, to store 12 characters, a computer uses 12 bytes of memory; one byte per character.[2]

Large data volumes, such as images, can require millions of bytes for storage. Therefore, binary system counts bytes in larger numbers: $2^{10} = 1024$ bytes correspond to one kilobyte (KB), 1024 kilobytes mean one megabyte (MB), and so on. Table 5.1 summarizes this count.

In reality, multiples of bytes are counted in two slightly different ways. Information technology (and DICOM) uses multiples of $2^{10} = 1024$, which makes perfect sense from the binary system perspective I just mentioned. Hardware manufacturers use Kilo, Mega, and the others in their metric meaning as multiples of 1000. When they sell you a 1 GB flash drive, it contains $10^9 = 1000^3$ bytes (*metric* GB), which according to our table is 7.37% less than $2^{30} = 1024^3$ bytes (*binary* GB) – certainly makes for a nice commission for hardware sales.

When lowercase *b* is used in Kb, Mb, Gb, it commonly stands for *bits*, not *bytes*. Consider networks: network bandwidth (unlike computer storage) is usually measured in *kilobits, megabits, and gigabits* per second (representing how much data the network can ideally transmit in 1 s). For example, dialup network speed is up to 56 Kbs (kilobits per second), which is identical to 56/8 = 7 kilobytes per second (7 KBs). A standard computer T1 line delivers 1.544 Mbs (megabits per second); DSL delivers on the order of 10 Mbs; and an average PACS network operates in the range of 10 Gbs (gigabits per second).

Hexadecimal is a shorthand representation of two consecutive bytes, leading to 65,536 ($256^2 = 65,536$) possible values. Because of their 16-bit (2-byte) nature, hexadecimal numbers can be written using a 16-base numerical system consisting

---

[2] But if you need to work in different languages, you will definitely need more than 256 character options – and multi-language Unicode uses 2-byte letters, just like advance monitors use 2-byte grayscale.

of digits 0–9 and characters A–F representing 10–15 respectively[3]: "digit" A stands for 10, "digit" B for 11, and so on up to F = 15. This is very similar to our common decimal numbers, except that now we need 16 symbols to represent a hexadecimal digit (so we add A–F for the new digits). We also prefix hexadecimal numbers with 0x to differentiate them from text or decimal numbers.

How can you read hexadecimal numbers such as 0x007F? Multiply the digits by the respective powers of 16 (just like you would with the decimal system using powers of 10). Thus, (ignoring the "0x" prefix) 0x007F in hexadecimal represents:

$$\mathbf{0} \times 16^3 + \mathbf{0} \times 16^2 + \mathbf{7} \times 16^1 + \mathbf{F} \times 16^0 = \mathbf{7} \times 16 + \mathbf{15} \times 1 = 127$$

in decimal. Many current calculators (including the one in Windows) offer binary-decimal-hexadecimal conversion functions, and would have A–F keys for typing the hexadecimal numbers.

In a decimal system, where we have 10 digits, 2-digit numbers can take $10^2 = 100$ possible values: from 00, 01, 02, and so on to 99. Similarly, in hexadecimal, with 16 possible digits (0–9 and A–F), 2-digit hexadecimal numbers range from 0x00 to 0xFF, covering $16^2 = 256$ possible values. But this 256-value range, as we already know, corresponds to a byte. For example, hexadecimal 0x7F represents a single byte, and hexadecimal 0x007F represents two bytes: 00 and 7 F. This is why leading zeros are always written in hexadecimal numbers: they do not change the number value (0 x7F = 0x007F = 127), but they show how many bytes of computer storage will be needed to store the number (one byte per two hexadecimal digits).

Interchangeably with the 0x prefix, DICOM may also label hexadecimals with an H suffix. For example, number 12 in DICOM would correspond to the decimal 12, while 12 H or 0x12 would mean hexadecimal 12, or $\mathbf{1} \times 16 + \mathbf{2} \times 1 = 18$ decimal. We will use H and 0x in this book only when necessary: omitting when hexadecimal is implied, and including when ambiguity needs to be avoided. Leading zeros and the A–F digits indicate hexadecimal format as well. As a general rule, remember that nearly all numerical data in DICOM is stored in hexadecimal (binary) format.

5.2 Text Versus Binary

Depending on its format, any data can be stored in either text or binary representations. The text format is typically used for names, dates, IDs, and other text strings. The binary format is used for encoding single numerical values or numerical sequences (image pixels and the like). As we learned in the previous section, binary format has the advantage of storing numbers in a more compact, *computer-oriented* manner, which makes it a more natural choice for digital data.[4] On the other hand, binary data encoding is associated with one serious inconvenience: it depends on the computer hardware.

---

[3]Case does not matter, so a–f and A–F are used with the same meaning.

[4]However, certain numerical data items routinely read by humans (such as patient weight or size) are stored as text.

Different computer systems use different byte orders to represent the same multi-byte number. While some systems record the numbers starting from the least significant byte (Little Endian order) others record the same numbers starting from the most significant byte (Big Endian order).[5] For example, what a Little Endian computer (such as Windows PC) stores in byte (binary) format as 0x007F, a Big Endian computer (Apple's Mac) would keep as 0x7F00, reordering the two bytes. When these numbers travel between the systems with different Endian types (for example, when you send a DICOM image from Mac archive to a Windows workstation), their Endian types must be properly converted (byte order reversed); otherwise the numbers will be read backwards, resulting in totally wrong values: 0x007F = 127 and 0x7F00 = 32,512. To avoid data transfer errors, DICOM applications always keep track of their Endian types, and any two connected DICOM units agree on the choice of Endian type during the initial network handshake between them, before they start transmitting any data (we will study this in Sect. 9.4). To make this agreement always possible, *DICOM reserves Little Endian as its default byte-ordering type* – meaning that all DICOM applications, whatever systems or hardware they are running on, must understand and process Little Endian byte order.

The Big Endian/Little Endian computer debate has much more to do with the history of computer hardware than technological merits. If you are involved in any DICOM development, dealing with different Endian types will be one of your responsibilities to ensure cross-platform compatibility of your product. If you are a DICOM user or administrator, bear in mind that byte-ordering problems could occur if you connect devices with different Endian types (PC and Mac, for example).

In comparison to numerical values, text data stores each character (byte) independently and therefore always remains in the same order regardless of the hardware.

Depending on data type, DICOM uses both text and binary formats. If you open a DICOM file in any word-processing application, you will see a strange mix of somewhat meaningful text strings and totally unreadable symbols – the latter being nothing more than the binary-encoded numerical pieces of DICOM data.

The screenshot in Fig. 5.1 shows a fragment of ACR-NEMA 2.0 file, opened in WordPad.

As a result, you will always need special DICOM software to read and interpret what is stored in your DICOM data. This differentiates DICOM from later, similarly organized standards (such as HTML or XML), which can be read and modified using any text editor.

Now I think it is high time that we see exactly how DICOM text and binary data is formatted.

---

[5]The names Big Endian and Little Endian originate from Jonathan Swift's *Gulliver's Travels* wherein the Blefuscudians' and the Lilliputians' are at war over the proper way to open soft-boiled eggs: on the *big end*, or on the *little end*.

5.3 DICOM Grammar: VRs

DS, Decimal String	A string of characters representing either a fixed point number or a floating point number Example: "12345.67", "-5.0e3"	0–9, plus (+), minus (−) E, e, and period (.)	16 maximum
Numbers in binary format (same as numbers in text format, but stored in binary)			
SS, Signed Short	Signed binary integer 16 bits long		2
US, Unsigned Short	Unsigned binary integer 16 bits long		2
SL, Signed Long	Signed binary integer		4
UL, Unsigned Long	Unsigned binary integer 32 bits long		4
AT, Attribute Tag	Ordered pair of 16-bit (2-byte) unsigned integers that is the value of a Data Element Tag		4
FL, Floating Point Single	Single precision binary floating point number		4
FD, Floating Point Double	Double precision binary floating point number		8
OB, Other Byte String	A string of bytes ("other" means not defined in any other VR)		
OW, Other Word String	A string of 16-bit (2-byte) words		
OF, Other Float String	A string of 32-bit (4-byte) floating point words		
Other			
SQ, Sequence of Items	Sequence of items		
UN, Unknown	A string of bytes where the encoding of the contents is unknown		

5.3.1 VR Length

VRs, as we all realize, define DICOM data types; and data size (VR length) is a very important part of this definition. DICOM keeps track of all data sizes in two ways. First, as we will soon see in Sect. 5.5.1, DICOM always records data sizes along with data values – this is how DICOM knows where each data element starts and ends. Second, for some VRs the data length is either fixed or limited – as you can see in the last column of our VR Table 5.2.

Data length limits, imposed by VR definitions, are sometimes overlooked in medical imaging software, which easily leads to incompatibility between programs that are "more or less DICOM-compliant." If you are in DICOM development, make sure that your product is *DICOM-compliant enough* to format all VR data with correct sizes, and *is smart enough* to understand improperly sized VRs when they come from another DICOM application.

Another reason for DICOM software developers to watch the VR lengths is related to the binary (numerical) VRs. Just like in the case of Big Endian and Little Endian, different computer systems use different sizes for the basic numerical data types (integers, floating point numbers, and such). Thus, the VR size specifications in DICOM also shield DICOM data from the differences in computer hardware and software design.

Even length is another fundamental rule of DICOM data encoding: whether fixed-length or not, all DICOM data elements are supposed to have even lengths; that is, they must contain an even number of characters (if text) or bytes (if binary). To ensure this, DICOM adds a single blank space character to any odd-sized text string (such as ST), and a blank NULL byte to any odd-sized binary string (such as OB[6]) to make their lengths even. For example, the name "Smith^Joe" will always be internally stored in DICOM as "Smith^Joe" with a trailing space added and length set to 10.

In one respect, even-length padding of DICOM data can be viewed as an advantage. One can always use it as a parity check to verify the validity of data strings and to mark anything odd-sized as corrupted. However, this approach is rather archaic and comes with the price of junk trailing spaces that any DICOM software should know to add and to trim. Moreover, because many DICOM applications are often used in conjunction with other software (PACS databases, radiology information systems, and such), the issue of ignoring and trimming the trailing blanks permeates the entire workflow chain. The safest approach is to trim DICOM data strings as soon as DICOM data is decoded to be sent to a non-DICOM application. When it is overlooked, what was stored in DICOM as "Smith^Joe" is retrieved as "Smith^Joe". This might look the same to many humans, but it can easily be misinterpreted as another name (or even another patient) by software that is not aware of the DICOM even-length padding.

---

[6]NULL byte padding is also used for the UI strings, although they are in text format.

5.3.2 Characters: Foreign and Wild

It is very natural to assume that users in different countries would prefer DICOM data in their native languages, and DICOM does in fact support *localization*. The language chosen (part of the system localization) also affects the choice of the letters, or characters, allowed in the VR data types. DICOM calls this selection "character repertoire."

Most current DICOM devices use the Latin alphabet (corresponding to the default DICOM character repertoire, labeled as ISO IR-6). It was the first repertoire used in the standard historically and it is quite adequate for many foreign languages. When it is not, transliteration is usually used as a simple shortcut for implementing non-Latin character sets. Instead of changing the Latin set of DICOM characters, foreign characters are mapped into the Latin set in some additional software patch based on their phonetic similarities. This approach is generic and allows users to deal with language-related problems whether they arise from the DICOM standard itself, or from somewhere else.

Transliteration might be abandoned as more countries accept regulations mandating the use of their native languages in clinical practices. However, this must be backed by all DICOM manufacturers, whose current support for language localization is far from perfect (as we will see later in Sect. 16.2).

> **Interface Localization**
>
> There was a story about an international research satellite lost in space because what one participating country wrote in millimeters, another country read in inches.
>
> Keep in mind that DICOM uses standard metric units: millimeters for sizes, kilograms for weights, and so on. These units are specified in the DICOM standard and should be displayed in any good DICOM interface to avoid ambiguity.
>
> DICOM date format has become the most common stumbling block in medical interfaces. The format used by the standard is YYYYMMDD – that is, "20110201" means "February 1, 2011." However, what is optimal for internal storage might not be optimal for display. Without a doubt, "February 1, 2011" works much better in any DICOM user interface than "20110201" or even "2011.02.01". When this is not done, or done improperly, the date could be interpreted differently by users from different countries.
>
> For example, I have seen 01.02.2011 in DICOM interfaces manufactured for US users, who would rather write this date as 02/01/2011.

In addition to various languages and formats, certain characters in DICOM have reserved meanings and should be used accordingly. In particular, DICOM allows for wildcard matches in text strings. The asterisk (*) wildcard represents *any character sequence*; the question mark (?) wildcard represents *any single character*; and the backslash wildcard (\) represents *or*. For example, if DICOM needs to search for either CT or MR studies it will search by a modality string *CT\MR* meaning "CT or MR" modality. In general, wildcards exist to your advantage. If you do not remember the complete patient name, you may enter the few first characters followed by an asterisk (*) to retrieve all similar matches. So entering "Smit*" in virtually any DICOM software should match Smith, Smithson, Smithsonian, and so on.

Nevertheless, wildcards can be confusing and lead to DICOM errors as well. DICOM software users can accidentally type question marks in DICOM reports, or include the backslash in a file name that later will be stored in a DICOM data element. As you might guess, such reports and file names can be easily misinterpreted as wildcard searches, resulting in incorrect or lost information.

5.3.3 Text VRs: CS, SH, LO, ST, LT, UT

Text VRs are easy: they are meant to store text strings. They are also the least-demanding data types, requiring minimal processing (except for trimming those pesky blank spaces at the end when exported to the other applications). The only important thing about the text VRs is that you know their size limits. For example, if CS can hold up to 16 characters, then going even a single character beyond this limit could cause a minor software error or a major PACS problem. Obviously, any length checks should be done by the DICOM software, and all strings exceeding their limits should be either trimmed or converted to longer VR types.

5.3.4 Dates and Times: DA, TM, DT, AS

DA, TM, and DT types are self-explanatory as well: they store dates and times in text (string) format. The most important thing about them is to know the right order of the date/time components. Also, older versions of DICOM and ACR-NEMA used slightly different date and time formats, with period (.) and colon (:) delimiters – for example, writing a time string as 18:32:00, instead of the current 183200. Good DICOM system developers should take this into account – backwards compatibility is very important.

Another problem with DA and TM types is that single attributes that really need to be DT types are often broken into DA and TM attributes. Take the Patient's Birth Date attribute for example, which is assigned the DA type and is complemented by the Patient's Birth Time attribute (TM type). It would make so much more sense just to merge the two attributes in one of DT type, storing the patient's birth date and time in a single attribute. Breaking a single piece of information across several attributes creates the problem of keeping the attributes in sync – when one is changed, the other(s) has to be updated as well.

Since 2008, DT format provides support for time zone information in its &ZZXX component – just in case you were thinking about using it. For example, the &ZZXX offset for United States Eastern Standard Time would be represented as −0500, for Japan Standard Time as +0900. Old "zoneless" timing was fine for local-area systems from the 1990s, when everything was happening on a couple of modalities in the same hospital. Now, as DICOM-based teleradiology starts spanning across multiple countries and continents, and because patients are less hesitant to travel, DICOM had to become more careful about handling time zone information. The next "DT challenge" would be providing a mechanism for synchronizing the time on different DICOM units – that is, keeping them in sync with each other and the universal world time.

If you ask me why DICOM needs the AS type, I do not really know. Out of the more than 2000 current standard DICOM attributes, only *one* (Patient's Age) uses it. However, the much more popular Patient's Birth Date attribute (with DA type) is definitely enough to find out the patient's age – and this is what all PACS rely on.

5.3.5 Numbers in Text Format: IS, DS

IS and DS data types store numerical values (integers and floating point) as text strings. Although less appropriate for computer storage compared to binary, text-formatted numbers are used in DICOM quite frequently. First of all, text-formatted numbers do not depend on Big/Little Endian byte order. Second, they are just easy to read – you can display them "as is" in any interface. For this reason, text-formatted numbers are commonly used for the data recorded from the real world, entered and interpreted by humans. Recording a patient's height or weight is a good example.

5.3.6 Numbers in Binary Format: SS, US, SL, UL, FL, FD, OB, OW, OF, AT

Essentially, these are the same numbers as IS and DS text types, but stored in binary format.

SS, US, SL, UL, FL, FD are used to represent single numbers (sometimes a few numbers of the same type are concatenated together).

OB, OW, OF are used for long numerical strings – think about storing a sequence of image pixels. In this case, each number in the sequence will have the same byte size (1, 2, or 4 bytes, respectively), and they all will be concatenated into a long binary series.

Note that while OB uses one byte per number, OW and OF use 2 and 4. Therefore, OW and OF will be affected by Big/Little Endian byte ordering.

Finally, AT stores a pair of 2-byte numbers. This data type corresponds to (Group, Element) tagging of all DICOM attributes, as we will soon see in Sect. 5.4. Thus,

AT type, unlike the other number types, is used strictly for enumerating DICOM data attributes.

5.3.7 PN – Storing Person's Names

The PN VR encodes the entire *Person Name*. Unfortunately, DICOM uses a single field to hold this value – that is, the entire name (first, last, middle, and so on) is recorded in a single PN-type VR. This definitely creates problems when *John Smith* can be written as "John Smith", "Smith John", or even "Smith, John". To eliminate this uncertainty, DICOM prescribes the following name order, known as "Person Name component group":

```
FamilyName^GivenName^MiddleName^NamePrefix^NameSuffix
```

All components are separated by the caret (^) character (see PN examples in Table 5.2). However, in a multifaceted medical environment this order is often permuted, resulting in permanently lost information or misidentified patients.

There are two remedies to this problem:
1. To identify patients, always use patient IDs (Medical Record Numbers) and not the patients' names. Using the patient ID leaves little room for spelling errors.
2. When searching for (patient) names on your PACS or any DICOM software in general, use wildcards such as the asterisk (*) meaning *any text*. As we already know from Sect. 5.3.2, wildcard searches are standard in DICOM. Typing "*Smith*" in the patient name search box will return all patients with "Smith" appearing somewhere in their names, including the names with incorrect component order. In fact, some DICOM programs automatically add wildcards to name searches, to return all similar-looking names.

Moreover, certain DICOM applications are smart enough to go beyond wildcard matching when they implement *phonetic matching* to find the names that sound similar, even with different spelling – for example, matching "Nelson" and "Neilsen." Features like this are very much appreciated in clinical workflow: they eliminate problems, instead of creating them.[7]

Recent DICOM editions had to stretch the definition of the person's name to accommodate a couple of new uses:
- Foreign names in ideographic transcription (such as Japanese or Chinese) can be accompanied by Latin phonetic transcription. In this case, different name transcriptions – that is, different component groups – are separated by the equals (=) character: "Wang^XiaoDong=王^小東". It is totally unclear how these names can be matched, so DICOM leaves this to software implementations.
- You do not have to be homo sapience to become a patient. Veterinary medicine enjoys DICOM in the same ways, so patient names like "ABC Farms^Running on Water" would most likely identify a horse, owned by ABC Farms, and called "Running On Water."

---

[7]Which is why "sounds like" phonetic matching is implemented in many other software applications, having nothing to do with DICOM – SQL server, for example.

5.3.8 AE – Naming Application Entities

The AE VR represents a DICOM *Application Entity*. AE is essentially the name of a DICOM device or program used to uniquely identify it (you cannot have two identical AEs in your PACS network). This makes AE one of the most important VRs for any DICOM network or PACS.

Even though DICOM does not have strict requirements for AE naming, Application Entities are typically labeled with numbers and uppercase characters only – no spaces, no punctuation signs, or other characters. In fact, it is not uncommon to see DICOM units that would accept only uppercase alphanumeric AEs. This brings us to the issue of case-sensitivity; simply put, avoid using case-sensitive names. Most DICOM devices will see no difference between Workstation1 and WORKSTATION1, but a few others can get picky. As far as the choice of AE names, it is totally up to you, but the rule of thumb is to use explicit and easy to understand titles, corresponding to the entity's function (CTARCHIVE) or location (MR1FLOOR).

We will look at AEs in more detail in Sect. 7.1.

5.3.9 UI – Unique Identifiers

The UI VR encodes a *Unique Identifier* primarily used to identify particular *instances* of DICOM data (objects). While AEs are expected to be locally unique (inside of your network, for example), DICOM unique identifiers (UIs or UIDs) must be globally unique, whenever and wherever used. For example, when you copy a DICOM study from one DICOM unit to another, the second unit should modify the Study UID attribute value to emphasize that it deals with another instance of the same study. Then, changing anything in the second study instance (e.g., reformatting some study images, for example) will not be confused with changes in the original.

As Table 5.2 indicates, UI names are built from groups ("components") of digits, separated by periods. There is a rather bizarre rule in DICOM, often overlooked by standard implementations: "The first digit of each component shall not be zero unless the component is a single digit." In other words, UI = 1.2.804.114118.2.0909 is illegal (we have a 0 after the period in component 0909), but UI = 1.2.804.114118.2.0 is OK.

We talk more about UIDs in Sect. 5.5.8.

5.3.10 SQ – Sequencing Data Sets

The SQ VR encodes a *SeQuence* of data sets, where each set may contain multiple data attributes. This VR provides support for the most complex DICOM structures, allowing VR *nesting* – placing some VRs inside others. This becomes really useful when you want to group several similar elements into a single data block (and keep them as such) instead of mixing them with other unrelated attributes. In this way, the entire block will be present (or not) and you do not have to worry about the individual block elements.

DICOM data fragment: data nesting with sequencing

Attribute Name
Referenced Series Sequence
>Series Instance UID
>Referenced Instance Sequence
>>Referenced SOP Class UID
>>Referenced SOP Instance UID

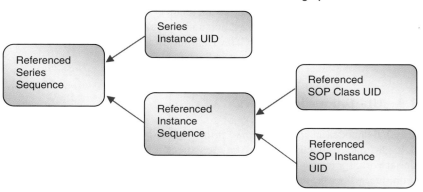

Fig. 5.2 Nesting DICOM data

In DICOM documents (our esteemed Conformance Statements included) sequencing is always indicated with the greater than (>) sign. For example, you could come across a piece of DICOM data looking like the example in Fig. 5.2.

In Fig. 5.2 data table, the first "Referenced Series Sequence" attribute is followed by two attributes with the greater than (>) sign, which means that the "Referenced Series Sequence" attribute has an SQ VR, and as a sequence includes the "Series Instance UID" and "Referenced Instance Sequence" attributes. What is even more interesting is that the "Referenced Instance Sequence" attribute is followed by two other elements with double greater than signs (>>), meaning that "Referenced Instance Sequence" in its turn is a sequence as well, and contains two attributes: "Referenced SOP Class UID" and "Referenced SOP Instance UID." In this way, "Referenced Series Sequence" contains four sub-elements: elements from its own first-level sequence, and elements from its subsequences.

Sequencing leads to a complex, nonlinear format of DICOM data when some VRs can branch out from the others producing intricate DICOM data *trees* – just like our branching in Fig. 5.2. Sequencing does pose some interesting problems for DICOM developers. For example, the VR (data) length for the *root* element "Referenced Series Sequence" in our example needs to be properly computed to include all nested element data. For this and similar reasons, SQ elements become harder to implement and to process, and often contain implementation bugs on the software level. If you are designing a DICOM product, handle SQ elements with particular care and use them with moderation.

Note that some DICOM data items (such as certain unique identifiers) are meant to be unique, and cannot be used in SQ elements by definition.

More details of SQ data encoding will be discussed in Sect. 5.5.5.

5.3.11 UN – Representing Unknown Values

The UN VR encodes *UNknown* values. In many ways, UN value representation is used for anything that does not fit in the other 26 VRs. Most commonly, UN is reserved for manufacturer-specific (proprietary) data, which is not meant to be standard interpretable anyway.

I would recommend that anyone working on DICOM application development avoid using the UN VR whenever possible. First, the other 26 VRs sufficiently represent nearly all data types. Second, labeling the attribute type as *unknown* seems more like an act of despair rather than a structured approach to defining data types. Consider Big/Little Endian byte reordering as one such example. You cannot perform this process for the UN attributes even when it is needed because you just do not know whether the data is binary or text – or for that matter, whether anything needs to be reordered at all.

So what did I hope you would learn from all that? Certainly, I do not expect you to have a sponge-like brain and photographic memory to recall every bit of VR grammar. But I do hope that you remember the basics: *VRs play the most essential role in DICOM data structuring. They connect DICOM to the outside world.* As we conclude our little VR excursion, we now know that VRs are word forms that DICOM understands and speaks. But how do we translate our real-world data items into VR? (Mental drum roll please. Open large velvet curtain.) Enter the DICOM Data Dictionary.

5.4 DICOM Data Dictionary

Part PS3.6 of the DICOM standard contains the complete DICOM Data Dictionary, used to encode all standard DICOM attributes. In addition to the standard dictionary, DICOM vendors can use their own dictionaries for their proprietary data attributes. In either case, the dictionary structure will follow the same rules. We review the rules in this section.

5.4.1 Standard DICOM Data Dictionary

In essence, the DICOM Data Dictionary is the registry of all standard data items (attributes) used in digital medicine. We now know that these items should be formatted into the 27 VR types.

Table 5.3 A few lines from the DICOM Data Dictionary

(Group, Element) tag	Attribute (data element) name	Keyword	VR	VM	Retired status
(0008,0001)	*Length to End*	*LengthToEnd*			*RET*
(0008,0005)	Specific Character Set	SpecificCharacterSet	CS	1-n	
...					
(0010,0010)	Patient Name	PatientName	PN	1	
(0010,0020)	Patient ID	PatientID	LO	1	
(0010,0021)	Issuer of Patient ID	IssuerOfPatientID	LO	1	
(0010,0030)	Patient's Birth Date	PatientBirthDate	DA	1	
(0010,0032)	Patient's Birth Time	PatientBirthTime	TM	1	
(0010,0040)	Patient's Sex	PatientSex	CS	1	
...					
(0010,1000)	Other Patient IDs	OtherPatientIDs	LO	1-n	
(0010,1001)	Other Patient Names	OtherPatientNames	PN	1-n	
...					
(FFFE,E00D)	Item Delimitation Item	ItemDelimitationItem		1	
(FFFE,E0DD)	Sequence Delimitation Item	SequenceDelimitationItem		1	

To put them in order in the more than 2000-item list, all items are first divided into numbered groups (based on loose similarity of the item contents). Groups are organized by individual elements. Thus, each item is numbered with its own *(Group, Element)* number, also known as element *tag*. The tagged elements are also called *attributes*, or DICOM *data elements*, or simply DICOM *elements*.

Group and element numbers are hexadecimal – as we saw in Sect. 5.1. Table 5.3 shows an excerpt of the DICOM Data Dictionary.

As you can see, the first column contains the hexadecimal (Group, Element) tag. The second "Attribute (data element) name" column – probably the most important to us at this point – explains what real-world data should be stored in this element. Because (Group, Element) tags uniquely correspond to the attribute names, we can refer to a data element by its tag (0010,0010) or attribute name ("Patient Name") interchangeably. This is a very important DICOM convention – (Group, Element) tags are shorter, with a fixed size and follow a very strict hexadecimal format. All DICOM applications refer to data elements using their (Group, Element) tags and not the descriptive attribute names.

The "Keyword" column is a recent addition to the standard. Looking very similar to attribute names, the one-word keywords provide descriptive element tags. These are textual alternatives to (Group, Element) pairs to be used in XML, HTTP (URL), and similar text-based standards, which are increasingly employed in DICOM interfaces.

The VR column in the dictionary specifies the format of each data element, as we learned in the previous sections (Fig. 5.3). For example, the "Patient's Birth Date" element (0010,0030) must be in DA format (that is, as an 8-digit, YYYYMMDD data string).

5.4 DICOM Data Dictionary

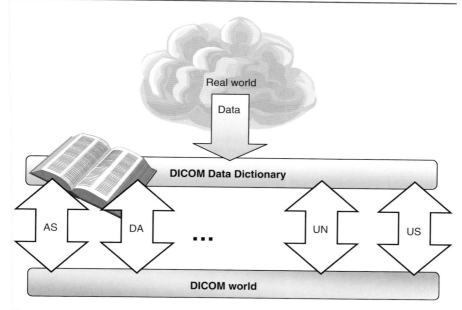

Fig. 5.3 From real world to DICOM world

Data element Value Multiplicity (VM) defines whether the related element may contain only one value of its type, or several. For example, the "Other Patient Names" element (0010,1001) can clearly include more than one name, so its multiplicity is marked as *1-n*, where n is any number. How do we put several values into a single element? DICOM concatenates multiple values into a single *multi-value* value. If these values are binary (have binary VRs), they are simply concatenated. The length of each single-value binary VR is known and fixed (for example, 2 for SS) and this is how they can be read back – in fixed-length pieces. Text values, on the other hand, usually do not have fixed sizes, so they are concatenated using the backslash (\) as the delimiter. For example, if our John Smith patient uses other names such as "Dr Jekyll" and "Mr Hyde", the (0010,1001) would contain something like "Dr^Jekyll\Mr^Hyde", corresponding to value multiplicity of $n=2$. As we already know, the backslash (\) has a very particular meaning in DICOM, which is "or" in multi-value attributes (see Sect. 5.3.2). For that reason, do not use the backslash (\) for any other purpose (file names, dates, and so on) because it will likely deceive your DICOM software.

The *RET* label in the DICOM Data Dictionary marks retired attributes – those from earlier versions of the standard that will not be supported in future DICOM releases. These elements cannot be redefined and their roles have been delegated to some new, better-designed dictionary elements. The retired items are also italicized. Practically, it takes several years for each new DICOM revision to spread through the industry, so items retired in 2010 will still be used in some DICOM units in 2015 or later. In fact, because all DICOM manufacturers prefer to remain backward compatible with their older models, retired items stay in the dictionary forever (getting less and less use), but are never completely ignored. Good DICOM applications must correctly process these items.

> **Retirement Plans**
> Updating and retiring DICOM elements may be far trickier than it sounds. I can borrow an example form David Clunie's blog (www.dclunie.com), discussing some problems with element "retirement plans." Imagine an old DICOM element – let's call it *XYZdata* – that used to be recorded as an integer, but as computer and modality precision progressed, required better decimal precision. Do you just change the attribute's VR from integer IS to decimal DS in the next DICOM Dictionary release?
> Not so fast! Think about all existing DICOM units, programmed to work with integer XYZdata values. When they start receiving newly-formatted decimal strings ("123.45" instead of "123", for instance), they would go nuts. So to keep them happy and sane, you will have to retain the old IS-formatted XYZdata in DICOM Dictionary for a long time, while adding a new *XYZdataDouble* attribute with proper DS VR. Problem solved?
> Still too fast! What happens now, if some DICOM unit receives both XYZdata and XYZdataDouble and they happen to be dramatically different, which one should be trusted? You may say "trust XYZdataDouble, it's the most recent type." But in fact, the original *true* data might have come from an older unit where XYZdata was recorded correctly, while XYZdataDouble was messed up later in some buggy integer-to-double conversion.
> The bottom line: DICOM element retirement can get quite complex and subjective, so you should *never ignore retired elements* if they are present in your DICOM data.

With some respectable knowledge of VRs and the DICOM Data Dictionary at hand, we can finally start *speaking DICOM*; at least on the very simple attribute level. For example, take a sentence such as:

"Patient John Smith, Male, born on August 6, 1954".

Looking at the dictionary excerpt in Table 5.3, we see that there are three data elements in this sentence: "Patient Name" (0010,0010), "Patient's Sex" (0010,0040), and "Patient's Birth Date" (0010,0030). These elements have value representations of PN, CS, and DA, respectively. Therefore, replacing names by their tags and applying VR formatting, we can say[8]:

(0010,0010)Smith^John (0010,0030)19540806 (0010,0040)M

This is our original sentence, DICOM-encoded. Quite simple, isn't it?

---

[8] As we will see later, DICOM sorts its data items in increasing (Group, Element) order.

5.4 DICOM Data Dictionary

Table 5.4 Making private data elements

(Group, Element) tag	Attribute (data element) name	VR	VM
(0009,0010)	Patient's Middle Name	PN	1

5.4.2 Private DICOM Data Dictionaries

I mentioned that the standard DICOM Data Dictionary contains some 2000 entries carefully compiled from the medical imaging industry. You might expect that this leaves a pretty slim chance of encountering an unlisted entry. But what if this happens anyway?

In fact, this does happen all the time with various DICOM and PACS manufacturers who need to add their proprietary DICOM attributes into DICOM-encoded data. Let's say that we designed some DICOM software, and would like to store the *patient's middle name* as a separate item. The standard DICOM Data Dictionary does not provide this attribute, so DICOM offers a very simple solution to the problem. All even group numbers are reserved for standard use in the DICOM Data Dictionary. All odd group numbers are reserved for *private use*.

In our "Patient's Middle Name" case, we can create our own private DICOM Data Dictionary and store an entry that looks like the example in Table 5.4.

We would use an odd "proprietary" group number such as 0009 and whatever element number we like.

Because our private dictionary is not standard, other DICOM applications would have no idea what our (0009,0010) tag means, but they will know – from the odd group number 0009 – that the tag is private. According to DICOM, unrecognized tags should be ignored; other applications will gracefully skip (0009,0010) when reading our DICOM data. Unfortunately, this is not so simple in reality. Another application may well have its own private dictionary with (0009,0010) being used for some other element (for example, "Physician's Last Name"). In this case, we run into the classical trap of private tag incompatibility. Our (0009,0010) tag will be accepted by another DICOM provider and will be completely misinterpreted. DICOM makes an effort to avoid this in PS3.5 (Sect. 7.8.1) by reserving certain tags as *private creator* elements, encoding the implementer of the particular private dictionary; but it always gets trickier in practical life.

For that reason, many smart people tried to keep track of at least the most well-known DICOM providers and their private dictionaries, but this is hard to do. These dictionaries are rarely published and change all the time – that's what "private" implies anyway. And it is not uncommon to open a DICOM file that contains mostly private data items – private tags are very heavily used; keep this in mind. If you do run into the private element situation one day, consult your DICOM vendor (Table 5.5).

5.4.3 Standard DICOM Command Dictionary

We know by now that all data items (elements) are listed in the standard DICOM Data Dictionary found in part PS3.6 of the standard. But these are *data* elements.

Table 5.5 Example of private Data Dictionary from TeraRecon Aquarius DICOM Conformance Statement (as you can see, odd group 0077 is used to store vendor-specific data elements)

Private groups table				
Module	Tag	Description	VR	VM
Aquarius Scene	Original Series/Study UID (0077, 0010)	Private	UI	1-N
Aquarius Scene	Original SOP UID (0077,0012)	Private	UI	1-N
Aquarius Scene	Referenced Volume ID (0077, 0014)	Private	LO	1-N
Aquarius Scene	Binary Data Name SCS (0077, 0014)	Private	CS	1
Aquarius Scene	Binary Data Name (0077, 0020)	Private	LO	1-N
Aquarius Scene	Number of SOP Instance UID (0077,0022)	Private	CS	1-N
...				

What if we need to encode *commands*? DICOM commands such as Print, Store, Move, or Get are used all the time in the medical imaging workflow, but they do not appear anywhere in the Data Dictionary.

DICOM encodes commands with the exact same format as data elements, using the reserved 0000 command group. For example, (0000,0100) element is commonly used to represent *command type* and (0000,0110) to represent *command message ID*. The DICOM standard does not provide a unified command dictionary (though it would be great to include it in PS3.6). Instead, it explains the use and contents of different command messages in detail in PS3.7 where command message objects are introduced. Annex E in PS3.7 gives the Command Dictionary itself, and we show it in Appendix A.1.

Unfortunately, unlike with data elements, DICOM does not support proprietary command attributes. As you will see later in this book, the current set of DICOM commands is rather limited, and was designed for local PACS architecture, which is becoming more and more outdated. Modern digital imaging projects such as teleradiology require more flexible DICOM command structures than the current standard can offer. Allowing proprietary tags in DICOM commands would be the first step in building this flexibility.

Meanwhile, this is all we need to know about the command dictionary for now. Chapter 7 provides ample examples of DICOM command objects, explaining commands in more detail.

5.5 DICOM Objects

Do you still remember our simple DICOM translation that we made at the very end of Sect. 5.4.1? Let's glance at it one more time; it was more than a trivial exercise because there you had just built your first DICOM data object. We used the elements:

5.5 DICOM Objects

"Patient John Smith, Male, born on August 6, 1954"

and replaced the names with their tags and applied VR formatting to say:

(0010,0010)Smith^John (0010,0030)19540806 (0010,0040)M

DICOM objects are the most essential part of the standard structure. They are the actual sentences of DICOM lingo that encode, convey, and store DICOM information and commands. All DICOM data (such as medical images, commands, and reports) is always wrapped in DICOM object format. In this format, it travels between various DICOM devices on a DICOM network and gets stored in DICOM files. In fact, even DICOM files can be viewed as memory dumps of DICOM objects to file media.

When we studied the DICOM Data Dictionary, we learned that DICOM breaks all real-world data into its building blocks: data elements, encoded with 27 available VR types. A *DICOM object is nothing but a collection of data elements*. For example, consider a digital medical image. It will have several attributes such as image width, height, colors (palette), date the image was acquired, and so on. All these attributes can be found in the standard DICOM Data Dictionary and will be translated into DICOM data elements, each with its own tag and value. The sequence of these translated elements, which describes the image in its entirety, becomes the image's DICOM object.

DICOM objects, however, can grow much more complex than simple element sequences. When we looked at VRs, I mentioned one particular VR type used for sequencing – SQ. The SQ VR is designed to hold a *sequence of data element sets* – each set being, in essence, a separate DICOM object. These DICOM objects in turn may also contain SQ VRs, meaning that *DICOM objects can contain sets of other DICOM objects*. This *recursion* or *nesting* of DICOM objects creates a more complex tree-like structure, making DICOM objects look like data trees, with DICOM objects being the branches and data elements the leaves (Fig. 5.4).

How does DICOM write all this complex branching data? It uses very basic data encoding rules that we are about to review.

5.5.1 Encoding Data Elements

Encoding in DICOM means writing attribute data in DICOM-specific format, converting potentially complex DICOM attribute values into a sequence of bytes. To write the entire data object one must know how to encode the individual data elements. Part PS3.5 of the DICOM standard defines two major encoding types: *implicit VR encoding* and *explicit VR encoding*.

Implicit encoding is the simplest one, and is used as the DICOM default. It is defined in Table 5.6.

As an example, consider our favorite patient, Joe Smith. The group number for the Patient Name entry in the DICOM Data Dictionary is 0x0010, and the element number is 0x0010. The original value length of the "Smith^Joe" text string is 9, but DICOM

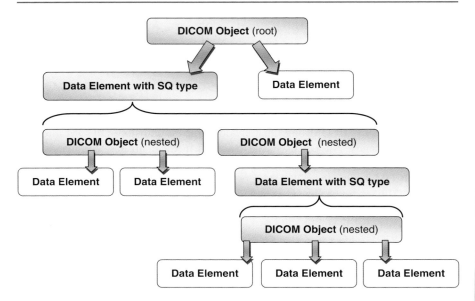

Fig. 5.4 DICOM object nesting

Table 5.6 Implicit VR encoding

Tag		Value length	Value
Group Number (2-byte unsigned integer)	Element Number (2-byte unsigned integer)	4-byte integer **L**	Even number **L** of bytes containing the data element value
2 bytes	2 bytes	4 bytes	**L** bytes

needs to make it even (VR length must be even, see Sect. 5.3.1), so it adds a trailing space, converting the name string into "Smith^Joe". The name length now becomes L = 10 = 0x0A characters, and we encode the patient name attribute as shown in Table 5.7.

Note one important detail: the default Endian type in DICOM is Little Endian (see Sect. 5.2), meaning that multi-byte numbers are written starting from the lowest byte. Therefore, for Group = 0010, the lowest (rightmost) byte 10 comes first, and the highest byte 00 is the next – the same applies to the Element and Length encoding. The 18 bytes that you see in the Binary line is exactly what DICOM will write as the encoded Joe Smith patient name.

To encode multiple data elements (which is always the case), DICOM will simply concatenate their individual encodings into a single binary string – we will see quite complex examples of this in Chap. 7. Because the length of each data item is included in the item's encoding – and Group, Element, and VR Length fields have a fixed size – you can always break concatenated elements into separate ones. For example, with our implicit Endian encoding in Table 5.7, just read the first 2 + 2 = 4 bytes for the (Group,Element) tag, then read length L from the following four bytes, and then read L bytes for the element value. After this, the next element starts, and the entire process repeats itself.

5.5 DICOM Objects

Table 5.7 Implicit encoding example

Byte #	1	2	3	4	5	6	7	8	9	10	11	12	13	14	15	16	17	18
Decimal	16	0	16	0	10	0	0	0	S	m	i	t	h	^	J	o	e	(space)
Binary	10	00	10	00	0A	00	00	00	53	6D	69	74	68	5E	4A	6F	65	20
	Group g=0010		Element e=0010		VR length L= 10=0x0000000A				VR value=Smith^Joe (with trailing space)									

Table 5.8 Explicit VR encoding (except OB, OW, OF, SQ, UT, and UN)

Tag		VR	Value length	Value
Group Number (2-byte unsigned integer)	Element Number (2-byte unsigned integer)	VR (2 characters)	2-byte integer L	Even number L of bytes containing the data element value
2 bytes	2 bytes	2 bytes	2 bytes	L bytes

Table 5.9 Explicit encoding example

Byte #	1	2	3	4	5	6	7	8	9	10	11	12	13	14	15	16	17	18
Decimal	16	0	16	0	P	N	10	0	S	m	i	t	h	^	J	o	e	(space)
Binary	10	00	10	00	50	4E	0A	00	53	6D	69	74	68	5E	4A	6F	65	20
	g=0010		e=0010		VR type		VR length L= 10=0x000A		VR value=Smith^Joe (with trailing space)									

Table 5.10 Explicit VR encoding (for OB, OW, OF, SQ, UT, and UN)

Tag		VR		Value length	Value
Group Number (2-byte unsigned integer)	Element Number (2-byte unsigned integer)	VR (2 characters) of OB, OW, OF, SQ, UT or UN	Reserved (2 bytes) set to a value of 0000	4-byte integer L	Even number L of bytes containing the data element value
2 bytes	2 bytes	2 bytes	2 bytes	4 bytes	L bytes

Explicit data encoding is very similar to implicit. It has two subtypes. The first is applied to all VRs *except* OB, OW, OF, SQ, UT or UN – as shown in Table 5.8.

As the name suggests, with *explicit* VR encoding we include 2-character VR types. What used to be a 4-byte VR length field in implicit encoding is split into a 2-byte VR type, and a 2-byte VR length. So the same example with the patient name will be now encoded as in Table 5.9.

For VRs *with* OB, OW, OF, SQ, UT, or UN an explicit encoding will use a slightly different method. Two reserved bytes (set to 0000) follow the VR name and allocate four bytes for the VR length (just like with implicit encoding) as shown in Table 5.10.

For example, to encode a pixel buffer for a 256×256 image with OB type (one byte per pixel, total of 256×256=65536=0x00010000 bytes), we would have Table 5.11.

Table 5.11 Explicit encoding example

Byte #	1	2	3	4	5	6	7	8	9	10	11	12	13	14	15	...	65547	65548
Decimal	224	127	16	0	O	B	0	0	0	0	1	0	0	3	0	...	10	10
Binary	E0	7F	10	00	4F	42	00	00	00	00	01	00	00	03	00	...	0A	0A
	g=7FE0		e=0010		VR type		Reserved		VR length L=0x00010000				VR value (pixels, one byte per pixel)					

One cannot mix explicit and implicit VR encoding in the same DICOM object – one type only must be used consistently. Even though explicit encoding seems somewhat redundant, it has its advantages:

1. Redundancy in VR names helps avoid data decoding errors.
2. As DICOM evolves, some VR types change and might not be the same in the present DICOM Data Dictionary as they used to be. In this case, explicit encoding preserves the original type names and provides additional backwards compatibility.
3. Explicit encoding is important for encoding nonstandard (proprietary, vendor-specific) VRs, which cannot be found in the standard DICOM Data Dictionary.

Nonetheless, DICOM defines implicit VR with Little Endian byte ordering as the *default* data encoding method. Because explicit and implicit VR encoding cannot be mixed, the decision regarding which technique to use must be made at the very beginning of any data transfer – DICOM applications can negotiate and agree on encoding types before they exchange any data. We will see more of this when we study DICOM Transfer Syntaxes in Sect. 9.4.

Explicit-Implicit Conversion

Often DICOM data will have to be converted from *implicit* to *explicit* VR representation and back – depending on the type required for current data transfer. Obviously, converting explicit to implicit is easy: just drop the VR types. Going back is trickier: you need to match each attribute tag in the DICOM Data Dictionary to find out its VR type. In some cases though, this wouldn't work. For example, if the attribute was proprietary (odd-numbered group number) it wouldn't exist in the standard dictionary. This is probably the only case when the UN (unknown) VR type comes in handy (see Sect. 5.3.11) – it can cover all unidentifiable VRs.

In any event, DICOM keeps the length of data items even – just as we did with encoding Joe Smith's name. VR length plays another important role in DICOM data reading (decoding) – it helps skip unknown elements. If your DICOM application encounters an element that it cannot understand, it should simply scroll the L=Length bytes and start reading the next element. The ability to gracefully ignore unknown data is quintessential for robust apps – they should not freeze or fail when they run into something they cannot interpret. Just skip to the next!

5.5 DICOM Objects

Finally, DICOM offers an option of using *undefined* length when data of unknown size is surrounded by standard delimiters. It happens mostly in SQ items, so we will consider it a bit later in Sect. 5.5.5.

5.5.2 Encoding Data Groups

We already know that all DICOM elements in the DICOM Data Dictionary are organized into groups and are labeled as (Group, Element) pairs. For example, group 0010 in the Data Dictionary gathers all elements related to a patient (name, ID, weight, size, age, and so on); group 0028 is dedicated to the information about the image (width, height, color depth); and group 7FE0 consists of only one element: pixel data. Groups with odd group numbers are not present in the Data Dictionary because they are reserved for manufacturers to store their proprietary data.

When DICOM data elements are encoded into DICOM objects, they are written there strictly in the order of their (Group, Element) tags, starting from the lowest. Thus, elements are sorted in ascending order within each element group, and groups are sorted in ascending group order. For example, element (0008,0012) would be recorded before element (0008,0014). Element (0010,0010) would be written after the first two because it has a higher group number.

> **DICOM Developers: Element Order in DICOM**
> Knowing that all DICOM elements in a DICOM object have to come in the well-defined ascending order of their element tags plays an important role in DICOM software design.
> First of all, this is a major validation tool. If, when reading a DICOM object, element (0010,0010) is encountered *before* element (0008,0012), then something went seriously wrong with the object. Most likely, the data was corrupted beyond recognition and needs to be rejected.
> Second, most basic data was historically placed into the groups with the lower group numbers, such as patient data in group 0010. This can help a DICOM application avoid reading the entire, potentially large, DICOM objects if it is only looking for a few basic tags. Start reading from the top. As soon as the required group is processed, stop and skip the rest.

Apart from (Group, Element) tag ordering, there is nothing of particular concern about encoding DICOM data groups, with one small exception: group length tag. Although this tag has been retired[9] in DICOM starting 2008, it still can be found in

---

[9]Group length was retired in DICOM data objects (gggg>0000), but still has to be present in DICOM command objects (gggg=0000), as we will see in Sect. 7.2.2. To justify this exception, DICOM declared that "elements in group 0000 are not standard elements", which sounds a bit funny for a standard.

(Group, Element)	VR	Length	Value
...... (data elements before group 0010)			
(0010,0000)	UL	4	*L* bytes
(0010,0010)	PN	10	Smith^John
(0010,0030)	DA	8	19540806
...... (more group 0010 elements)			
(0010,4000)	LT	12	No_comments_
(0012,0000)	UL		
...... (remaining data elements)			

The rows from (0010,0010) through (0010,4000) are bracketed as *L* data bytes.

Fig. 5.5 Example of group length element: element (0010,0000) at the very beginning of group 0010 contains data value equal to L, where L in the total number of bytes in the encoded group 0010 data elements (following right after element (0010,0000)). The number of bytes in (0010,0000) is not included in L

many implementations, and is worth looking at. For each DICOM group gggg, its very first element (gggg, 0000) is reserved to hold the entire length L (in bytes) of all following gggg data elements present in the given DICOM object. Because all data and tag lengths in DICOM are even, L is the even number of bytes from the end of the (gggg,0000) element to the beginning of the next group in this object. When a DICOM object is written, element (gggg, 0000) must be placed in the beginning of each new group gggg in UL VR format, recording the entire length of all group gggg elements up to the beginning of the next group (Fig. 5.5).

The reason for group length encoding is exactly the same as it is for element length encoding. If your application does not need to read the group gggg data, it might read only the group length L from the (gggg,0000) tag, and then fast-forward L bytes, proceeding to the next available group. Because the number of elements in gggg can be large, this forwarding can substantially speed up DICOM object reading (a technique known as partial parsing). This becomes particularly handy when dealing with proprietary, odd-numbered groups. Such groups can be correctly interpreted only by their manufacturers and have to be ignored by everyone else. If group length is provided in element (gggg,0000), skipping such groups becomes a very easy exercise.

Group length can also be viewed as a basic security feature. Group length (just like data checksums) makes it harder to modify something in part of a DICOM object without destroying the entire object structure.

5.5 DICOM Objects

There is no free lunch, however, and this method has its own principal drawbacks. To be able to write the (gggg,0000) tag, DICOM software applications must know the length L of all data elements from the gggg group that are present in the DICOM object. That is, it needs to know the total length of all gggg elements, which will be written *after* the very first (gggg,0000) tag. This implies that all gggg elements must already be available to you with their final values and encoded ahead of encoding the (gggg,0000) element. To DICOM software developers, this means two things:
1. Writing DICOM objects on-the-fly becomes practically impossible because all data must be collected first.
2. Modifying any data element in DICOM objects (for example, replacing Patient Name with another name) inevitably affects the length of the related element's group, which also needs to be updated accordingly.

This additional processing proved to be too much for those of us living in the lazy world of software developers. Consequently, most DICOM software ignores (gggg,0000) group tags, or worse, writes them incorrectly. This might have been the final straw behind retiring group element tag in post-2007 DICOM: the honorable (gggg,0000) group tag is now destined to fade away, and will eventually disappear from future standard releases. However, DICOM apps still must be able to read group length tags, if they are provided: "All implementations shall be able to parse group length elements, and may discard and not insert or reinsert them... No implementation shall require the presence of group length elements."

As a result, most DICOM software reads (gggg,0000) tags, but makes absolutely no use of them. This certainly works as the best defense against inconsistently written or incorrectly updated group length values.[10]

5.5.3 Example: Element and Group Lengths

Encoding element lengths is a very important part of DICOM data representation, and deserves an illustration. Let's consider a simple C-Echo-Request object used in the DICOM standard to verify DICOM network connectivity. I will talk more about C-Echo when we study DICOM services in Sect. 7.2.2, but for now all we need to know is what this object contains. The data encoded in a C-Echo-Request is shown in Fig. 5.6. C-Echo-Request is a DICOM command object, which also means that it contains attributes from group 0000 only (DICOM command attributes) and is encoded with implicit VR encoding(mandatory for all DICOM command objects).

As the table in Fig. 5.6 shows, the object contains only five elements from group 0000: elements 0000, 0002, 0100, 0110, and 0800. I did the length math under each element in the table. Element tag (group and element numbers such as (0000,0002)) will always be encoded with 2+2=4 bytes, and the length of the data field will always be encoded with four bytes.

---

[10]Despite the retirement, references to group length tag can be still found in many parts of DICOM standard – in particular with command objects encoding (gggg=0000) in PS3.7.

Element Tag	Value Length	Value		Element length
(0000,0000)	4	56		
2+2 bytes	4 bytes	4 bytes		=12 bytes
(0000,0002)	18	1.2.840.10008.1.1		
2+2 bytes	+4 bytes	+18 bytes		=26 bytes
(0000,0100)	2	0030		
2+2 bytes	+4 bytes	+2 bytes		=10 bytes
(0000,0110)	2	0001		
2+2 bytes	+4 bytes	+2 bytes		=10 bytes
(0000,0800)	2	0101		
2+2 bytes	+4 bytes	+2 bytes		=10 bytes

Fig. 5.6 Doing length math for C-Echo-Request object

The total of all four elements *following* element (0000,0000) is 26 + 10 + 10 + 10 = 56 bytes. Therefore, 56 will be stored as the value of the (0000,0000) element. If there was another group after group 0000, we could have skipped 56 bytes right after the end of the (0000,0000) element and this would have taken us to the next group available.

5.5.4 Encoding DICOM Data Objects

If you, my dear reader, have made it through the data element encoding part, you have really nothing else to fear. DICOM objects are sequences of DICOM data elements (Fig. 5.7), and therefore are encoded in a straightforward element-wise fashion.

Sure, a data element may contain an SQ item, which would correspond to a nested DICOM object as we discussed earlier. This adds complexity, but does not change the principle. A single rule determines the element order: all data elements inside DICOM objects must be ordered by their tag (Group, Element) number. This ordering serves at least two practical purposes:

5.5 DICOM Objects

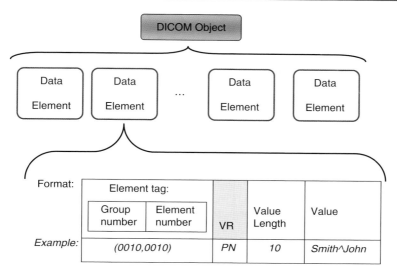

Fig. 5.7 Object without SQ elements – simple sequence of data elements

1. *Helps verify data integrity (similar to what even data length does).* If, when reading a DICOM object element after element, you run into an element with a smaller tag number than the one you read before, the object is corrupted.
2. *Helps put data in the order in which it should really be interpreted.* For example, image width and height have lower tag numbers than the actual image pixel buffer. This means that width and height are read first, and only after will you read the pixels, already knowing how to group them into the width-by-height pixel matrix.

5.5.5 SQ: Encoding DICOM Object Sequences

As we have already seen, one VR type – SQ (sequence) – plays a very special role in DICOM data encoding. It allows us to store entire sequences of DICOM objects in a single SQ VR (see Sect. 5.3.10). With the introduction of the SQ type, DICOM object layout changes dramatically. The SQ element has no data of its own. Instead, *it contains a sequence of DICOM objects*. These objects become nested in the parent DICOM object (the object containing the SQ element). Moreover, because the DICOM objects in the SQ sequence obey the same DICOM object format, they can also contain SQ elements. As a result, we could have multiple nesting levels as shown in Fig. 5.8. The nesting stops at the level where nested DICOM objects have no more SQ elements.

Thus, the entire concept of object sequencing comes quite naturally. If it looks thorny to you, think about the structure of this book. The book has chapters (data

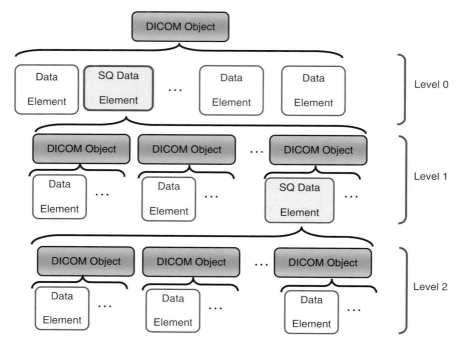

Fig. 5.8 Object with SQ elements – nesting DICOM objects

elements), but some of these first-level chapters have second-level chapters (subsections) inside them, and some second-level chapters have their own subchapters as well (third level), and so on. So, if we consider this book as a large DICOM object, chapters with subchapters would be our SQ elements. In fact, many current data representation languages (XML, for example) make full use of data nesting just like DICOM does.

How do we encode SQ elements though? Without SQ everything is easy. A DICOM object is a list of its data elements, so we encode it as a list as well. For SQ elements, DICOM provides a special SQ encoding scheme that *encapsulates the DICOM object sequence within a single VR*. This is similar to what we learned in Sect. 5.5.1 and depends on the VR encoding method (explicit or implicit) and our choice of data SQ item delimiters (known or unknown length). The following three examples in Table 5.12 cover all possible SQ encoding methods (nested DICOM objects are in gray cells):

If you compare the three examples, you might discover the SQ encoding rules on your own. The rules include:
1. DICOM objects in SQ sequence are encoded as sequence items.
2. Each object-item in the SQ sequence is preceded by the (FFFE, E000) tag (known as *item delimitation* item). This item is followed by one of the following:

5.5 DICOM Objects

Table 5.12 SQ encoding

Example 1: SQ data element with explicit VR defined as a sequence of items (VR = SQ) of undefined length, containing two DICOM objects (items) of explicit length

Tag	VR	Value length	Value (sequence of DICOM objects)									Sequence Delimitation Item	
			First Item				Second Item						
			Tag (FFFE, E000)	Length: 0x1234	Value: DICOM object		Tag (FFFE, E000)	Length: 0x1000	Value: DICOM object			Seq. Delim. Tag (FFFE, E0DD)	Seq. Delim. Item Length 00000000
(gggg, eeee)	SQ	FFFFFFFF (undefined length)											
4 bytes	2 bytes	2 bytes	4 bytes	4 bytes	0x1234 bytes		4 bytes	4 bytes	0x1000 bytes			4 bytes	4 bytes

Example 2: SQ data element with implicit VR defined as a sequence of items (VR = SQ) with three items of explicit length

Tag	Value length	Value (sequence of DICOM objects)								
		First Item			Second Item					
		Tag (FFFE, E000)	Item Length: 0x000004F8	Value: DICOM object	Tag (FFFE, E000)	Item Length: 0x000004F8	Value: DICOM object			
(gggg, eeee)	0x00000A00									
4 bytes	4 bytes	4 bytes	4 bytes	0x04F8 bytes	4 bytes	4 bytes	0x04F8 bytes			

Length math: 0x04 + 0x04 + 0x04F8 + 0x04 + 0x04 + 0x04F8 = 0x0A00

Example 3: SQ data element with implicit VR defined as a sequence of items (VR = SQ) of undefined length, containing two items where one item is of explicit length and the other item is of undefined length

Tag	Value length	Value (sequence of DICOM objects)									Sequence Delimitation Item	
		First Item				Second Item						
		Item Tag (FFFE, E000)	Item Length 0x0000 17B6	Value: DICOM object		Item Tag (FFFE, E000)	Item Length 0xFFFFFFFF (undefined length)	Value: DICOM object	Item Delim. Tag (FFFE, E00D)	Length 0x00000000	Seq. Delim. Tag (FFFE, E0DD)	Seq. Delim. Item Length 0x00000000
(gggg, eeee)	FFFFFFFF (undefined length)											
4 bytes	4 bytes	4 bytes	4 bytes	0x17B6 bytes		4 bytes	4 bytes	Undefined length	4 bytes	4 bytes	4 bytes	4 bytes

i. Explicit length of the DICOM item (for example, first and second items in example 1). This length defines the number of bytes to be read to get the following DICOM object.
  ii. Implicit (*undefined*) length set to hexadecimal FFFFFFFF (second item in example 3). In this case, we need to mark the end of the DICOM object item with (FFFE, E00D) tag. This delimiter is followed by its zero length because it only marks the end of the DICOM object and has no data of its own.
3. Similar to item 2, the entire SQ sequence can have explicit or undefined length:
  i. If explicit length is used (example 2, length 00000A00), this length is equal to the total length of the encoded DICOM object sequence (immediately following the length tag). In example 2, we read 00000A00 bytes and start breaking them into DICOM objects based on (FFFE, E000) tags.
  ii. We could use implicit (undefined) length instead, which in DICOM is marked with FFFFFFFF. Because the length is not known, we have to mark the end of the SQ sequence with the sequence delimitation tag (FFFE, E0DD) followed by its zero length.

If you think about this, the undefined length is identical to the XML approach with the (gggg,eeee) SQ tag playing the role of the XML "<" marker and the (FFFE, E0DD) delimiter playing the role of the XML ">" marker. Similarly, on the object/item level (FFFE, E000) works just like the XML "<" marker and (FFFE, E00D) corresponds to the XML ">"marker. Apart from this XML analogy, the principal beauty of undefined length delimiters is that *you do not have to compute the total length of your DICOM objects or sequences*. If you make a tiny error in this rather complex length value (example 2) the entire sequence will become unreadable. Therefore, undefined-length delimiters are more reliable and easier to implement.

On the other hand, explicit length (example 2) permits you to skip the entire SQ elements or their individual items if you are not interested in reading them. For example, after you have read the 00000A00 sequence length in the example 2 object, you may fast-forward past 0x00000A00 = 2560 bytes to the next element, ignoring the entire SQ element if, for whatever reason, you do not need those bytes for your processing. In short, you gain performance, which probably was a big deal in 1983, but not so much now. These days, carefully written DICOM software reads the most complex DICOM objects in fractions of a second, and the performance would be much more affected by network speed or image encoding than by the use of implicit length items. Therefore, if you implement DICOM software, I would recommend staying with implicit (undefined) length delimiters; they are simple and straightforward for writing your DICOM objects.

However, bear in mind that if you *can* choose between explicit and delimited lengths while *writing* your own DICOM sequences, you *must* implement both length types to *read* DICOM objects. In other words, write as you like, but be polite to other DICOM manufacturers who might have used the opposite length encoding type. You are still responsible for being able to read their objects.

Lastly, keep in mind that each DICOM object item in our three examples could in turn contain SQ items and therefore would be encoded with the same rules as we just discussed. Let's review the nested object from Sect. 5.3.10 in the way it will be stored, using SQ elements, as shown in Fig. 5.9.

5.5 DICOM Objects

DICOM data fragment

Attribute Name	Tag
Referenced Series Sequence	(0008,1115)
>Series Instance UID	(0020,000E)
>Referenced Instance Sequence	(0008,114A)
>>Referenced SOP Class UID	(0008,1150)
>>Referenced SOP Instance UID	(0008,1155)

its SQ graph:

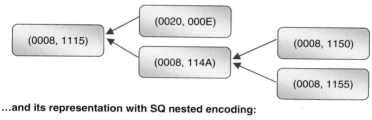

...and its representation with SQ nested encoding:

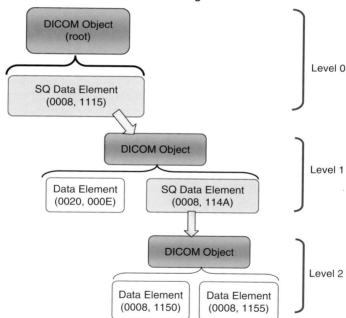

Fig. 5.9 Object with SQ elements

In the example shown in Fig. 5.9, each SQ element contains only one DICOM object. Each of our three encoding examples can be applied with different length explicitness and encoding starts from the bottom. First, we encode a DICOM object at level 2 (it does not have SQs and we encode it as a plain VR sequence). Then the encoded object is placed in the (0008, 114A) SQ element with explicit or undefined length and we arrive at level 1. Finally, the entire encoding process is repeated to create the level 1 DICOM object and to put it inside (0008,1115); (0008,1115) becomes the only element in the root (parent) DICOM object, ready to be stored or networked. If you are programming SQ encoding, you can easily implement it with recursion, just like you would for any tree-like data structure.

5.5.6 Required and Optional Data Elements

Notice that, despite the flexibility of DICOM objects, you should still be very careful with what you put into them. Storing an ultrasound image along with the Hounsfield grayscale CT calibration in the same DICOM object would hardly make sense. PS3.3 (Information Object Definitions) goes into great detail describing the tags and elements required for each particular DICOM object type, such as particular modality images.

This leads to another classification of all data elements: required, conditional, or optional (Sect. 7.4 in PS3.5). To be exact, DICOM defines the following attribute types shown in Table 5.13.

For example, patients in a DICOM workflow are identified by their IDs rather than their names. Therefore, the "Patient ID" attribute (0010,0020) would be Type 1 in virtually any DIOM data object. Consequently, the "Patient Name" attribute (0010,0010) can often be Type 2. The "Image Lossy Compression" attribute (0028,2110) is often Type 1C – it must be specified only if the images have undergone lossy image compression.

While pure DICOM devices such as digital modalities automatically include all required elements in the objects they produce, be careful when you use less-standard DICOM conversion software. It is not uncommon to see a film digitizer encapsulate your scanned film into DICOM format and totally forget to enforce the presence of required tags. DICOM objects (including DICOM files) missing required elements will be considered illegal, and could be rejected or totally misinterpreted by other DICOM devices. Take missing Patient ID as an example: if it is not specified, the object becomes invalid. Worse, if it is specified but left blank, it could be interpreted as "any" (blank elements can be interpreted as wildcards). This means that you can scan several different patients on your digitizer and they will all be merged into one single patient! Believe it or not, this is one of the most widespread errors found in medical data archives.[11]

5.5.7 Storing Image Data

Images follow the same data encoding rules and therefore can easily be put into DICOM objects. As you might imagine, each medical image has several important

---

[11] There are nice public tools for checking DICOM attribute compliance. For example, the DVTk (DICOM Validation Toolkit) is available at http://www.dvtk.org.

5.5 DICOM Objects

Table 5.13 Data element types

Attribute type	When to use
1	Such attributes shall be present with an explicit value, and shall be supported by DICOM applications and services
1C	Such attributes shall be present with an explicit value *provided the specified condition is met*. They shall be supported
2	Such attributes shall be present with an explicit value *or with a zero-length value if unknown*. They shall be supported
2C	Such attributes shall be present with an explicit value *or with a zero length if unknown, provided the specified condition is met*. They shall be supported
3	Such attributes *may be present* with an explicit value or a zero-length value. They may be supported or ignored

elements that correspond to attributes in the standard DICOM Data Dictionary. A few of these include:

- *Image height* – corresponds to the "Rows" attribute (0028,0010).
- *Image width* – corresponds to the "Columns" attribute (0028,0011).
- *Image pixel data* – corresponds to the "Pixel Data" attribute (7FE0,0010).

The latter contains the actual image and in many cases takes some 95% of the DICOM object size (medical images are large).

Moreover, you can put sequences of image frames into a single DICOM object, which is how DICOM stores digital video such as ultrasound cine loops. In fact, we can look at this process from a wider perspective: interpreting digital images as digitized signal sequences. This makes them similar to any other signal data – audio, for example – that you might want to record and put into DICOM objects. With sensible use of the Data Dictionary it all becomes very possible and you can easily encode your favorite movie as a single DICOM object with multiframe image and audio.

I Want My MTV!

As I just said, DICOM stores videos as sequences of individual image frames. For example, a single ultrasound cine loop, 10 s long, recorded at 25 frames/s will be digitized in DICOM as $10 \times 25 = 250$ consecutive image frames stored in a single DICOM object.

When these are displayed in DICOM software, they still will be displayed as a series of 250 still images. In other words, you always have to push some "Play" button to make them run as a video. I have seen several people puzzled by this concept: if this cine loop is a video, why does not it play automatically? Simply because the playback is a function of your viewing software and not the function of DICOM. DICOM stores 250 still video frames accompanied by the (0018,0040) "Frames Per Second" attribute value just to indicate that these frames *should be played* as a video.

5.5.8 Unique Identifiers

Whether you ever played with object-oriented applications or not, you should be familiar with the notion of *an instance*. In brief, an instance is a *snapshot of an object in time* with all its current data values. Changing an object's data always produces another instance of the object. Consider a medical image; say the head X-ray of John Smith, stored in a DICOM object. If you make a copy of this DICOM object, you essentially create another image instance. The original image (instance) remains unchanged; the new copy can be cropped, color-edited, annotated, and more. In short, it can be modified to become very different from the original. Yet it will still be labeled as "head X-ray of John Smith." Which instance should be used by your radiologist? When you work in healthcare, you realize that it is in your best interest to be able to differentiate between the instances. In DICOM, this is achieved with Unique Identifiers (UIDs).

Look at Fig. 5.10. It illustrates how one original image can produce multiple instances, some of them still being identical to the original, yet residing in different locations or serving different purposes. It also explains why UIDs, used to label those instances, must be globally unique. Image instances can be sent far away from the original (for example, for teleradiology reading in another country) where they will be stored with many other images in other archives. DICOM UIDs, just like human DNAs, work as unique markers that are always capable of identifying a particular instance wherever it might be (Fig. 5.10). For the same reason, unique identifiers are used in DICOM to tag not only individual images, but also image series, studies, devices, syntaxes in data exchange protocols, and many other things that you do not want to confuse.

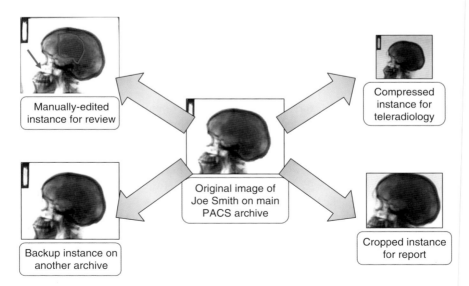

Fig. 5.10 Instances of the same image; each needs a different UID

5.5 DICOM Objects

DICOM unique identifiers are strings such as "1.2.840.10008.1.2" built from numerical components separated by periods; that is, they conform to the UI type (see UI type in our VR table, Sect. 5.3). UID strings are supposed to be *globally* unique to guarantee distinction across multiple countries, sites, vendors, and equipment. In our globalized universe, this is the only way to ensure that your image or transaction does not run the risk of being confused with any other – no matter where it comes from. Therefore, DICOM uses the following UID encoding convention:

$$UID = <org\ root>.<suffix>$$

Here, the <org root> portion of the UID uniquely identifies an organization, (that is, manufacturer, research organization, NEMA, and so on). Ideally, each organization is supposed to apply and receive its own root ID (which does not always happen) to guarantee that this root is not in use (see Annex C, DICOM PS3.5, for the root registration rules). Also, the 1.2.840.10008 string is reserved as the universal <org root> for all DICOM transaction UIDs, and cannot be used elsewhere.

> **Tip: Recognizing DICOM Files**
> Open an unknown file in WordPad, and search it for 1.2.840.10008. If this string is found, you are likely dealing with a DICOM file.
> The four DICM letters at the very top of the file (characters 129–132, counting from the file start) are another way of identifying DICOM files. However, some old or incorrect DICOM implementations might not write them, while multiple UID prefixes like 1.2.840.10008 should be easier to spot.

The <suffix> portion of the UID is also composed of a number of numeric components, and "shall be unique within the scope of the <org root>" (see section 9 in DICOM PS3.5). While roots are relatively short, these are the suffixes that are used to capture the *uniqueness* of the instance. For example, if you build a suffix like:

<patient ID>.<study ID>.<current date>.<current time in milliseconds>

you could be pretty sure that no one in your enterprise will have the same UID. This is why all 64 UI-type characters come in so handy; the more characters you use, the fewer your chances of having two equal UIDs.

For the same reason, UIDs are often used as DICOM file names. This is not really DICOM-compliant (see Sect. 10.1.4). True DICOM file names should come from 8-character components containing only capital letters, digits, and underscore characters (for example, DIR1\SKW_12AB5). However, if the 8-character format is mandatory for file-exporting applications (writing DICOM files to external, removable media such as CDs/DVDs or flash drives – see Chap. 10), UID-based names are widely used internally by nearly all DICOM applications to store their images on local hard drives. The UID-based DICOM file naming is justified: each DICOM image object includes the Image "SOP Instance UID" attribute (0008,0018). This makes it a good name for a DICOM image file, associating it with the unique object instance within. When you see file names such as:

```
1.2.804.114118.2.20040909.125423.3692976692.1.1.1
```

you are likely dealing with DICOM files. In essence, DICOM files are nothing more than DICOM objects stored on your hard drive – DICOM object memory dumps, if you wish.

> **UID Parsing?**
> Even though UID names are always built with certain logic in mind, do not try to parse them or use their names to convey additional information. For example, even if you know that a UID name might include patient ID or study date, do not try to extract this data. DICOM explicitly warns against this.
>
> UID names are not meant for any data exchange and their sole purpose is to distinguish between multiple object instances. As long as this is guaranteed, the DICOM application is free to change or update UID names as it finds appropriate with whatever additional naming logic it might be using. In addition to what DICOM prescribes, correct UID-issuing policy always remains on your DICOM manufacturer's mind. They – through their DICOM-compliant software – must track image changes and create a new UID for each clinically different instance of the same image.

5.6 DICOM Information Hierarchy

Before we continue with our review of DICOM data, it is worth having a quick look at how DICOM structures its information. Certainly, DICOM Data Dictionary attributes play very important roles in mapping real-world data into the DICOM standard. But still, these attributes are many. Don't we need to put them in some order?

This order is achieved in DICOM with the *Patient-Study-Series-Image* hierarchy (Fig. 5.11):
- One patient may have multiple studies.
- Each study may include one or more image series.
- Each series has one or more images.

This hierarchy naturally reflects what happens in the real world when a patient needs to have some medical imaging done. John Smith comes to a hospital where several studies may be scheduled (for example, MR, CT, and US exams). Several follow-up studies could be needed later. Each study may have multiple image series (CT, ultrasound, 3D reconstructions, with varying imaging protocols, and so on). And each series, quite naturally, will have one or more images. Now, if we need to find or sort images for this patient, requirement seriously. If you are planning on buying one, please verify that it has ample support for entering DICOM data, and for assigning the images to the same Patient, Study, or Series groups.

5.6.3 Hierarchical and Relational Data

To wrap up our discussion on the DICOM Patient-Study-Series-Image information model, let us briefly mention that it represents a central part of a more complex *DICOM model of the real world*. This model can be found in the standard (section 7 in PS3.3) adding more items to the basic Patient-Study-Series-Image hierarchy without changing its essence. Virtually all DICOM devices function on the Patient-Study-Series-Image steps, performing *hierarchical* data searches, retrievals, and transactions.

To identify a series, you will need first to find the patient and the study the series belongs to. This logic is clearly reflected in all DICOM interfaces. They always start browsing their data from the top, from the highest Patient (sometimes Study) level, then gradually descend to Series and Images. Moreover, hierarchical DICOM queries and data retrievals will fail on any of the four Patient-Study-Series-Image levels if the information about the higher level IDs is not known. For example, a hierarchical search for a particular series will fail if its study and patient IDs are not known beforehand.

The only DICOM alternative to hierarchical data processing is known as relational data processing (Fig. 5.12). Unlike hierarchical processing, relational data processing does not break data into the four levels, and it permits you to search data in any way possible (provided that the data is somehow related). For example, you can search for a particular series not knowing its Study and Patient IDs as long as you provide other data to identify the series (such as modality, date/time, UID, and so on).

DICOM supports relational (nonhierarchical) data processing as an option. While hierarchical data processing is mandatory on any DICOM unit, relational data processing may or may not be provided in addition – and more often it is not. Whether relational data processing is available should be specified in the device's DICOM Conformance Statement.

5.7 Modules, IODs and IEs

Building DICOM objects from data elements is the only way to do it right, but with some 2000 data elements in the DICOM Data Dictionary, we would like to have a bit more structure. You cannot really get a few MR-specific elements (such as (0018,0087) magnetic field strength), add a few CT tags (such as kvp in (0018,0060)), insert ultrasound images, and call this a DICOM object. The chimera will be rejected by most DICOM devices and even the remaining ones – marvels of DICOM data processing flexibility that they are – won't have any idea how to process such a jumble.

Data elements are the smallest building blocks, and they might not necessarily fit together. To put this in a better order, we need to group data elements into larger

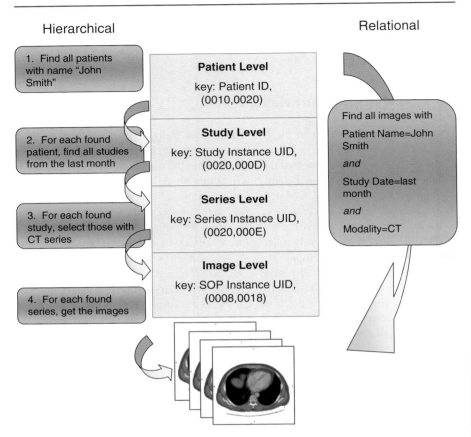

Fig. 5.12 Example of hierarchical (*left*) versus relational search for "images of last-month CT study for John Smith." Hierarchical searches are simpler. This makes them more efficient, but it requires more steps

building blocks, and use them to build more meaningful and more defined DICOM objects.

DICOM calls these blocks *Information Modules*, *Information Entities* (IEs), and *Information Object Definitions* (IODs). Like many things in DICOM, they are related hierarchically. Modules form IEs, which in turn are used to build IODs. Because DICOM data is defined for each image modality the proper choice of modules, IEs, and IODs depends on the modality. Let us have a closer look at how it all works.

5.7.1 Attribute Macros: Making It Easier

Often, you might prefer to group similar attributes to shorten their referencing in other modules. DICOM calls these groups of common characteristics *macro attributes* (Table 5.14).

5.7 Modules, IODs and IEs

Table 5.14 Series and instance reference macro attributes

Attribute name	Tag	Attribute description
Referenced Series Sequence	(0008,1115)	Sequence of Items each of which includes the Attributes of one Series. One or more Items shall be present
>Series Instance UID	(0020,000E)	Unique identifier of the Series containing the referenced Instances
>Referenced Instance Sequence	(0008,114A)	Sequence of Items each providing a reference to an Instance that is part of the Series defined by Series Instance UID (0020,000E) in the enclosing Item. One or more Items shall be present
>>Referenced SOP Class UID	(0008,1150)	Uniquely identifies the referenced SOP Class
>>Referenced SOP Instance UID	(0008,1155)	Uniquely identifies the referenced SOP Instance

Table 5.15 Patient identification module

Attribute name	Tag	Value/description
Patient Name	(0010,0010)	Patient's full name
Patient ID	(0010,0020)	Primary hospital identification number or code for the patient
Other Patient IDs	(0010,1000)	Other identification numbers or codes used to identify the patient
Other Patient Names	(0010,1001)	Other names used to identify the patient
Patient's Birth Name	(0010,1005)	Patient's birth name
Patient's Mother's Birth Name	(0010,1060)	Birth name of patient's mother
Medical Record Locator	(0010,1090)	An identifier used to find the patient's existing medical record (for example, film jacket)

Note the possible use of sequencing (see Sect. 5.3.10). The "greater than" sign (>), as always, indicates that the next element is embedded into the previous one with the SQ VR. But even without sequencing some macros can be pretty large and can take several pages in PS3.3 (Image Pixel macro, for example). As far as information structuring is concerned, macros do not correspond to any particular object or data block; they help us avoid repetitive element tables.

5.7.2 Information Modules: Basic Data Blocks

Modules, as I just said, provide the very first and the most essential level of data element organization. For example, Patient Identification Module (Table 5.15) groups all patient-identifying information: data tags for patient name, ID, birth name, maiden name, and more.

The contents of this module are self-explanatory: they capture all possible attributes (data elements) related to patient identification. Clearly, not all of them can be

Table 5.16 Clinical trial module

Attribute name	Tag	Attribute description
Clinical Trial Sponsor Name	(0012,0010)	The name of the clinical trial sponsor
Clinical Trial Protocol ID	(0012,0020)	Identifier for the noted protocol
Clinical Trial Protocol Name	(0012,0021)	The name of the clinical trial protocol
Clinical Trial Site ID	(0012,0030)	The identifier of the site responsible for submitting clinical trial data
Clinical Trial Site Name	(0012,0031)	The name of the site responsible for submitting clinical trial data
Clinical Trial Subject ID	(0012,0040)	The assigned identifier for the clinical trial subject. Shall be present if Clinical Trial Subject Reading ID (0012,0042) is absent. May be present otherwise
Clinical Trial Subject Reading ID	(0012,0042)	Identifies the subject for blinded evaluations. Shall be present if Clinical Trial Subject ID (0012,0040) is absent. May be present otherwise

collected for a given patient, and in some cases none can be known at all (unconscious patients, for example). However, modules are not meant to contain complete values for all their attributes. Unknown fields can be left blank or even omitted if not required. The main purpose of modules is to gather related data attributes (elements) in a consistent, structured manner. For example, if our patient becomes a subject of a clinical trial, we add a Clinical Trial module to record all trial attributes (Table 5.16).

To give you a slightly different module example, let's look at the Cine module in Table 5.17, which defines playback parameters for multiframe images.

If a DICOM object contains a sequence of video frames (a sequence of images that are consecutive frames of a digitized video), a Cine module stores the information on how this sequence needs to be played. The most essential parameter here would be "Frame Time" (0018,1063), representing the time delay in milliseconds between the frames. For example, a 25 frames per second average video rate corresponds to $1000/25 = 40$ milliseconds in (0018,1063). However, as you can see, a number of other attributes can be supported depending on the data content. Note that the Cine module uses the Code Sequence macro.

Just like almost anything in DICOM, information modules can be *mandatory* (indicated in DICOM by a capital M); *conditional* – required if other specific modules are present (indicated by a capital C); and *user-defined* – think about proprietary data elements (indicated by a capital U).

The proper selection of modules depends on the type of data stored in the DICOM object. In most cases, this type corresponds to the image modality (CT, MR, CR, and so on); but there are also non-modality object types (think about ECG, reports or voice recordings). For example, Patient Identification Module is always mandatory for any DICOM modality; we cannot have a digital image without knowing who it belongs to. The Cine module, as you would imagine, is required

5.7 Modules, IODs and IEs

Table 5.18 CT IOD

IE	Information module	Usage
Patient	Patient	M (mandatory)
	Clinical Trial Subject	U (user-defined)
Study	General Study	M
	Patient Study	U
	Clinical Trial Study	U
Series	General Series	M
	Clinical Trial Series	U
Frame of Reference	Frame of Reference	M
Equipment	General Equipment	M
Image	General Image	M
	Image Plane	M
	Image Pixel	M
	Contrast/bolus	C (conditional) – Required if contrast media was used in this image
	CT Image	M
	Overlay Plane	U
	VOI LUT	U
	SOP Common	M

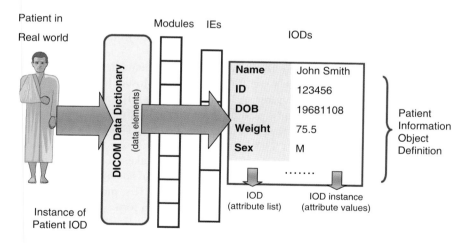

Fig. 5.14 From patient to patient object

Furthermore, DICOM breaks all IODs into Normalized and Composite. A normalized IOD represents a single, real-world entity just as our Patient IOD represents a patient; all attributes of a normalized IOD are inherent in the real-world entity it represents. The DICOM Study IOD, for example, is normalized and contains only inherent study properties such as study date and time. Patient name, for example, being a property of a patient rather than a study, would not be present in the study IOD.

Composite IODs are mixtures of several real-world entities or their constituent parts. Consider a CT image IOD, for example: in DICOM, this IOD will contain some of the patient attributes (name, ID, and so on to identify the patient the image belongs to) along with attributes of the CT scanner, patient study, and more. This blend from several real-world entities makes a CT image an IOD composite. As you might guess, composite IODs work better for capturing relationships, associations, processes, and contexts. Normalized IODs are meant to represent single objects. However, the line between *composite* and *normalized* is often blurred, and as far as we are concerned they all remain IODs, equally treated by DICOM.

To summarize, IODs are abstract representations of real world objects – patients, CT images, and more. In terms of object-oriented design, IODs are objects, or classes. Any actual DICOM objects that we discussed earlier (Sect. 5.5) are nothing more than IOD instances recorded in DICOM format where VRs are used to record data element names and values.

5.7.6 Learning More

I presented you with the basic concepts of DICOM data organization. Now you know enough to be able to understand DICOM from VRs to IODs. If you want to go any further, part three of the DICOM standard (PS3.3) is your ultimate reference. It applies the principles you have learned to define all particular objects and data types used in DICOM. It will also give you more details on DICOM information models and the way DICOM structures radiology workflow by binding it with IODs and IEs.

Bear in mind that part three is the largest part of the standard; it is well beyond 1000 pages already and grows by some 100 pages a year. Most of the changes in this document are recorded in its annexes: A (composite IODs), B (normalized IODs), and C (information modules). Just reading them continuously could probably get you into the *Guinness Book of World Records*; they go on and on with specific IOD types. Instead, try to *data mine* PS3.3, searching by your keywords. Unfortunately, the evolutionary approach to DICOM writing sometimes takes ill turns; one cannot indefinitely improve the standard by growing the number of its object definitions. If DICOM 4.0 ever happens, maybe the entire assembly of IEs, modules, and IODs will be restructured into a more normalized and condensed form.

Medical Images in DICOM 6

Let me assume, my dear reader, that the time we used to wander in the land of VRs and DICOM objects has been well spent, and that you have a much better idea of how DICOM deals with medical data. This prepared you for the next important step in your voyage: looking at how DICOM works with medical images. Certainly, images possess some well-known properties (width, height, bits per pixel), which can be found in the DICOM Data Dictionary, and which DICOM encodes with explicit or implicit VRs, as you have already learned. But the most interesting image attribute is the image itself – the sequence of image pixel values – that DICOM stores in the standard (7FE0, 0010) Pixel Data tag, using either OB (for 1-byte pixel samples) or OW (for 2-byte pixel samples) encoding.

DICOM supports a wide range of image formats for storing these (7FE0, 0010) pixels. The formats can be loosely broken into two main groups:

1. *DICOM-specific*: the formats that are used by DICOM only. They are typically the oldest ones, introduced at the dawn of the computer era before better image-storing approaches had been developed. They resemble raw bitmaps with varying ways of packing the pixel bytes.
2. *Independent standard formats accepted by DICOM*. These include such well-known formats as JPEG, RLE (run-length encoding), ZIP, and the less known (but getting more and more popular) JPEG2000, and JPEG-LS. All these standards are also associated with various image compression techniques, reversible and not, which makes them particularly useful in medical imaging (reducing image data size *is* important). When DICOM includes other standards to be used for particular tasks (such as JPEG for image encoding), the embedded standard approach is very convenient, consistent, and makes good practical sense.

Let us start with the first type, because it is the easiest and the oldest, and because it is still used most of the time as the DICOM default. Then we'll review the most important points of the independent standards. You can read more about them elsewhere, but some of their properties have tremendous effects on medical imaging storage and analysis, so I will try not to miss them.

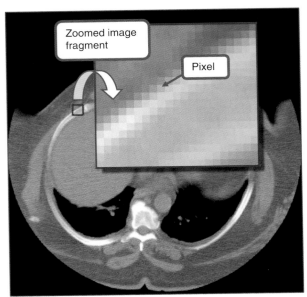

Fig. 6.1 Zooming into digital image

6.1 DICOM Bitmaps

A digital image, as you might already know, is a rectangular matrix of pixels (*picture elements*) – tiny dots of different colors that form the actual picture. For example, a typical CT image is 512 pixels wide and 512 pixels high; that is, it contains $512 \times 512 = 262144$ pixels. If you write these pixels line-by-line starting from the top left corner you will have a sequence of 262144 pixel values, which you can store in a file. Essentially, this file is your raw bitmap image (Fig. 6.1).

Now close your eyes and make a mental list of all digital image attributes that you consider important. Are you done? Compare yours to DICOM's:

- *Image width and height* – Definitely, you need to know them. Their product is often referred to as *spatial image resolution* and equals the total number of pixels in the image.
- *Samples per pixel* – Each image pixel can be a blend of several sample values. The most typical case is a color pixel, which comprises three independent color samples: red, green, and blue (known as the RGB color space). While the value of each sample contributes to the pixel's brightness, their mixture creates the color. For example, mixing equal quantities of red and green produces shades of yellow and equal quantities of red, green, and blue correspond to grayscales. Grayscale images, however, are usually stored with one monochrome sample per pixel, corresponding to the pixel's grayscale luminance. When 2-byte (16-bit) samples are used (OW VR), this provides for $2^{16} = 65536$ possible grayscales – the source of DICOM support for deep grayscales in CT, MR, CR (X-ray), and many other modalities.

In any event, the choice of pixel sampling remains constant for all pixels in an image, depending only on the imaging technique.

6.1 DICOM Bitmaps

- *Bits used to store a pixel sample, B_s* – DICOM calls this parameter "bits stored." For example, if you have a grayscale image where each pixel (sample) uses eight bits, then $B_s=8$, and the number of grayscale shades in this image will be $2^{B_s}=2^8=256$. If you increase the number of stored bits to $B_s=10$, you will have $2^{10}=1024$ shades per sample, and so on. As you can see, the *bits stored* number is responsible for the color depth[1] of the image; it shows how rich your image is. In this respect, this attribute is similar to spatial resolution (image width and height), but in the luminance domain – the more, the merrier. It is particularly valuable and important in digital medicine where you often need to see minute changes in colors and brightness.
- *Bits allocated per pixel sample, B_a* – essentially, B_s, rounded up to a multiple of eight (to fit into whole bytes). This is how much computer memory will be used to store a pixel sample. Clearly, $B_s \le B_a$.
- *High bit, B_h* – as we will see in a minute, this bit corresponds to the end of the B_s pixel sample within the B_a segment.

Figure 6.2 summarizes the structure of a multi-sample DICOM pixel. The example pixel comprises three samples: red, green, and blue. In this particular example, each sample has $B_s=12$ bits. Because all computer data is stored in bytes (1 byte = 8 bits), the 12 bits are rounded up to $B_a=16$, and $B_h=11$. Usually $B_h=B_s-1$. The same 16-bit storage is allocated for the other samples (red and blue in this case), and the entire image is written as a sequence of its pixel samples.

I hope this does not seem difficult, but to make this picture complete, let me show you another example of pixel sample encoding in Fig. 6.3.

In this case, a sample was stored in $B_s=10$ bits, but counting from bit two. Because DICOM stores the values of high bit B_h and bits stored B_s, we can recover the first "low bit" position as B_h+1-B_s and the rest will follow.

The trickiest part in all "old school" pixel encoding is how DICOM can take advantage of the unused bits. If we look at the second example, we see

$$B_a - B_s = 6 \text{ bits}$$

(bits 0–1 and 12–15) not containing any pixel data; so we wasted $6/16 = 37.5\%$ of the storage space. To recoup this space, DICOM used to store additional information there, such as image overlay pixels (which are not particularly related to the original image pixel data). In essence, pieces of one information stream were jammed between the pieces of others just to use all the bits in every byte.

This approach was popular in the early DICOM days when image compression was still in its cradle, and storing other data between the pixel samples was considered a cool way of optimizing the storage. As you can imagine, in reality it lead to rather confusing bit mixtures that eventually made themselves obsolete. These days, one can achieve much better memory usage with image compression than with chasing stray inter-pixel bits. Nevertheless, "bit squeezing" techniques are still standard

---

[1] By *color depth*, I mean both the number of colors available in the color image and the number of grayscale shades available in the grayscale image.

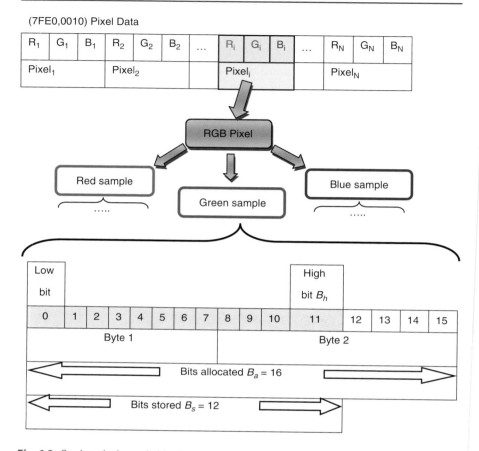

Fig. 6.2 Storing pixel sample bits: basic

in DICOM, and can be found in some applications and data, especially if you deal with an older DICOM unit – be aware of them. Annex D in DICOM PS3.5 of the standard explains other possible sample encoding schemes.

If you can deal with the various ways of recording image pixels (samples), you know how to read and write DICOM bitmaps. As I have mentioned, DICOM treats image information like anything else and all important image attributes are translated into DICOM VRs stored in DICOM objects. These attributes must be present in any image-containing DICOM object. In DICOM parlance, these attributes are *required*. Table 6.1 provides a more detailed snapshot of some important image attributes, taken from the DICOM Data Dictionary.

This is but a fraction of all DICOM pixel-related tags, but if you have any experience working with other image formats, you should appreciate the completeness of DICOM. For example, as (0028,0008) suggests, you can store a sequence of frames

6.1 DICOM Bitmaps

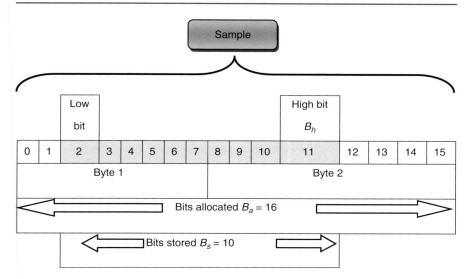

Fig. 6.3 Storing pixel sample bits: more complex

Table 6.1 Important image attributes in DICOM Data Dictionary

Tag	Name	VR	VM
(0018,0050)	Slice Thickness	DS	1
(0018,0088)	Spacing between Slices	DS	1
(0020, 0032)	Image Position	DS	3
(0020,0037)	Image Orientation	DS	6
(0028,0002)	Samples per Pixel	US	1
(0028,0004)	Photometric Interpretation	CS	1
(0028,0008)	Number of Frames	IS	1
(0028,0010)	Rows	US	1
(0028,0011)	Columns	US	1
(0028,0030)	Pixel Spacing	DS	2
(0028,0100)	Bits Allocated B_a	US	1
(0028,0101)	Bits Stored B_s	US	1
(0028,0102)	High Bit B_h	US	1
(0028,0103)	Pixel Representation	US	1
(7FE0,0010)	Pixel Data	OW/OB	1

(essentially, a digital video) in a simple DICOM *image*. You can specify the physical dimensions of pixels in (0028,0030) – for example, 0.7×0.7 mm in CT image – which allows you to measure the image objects in their physical units, such as millimeters. Knowing pixel spacing, spacing between the images (0018,0088), image position (0020, 0032), and orientation (0020,0037) allows for the most elaborate 3D reconstructions because we can preserve the correct sizes and locations of the objects.

I could go on with this list almost indefinitely, but let me stop here and conclude the overview on DICOM bitmaps; after all, we do have bigger fish to fry.

Just keep in mind that DICOM provides extremely rich support for storing image data and all related parameters, which no other image format can provide. This explains the success of DICOM in medical imaging. This also explains why exporting DICOM images in other "conventional" formats (such as 8-bit JPEG) always leads to losing critical image data and can result in potentially dangerous image misinterpretation. Besides, exporting in this manner simply does not make any sense. DICOM supports JPEG and other compression methods internally to compress pixel buffers in the (7FE0,0010) "Pixel Data" attribute within DICOM objects without sacrificing any other attribute data.

Let us take a look at all this image compression stuff; maybe I can show you what all the hubbub's about.

6.2   Image Compression

Consider a typical CT image with width=height=512, grayscale (one sample per pixel), and bits stored=12. How much computer memory would it take to store this image?

Well, let us do the math. For storing 12 bits, we need to allocate two full bytes (16 bits). The total number of pixels is 512×512, so the total number of bytes to store them will be:

$$512 \times 512 \times 2 = 524,288$$

That is, we would need half a megabyte for the pixel data stored in the (7FE0,0010) "Pixel Data" attribute of the DICOM CT object.

However, the CT images do not come alone; they come in series and studies, each containing anywhere from a few hundred to a few thousand images. In our case, a mere 200 CTs will occupy 100 megabytes. This will take nearly 6 h to download on a dial-up network, or several boring minutes on a broadband. A few days of studies like this can easily fill your hard drive. How do you deal with such data volume (Table 6.2)?

Typical replies might be "*Buy a better computer,*" or "*Get a faster network.*" While upgrading system hardware is always a good idea, in this case it actually solves only one problem: how to spend your money. Look at the tremendous progress in the quality and resolution of digital image acquisition devices. DRs and CRs, multi-slice CTs, enhanced (higher-resolution) imaging, digital mammography, and ultrasound devices keep increasing the resolution and the number of images produced, which inevitably translates into larger image and study sizes (Branstetter 2009). If you plan to run a competitive and scalable medical enterprise, and you look into applications such as teleradiology, you won't be able to survive without image compression (Huang 2004).

Given this, image compression has been included in the DICOM standard since its inception. Image compression targets the (7FE0,0010) image pixel bytes, and

Table 6.2 Typical sizes of digital images and studies

Image modality	Typical image matrix (height width, bytes per pixel)	Image size, kilobytes (KB)	Typical number of images in a study[a]	Typical study size, megabytes (MB)
Nuclear medicine, NM	128×128×1	16	100	1.5
Magnetic resonance, MR	256×256×2	128	200	25
Computed tomography, CT	512×512×2	512	500	250
Color ultrasound, US	600×800×3	1400	500	680
Computed radiography, CR	2140×1760×2	7356	4	30
Color 3D reconstructions[b]	1024×1024×3	3000	20	60
Digital mammography, MG	Up to 6400×4800×2	60000	4	240

[a]Because this varies greatly depending on facilities, studies, and protocols, I provide the most general "order of magnitude" numbers
[b]"Secondary capture" (SC) reconstructions; offered more often nowadays by CT and MR modalities

cleverly rearranges them into a much shorter form. This significantly reduces the original image size (much better than old style *bit squeezing*), which in turn saves storage space and often reduces image download time. I have already mentioned that DICOM does not invent image compression techniques of its own. Rather, DICOM includes nearly all well-known image compression algorithms including RLE, JPEG, JPEG2000, JPEG-LS, and ZIP. All these algorithms have been developed separately, resulting in separate ISO[2] standards and applications; DICOM simply adopted them. All DICOM data objects with compressed (7FE0,0010) pixel buffers are encoded with an explicit VR Little Endian type (see Sect. 5.5.1).

The use of image compression could have a significant effect on the image appearance and on the overall performance of PACS, so you need to know compression basics regardless of your current role in your medical enterprise. The main idea of data compression is not difficult at all. *Any compression algorithm will try to find and trim the most redundant and repetitive information, thus making the data shorter*. The efficiency of this trimming is quantified by the following compression ratio:

$$R_{comp} = \frac{Original\,data\,size}{Compressed\,data\,size}$$

The higher the ratio, the better compression is achieved. Each compression algorithm offers it own strategy to maximize R_{comp}, but conceptually and practically, all compression techniques can be assigned to one of two categories: *lossless (reversible)* and *lossy (irreversible)* compression.

---

[2]International Organization for Standardization.

6.2.1 Lossless Compression

Lossless compression *does not change the image*. After you compress and uncompress an image, you always get the original – pixel by pixel. This is done with clever regrouping and renaming of the pixel bytes. Just to grasp the general idea, consider the following sequence of pixel values:

```
1000, 1001, 1002, 1002, 1000, 1000, 1001, 1057,….
```

A typical lossless compression algorithm will try to explore the repetitiveness of the most frequent values like 1000 and replace them with shorter symbols. For example, if we replace "1000" by "a", the original string turns into:

```
a, 1001, 1002, 1002, a, a, 1001, 1057,….
```

Because "a" is shorter than "1000," our entire data string has become shorter, and as long as we remember that we used "a" to *compress* the value of "1000," we can always *uncompress* this string to its original value. This compression approach is known as "variable length coding." Now think about this: if we take the most repetitive elements in the original data, and replace them with the shortest possible symbols, we could achieve substantial data size reduction, but we will always be able to recover our data. Well then, we just rediscovered the Huffman compression algorithm – the most popular algorithm in variable length coding (Oakley 2003). All *natural* images always have something repetitive to compress. First, neighboring pixels often tend to have similar values; second, an image can have large areas with the same pixel value (such as a black background). This intrinsic redundancy leads to successful lossless compression. When this redundancy is explored in an increasing number of available image dimensions – in x and y for a regular 2D image, or in x, y, and z for a 3D image set (such as CT slice sequences) – then more substantial compression can be achieved.

Nevertheless, pixel repetitiveness can be exploited only to a certain extent, and for an average medical image R_{comp} will be somewhere between two and four; meaning that the compressed image size will be between one-half and one-quarter of the original. This is already good, but not impressive if you have a lossy compression option.

6.2.2 Lossy Compression

Lossy compression, as its name suggests, *sacrifices some of the original information* to achieve a much higher compression ratio R_{comp}. This sacrifice is made to force additional data redundancy so it can be efficiently complemented with the lossless compression step. Let us take the same pixel sequence as before:

```
1000, 1001, 1002, 1002, 1000, 1000, 1001, 1057,….
```

6.2 Image Compression

If the pixel intensity is about 1000, would you be able to visually perceive the difference between 1000 and 1001? Probably not because this is only a 0.1% change in the pixel brightness. Therefore, we can slightly modify this sequence by choosing one grayscale level as an acceptable error margin and replacing 1001 with 1000:

    1000, 1000, 1002, 1002, 1000, 1000, 1000, 1057,….

If we apply the lossless compression to this modified sequence, as we discussed earlier, we would get:

    a, a, 1002, 1002, a, a, a, 1057,….

The result is much shorter than with pure lossless compression. In other words, if lossless compression is taking advantage of the *equal* pixels, lossy is extending this to the *nearly equal* pixel values within a hard-to-notice error margin.

Believe it or not, current state-of-the-art lossy compression algorithms can have R_{comp} as high as 100 – that is, reducing data to 1% of its original size! For average medical images, reasonable R_{comp} values would be around 10 and sometimes up to 20. The value of R_{comp} in the lossy compression entirely depends on the value of the perceptually-acceptable error. In the above example, we compromised one grayscale, but using 2-grayscale error would produce an even better compression result of:

    a, a, a, a, a, a, a, 1057,….

Obviously, this error margin cannot be increased indefinitely. At some point it does become perceivable, introducing visible artifacts in the lossy-compressed image. Balancing lossy compression between high R_{comp} and visible image degradation has become an art in itself, but remember the following:

1. *Lossy compression could lead to legal disputes.* If lossy compression is used in the program, DICOM (and FDA) require that all lossy-compressed images be labeled as such.
2. *Computer-Aided Diagnosis (CAD) issues.* As CAD gains more popularity, computers and computer software become more involved in medical image analysis. Errors invisible to human eyes will be visible to CAD software and can become destructive.

CAD and Lossy Compression

Your CAD program, if you have one, can become an objective tool for evaluating the appropriateness of lossy compression. If it produces the same outcomes on the original image and the image after lossy compression, then you may use it as a good indication that the images were not over-compressed, and the lossy compression ratio you use at least does not interfere with your CAD analysis.

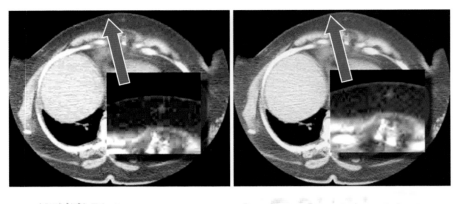

Fig. 6.4 Illustrating excessive lossy compression with images and text patterns. Overdone JPEG creates highly visible blocking artifacts; overdone JPEG2000 creates blur

At the present time, lossy image compression has become popular in various teleradiology systems where images must be transmitted over long, sometimes bottlenecked networks with unpredictable bandwidth. But even there, it should be used with moderation. Last year, I saw one teleradiology service using lossy JPEG with 70% quality for medical image exchange. In case you do not know, you wouldn't use 70% JPEG even for your pets' pictures. The lossy compression artifacts at this quality level can become very apparent.

If you plan to use lossy compression in your enterprise, always evaluate it with a trained radiologist for each image type/modality and make sure that the loss is indeed invisible.

Too much lossy compression will produce highly visible image artifacts – as you can see in Fig. 6.4.

The image on the left has been *overcompressed* with JPEG, which lead to the notorious JPEG *checker* artifacts – easily perceptible, rectangular blocks with constant color. The same image on the right has been exposed to large doses of JPEG2000 lossy compression; instead of checkers, this led to the image blur. The R_{comp} for both images was about 70. Compressing them to a tenth of the original size would have produced a much better result, visually identical to the original image.

Bear in mind that responsibility for using lossy compression rests on the radiologist's shoulders; and the radiologist will be to blame if something is misinterpreted due to image quality loss. PACS manufacturers are only responsible for:

1. Consistently providing noncompressed images and providing compression as an *option*. Using the lossy option is *your choice*.
2. Clearly labeling lossy-compressed images as such when they are displayed on the viewing workstation. In this case, if you are not satisfied with the image quality, you should be able to reload the images as uncompressed (always confirm this with your PACS vendor).

6.2 Image Compression

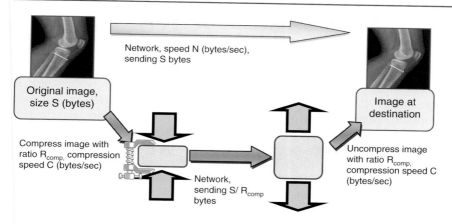

Fig. 6.6 Using image compression on networks

If we consider a moderate lossless compression ratio of $R_{comp}=3$ and we want to achieve a reasonable twofold transmission speed-up of $K=2$ we get:

$$C > 2N \;/\; (1/2 - 1/3) = 12N$$

The image-compressing algorithm must process data at least 12 times faster than the network speed. Even if you have a relatively slow 10 Mbit/s network, you will need a 120 Mbit/s = 15 MByte/s compression algorithm to make your images travel twice as fast. Current compression algorithms, however, usually work on the 1–2 MByte/s level. As you can see, on reasonably fast networks they will actually slow you down rather than speed you up. On the other hand, in distributed clinical networks like those used for teleradiology, overall network speed tends to be low,[3] and compression can noticeably improve image transmission rates.

---

[3] Often due to the "last mile" problem.

Third, compression ratio R_{comp} always depends on the image and cannot be known before the image is compressed. For example, images with large monotone backgrounds (such as mammograms) generally compress better than images with substantial noise (such as nuclear medicine) simply because *monotone* translates to *redundant and compressible*. These days, increasingly higher performance is expected from 3D compression techniques – we can use 3D JPEG2000 as one good example. 3D compression explores the additional dimension of inter-image redundancy, which allows us to achieve higher compression ratios. Also, each compression algorithm has its own class of medical images for which it will perform best. For example, 8-bit lossy JPEG, completely inappropriate for CT or MR images,[4] works great with ultrasound and is commonly implemented on ultrasound devices.

Finally, although the images account for the bulk of DICOM data, TCP/IP networking in general and DICOM networking in particular work in their own ways, taking additional time to establish connections, communicate protocols, and to break and assemble data into smaller packages. Therefore, even with the packing and unpacking time excluded, do not expect your network to transmit the compressed image exactly R_{comp} times faster – some aspects will surely require more time.

We have to leave the in-depth compression discussion for another time because it is beyond the scope of this book; but if you have the time, I suggest you do a little reading on modality-specific compression ratios (Branstetter 2009), and consult with an expert before implementing any particular image compression type at your medical enterprise.

Low-Hanging Fruits

Sometimes compression can be much easier to implement than it sounds. For example, Microsoft Windows supports built-in file compression – you can always right-click on a folder and set it as compressed. This means that all files, stored in this folder will be compressed with lossless, native Windows compression, regardless of what program you use to handle these files.

What if this folder happens to be your image storage folder? Then all images, stored in this folder will be compressed automatically and losslessly, regardless of your archiving software.

We once tried to use this method for our CT image archive, and it gave us an average $R_{comp} = 1.6$. Not the most impressive result, but hey, we reduced image storage by 1.6 times by doing absolutely nothing!

With the 10–20 cents/MB that many current PACS charge for image storage, you can buy several new imaging servers if you only compress data on one of them.

---

[4] 8-bit JPEG can handle only 8 bits per pixel, and CT or MR images have up to 16. The last thing you want to lose is the color/grayscale depth of the image. Always favor the compression algorithms that do not have any color depth limits.

6.3 Working with Digital Medical Images

6.3.1 Image Interpolation

With so many legal and clinical arguments spent on lossy image compression, the entire subject of image interpolation (digital zoom) seems to be totally ignored. Some time ago I wrote a program to export DICOM images into conventional image formats such as JPEG and BMP. Many radiologists still like to do this if not for medical purposes (which I strongly discourage), but for other work such as writing research papers and keeping teaching files. Soon after, one of my colleagues (an experienced radiologist) called me to ask why her MR images had become so small when exported – much smaller than she used to see on her PACS workstation. What was wrong?

The answer was "Absolutely nothing." When dealing with digital imaging data, what you see is more likely *not* what you have. A standard 256×256 MR image *does* look small on a typical 1024×1024 monitor, and looks minuscule on a good radiological one. For this reason, all PACS application do something that other imaging programs do not: they always *interpolate* the small images to make them larger so they can take advantage of the entire monitor area.

Interpolation (digital zoom) is the process of changing the original resolution of a digital image, artificially increasing its pixel count. If you have a 256×256 image you have only $256 \times 256 = 65536$ pixels. If you want to show this image full screen on a 1024×1024 monitor, it must be converted to a 1024×1024 image with $1024 \times 1024 = 1048576$ pixels. So, when you zoom this image to full screen, where do the extra $1048576 - 65536 = 983040$ pixels come from? They are generated by an interpolation algorithm[5] and inserted between the original image pixels, thus making the image matrix larger. As a result, when you zoom in on a digital image, you see progressively more pixels that *were not present in the original data but are added by the interpolation*. Thus in a 4X-zoomed image, only *one* pixel out of every $4 \times 4 = 16$ pixels comes from the original image, and the other 15 are essentially created by a program (Fig. 6.7). A substantial addition, isn't it? Much more substantial than any reasonable lossy compression would do.

This dominance of the artificial pixels explains why image interpolation should be taken very seriously by all PACS developers and users, and a good amount of research continues in this area. Because the interpolating program has no access to the original object (patient) to make a better image, it has to *cleverly fake* all the extra pixels so that they look as natural as possible. The quality of this faking should be extraordinary and can always be used to judge the quality of image viewing software. To test a PACS viewing workstation that you might consider buying, load a small image (such as MR or NM), zoom in on it and check for tiles, jaggies, broken lines, and other unnaturally looking artifacts. If you see any of these problems, they

---

[5] Bicubic interpolation is usually used.

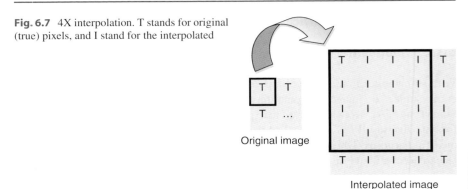

Fig. 6.7 4X interpolation. T stands for original (true) pixels, and I stand for the interpolated

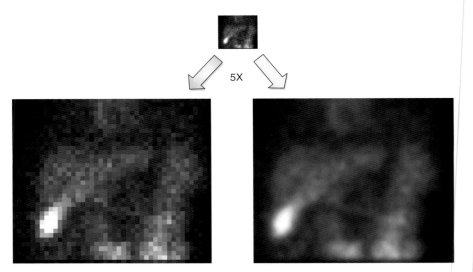

Fig. 6.8 (*Top*) The original small nuclear medicine image. (*Left*) Poor *nearest neighbor* image interpolation. (*Right*) Much better *bicubic* interpolation. The snapshots were taken from two different commercial image viewing programs

are most definitely coming from poor interpolation, and you are looking at a very cheap approximation of the required standard quality. Figure 6.8 demonstrates this difference for a small nuclear medicine image, and Fig. 6.9 gives a more subtle example. As you can see, the interpolation on the left is extremely poor and the one on the right is much more natural.

Interpolation does have another artifact that is impossible to avoid. When an image is zoomed in too much (such as 5X in Fig. 6.8) you will start seeing some blur. This merely reflects the fact that interpolation does not add information to the image and cannot add any finer, sharper details. Hence another conclusion: do not spend your money on an expensive, super-high resolution monitor if you mainly deal with

6.3 Working with Digital Medical Images

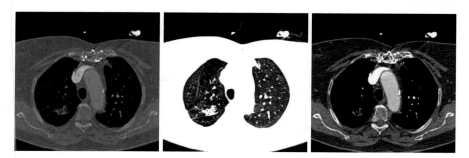

Fig. 6.12 Same CT image, shown at different window/level settings: overall view (*left*), lungs (*middle*), soft tissue (*right*)

original DICOM format, it will keep all its 1024 shades, so they can be displayed and viewed with proper software or monitors. On the other hand, as soon as the image is exported into a non-DICOM format such as BMP or JPEG, supporting only 256 shades of gray, or compressed with the wrong compression technique, there is no way to preserve the original 1024 gray levels. No software or hardware in the whole wide world will display a degraded image with the original quality: what is lost is lost (same story as with overused lossy compression).

This is the principal reason why any teleradiology project (often falling for simple image formats and exports) should maintain the original image format rather than try to "recover" permanently lost quality with overpriced viewing workstations. This is also the reason why many official radiology project guidelines (including those for teleradiology) insist on preserving the original image quality more than mandating image viewing options[7] (TeleradUSA). *Preserving diagnostic image quality is a must.* Everything else is simply subjective; mattering only for personal viewing comfort.

Consider the window/level (W/L) function – available in absolutely all PACS or DICOM software – that is used to adjust the currently visible grayscale range. For example, if you are viewing a CT image with 1024 shades of gray on a conventional off-the-shelf display (capable of 256 grayscales only), you still will be able to navigate in the original 1024 range with your "bone," "liver," "brain," and other windows (Fig. 6.12). Each of these windows would simply take the corresponding [C0, C1] subrange from the original 1024 CT shades and map it into the 256 available to you on the monitor. In other words, this is very similar to zooming and panning the image, but now you "zoom" (window) and "pan" (level) in the grayscale range. *If the original image quality was preserved, you would be able to see all image shades on any monitor* – ranging from your cell phone display to your radiological 10-megapixel monster. Simply put, on a 1024-bit radiological monitor you will see them at once, and on a 256-bit conventional monitor you will have to navigate between them.

---

[7]The only exception is made for mammography displays: they are expected to have impressive 5-megapixel resolution (typically $2,048 \times 2,560$ pixels), and current models deliver high 750 cd/m^2 luminance with 4,096 supported grayscales.

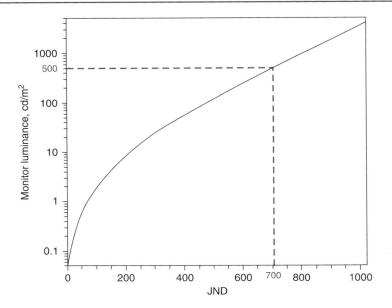

Fig. 6.13 JND curve. Note that the luminance axis is logarithmic

With all this being said, we can only debate the affects of different monitor properties on the optimal image grayscale display. By far, the most important properties would be monitor *luminance* and *contrast ratio*. Contrast ratio is the ratio between the brightest white and the darkest black that the monitor can reproduce. For example, a contrast ratio of 1000:1 means that the brightest monitor shade is 1000 times brighter than the darkest. Monitor luminance, typically expressed in *nits* (candelas per square meter, cd/m^2), measures the amount of light produced by the monitor. Naturally enough, higher contrast and luminance come together and mean better differentiation between the image shades, which translates into better image interpretation quality.[8] DICOM describes this differentiation with the concept of *Just Noticeable Difference (JND)* – *the smallest difference in grayscale that the average human observer can perceive under given viewing conditions.* Theoretically, JND depends on monitor luminance – you can find a really impressive empirical formula in DICOM PS3.14, corresponding to the curve shown in Fig. 6.13.

For example, if you pick a pretty good 500 cd/m^2 luminance monitor, your eyes would be expected to see some 700 different shades of gray – provided, the monitor and its graphics card are capable of supporting those 700 shades (see Annex B in DICOM PS3.14 for a more complete JND value table). Moreover, if the monitor can display 1024 shades, you still won't perceive more then 700 at 500 cd/m^2. Apart from these averaged and theoretical expectations, the JND function is used for one

---

[8]Because of this, luminance and contrast numbers turned into pure sales pitches with many display manufacturers – sometimes claiming much higher values than they can actually deliver. It is always worth the time to evaluate the monitor display quality visually, preferably with side-by-side monitor comparison.

very practical purpose: calibrating radiological monitors. The entire purpose of calibration is to tune monitor luminance at different levels in such a way that JNDs would be uniformly distributed. Your ability to differentiate between darker shades will be the same as your ability to differentiate between the lighter ones. That provides the sense of not favoring certain intensity ranges at the expense of others – for example, in the CT case, not making Hounsfield units more visible in one density range compared to the others.

The rest of the perfect monitor debate gets extremely vague and subjective – especially when we get into the area of *diagnostic* display quality. Even the most perfect JND calibration cannot guarantee optimal viewing – the human vision system is very complex. For example, your ability to perceive certain shades will be affected by image noise, distribution, shape, and position of the objects you are looking at. Your perception is also affected by the ambient light and by a host of other factors – possibly including the height of your chair and the quality of your diet. In some hospitals, reading rooms are not just dark, they are painted black, and radiologists cannot wear bright coats while working there. Finally, experience shows that mere image reading *comfort* sometimes means much more to quality image interpretation than the most technologically advanced solutions. For example, seeing the maximum number of grayscales at once can still make image reading easier (Kimpe and Tuytschaever 2007), but it also translates into increased monitor luminance (as shown on the JND curve in Fig. 6.13). According to some reports, this can become a distraction in itself if above 600 cd/m^2. But 600 cd/m^2 correspond to only 730 JNDs – well below our 1024 shades in an average CT or X-ray image; and 1024 JNDs would require blasting 4000 cd/m^2, which is quite likely unbearable to look at. As a result, current 300–400 cd/m^2 radiological monitors provide comfortable luminance, but do not get anywhere near the original image grayscale depth.

This analysis sets limits to the clear-cut JND theory, which is why more and more institutions try to solve the display "grayscale depth" puzzle from the empirical point of view. How many monitor shades would be enough for a radiologist to read images with maximum comfort and minimum errors? In one experiment Bender et al. 2011, the images with low-contrast pathologies (small lung nodules, little bone fractures, low-contrast tumors, and such) were presented to radiologists with conventional 8-bit and advanced 10/11-bit technology. The radiologists were asked to select the best image quality, and the results were quite surprising: in the majority of cases, the radiologists did not appreciate the deeper 10/11-bit grayscale and were as productive and accurate with the usual 8-bit displays. Moreover, in some cases the deep 11-bit monitor grayscale was perceived as "less sharp"; the higher number of shades was creating an illusion of a visibly smoother image, which was perceived as degraded, blurred quality (Fig. 6.14). How ironic! Humans are amazing creatures. You can never tell what will make them happy; and sometimes the simplest things work best.

Bottom line: The original DICOM image quality is all that matters. It was meant to be diagnostic, so let's keep it that way. I am typing this book using a new, off-the-shelf monitor that has 500 cd/m^2 brightness, 1000:1 contrast ratio, and 1200×1900 pixel resolution – nearly the same as or even better than many current PACS monitors produce. The real difference is that the PACS monitors are ten times more expensive (Hirschorn).

Monitor Placebo

A most interesting case of "expected vs. practical" monitor use happened to me a couple of years ago in a well-recognized international hospital using PACS from a well-respected PACS vendor. Because the PACS came equipped with high-resolution, dual-monitor radiological displays (from a well-respected display manufacturer), everyone was absolutely certain that they were 10 bits per pixels, thus capable of $2^{10} = 1024$ simultaneous grayscales. Moreover, the PACS company confirmed that their PACS software was also 10-bit capable.

After 2 years, by sheer accident we discovered that the monitors were only eight bits per pixel – in other words, providing only of $2^8 = 256$ grayscales, which any conventional monitor would deliver! It just turned out that although the monitors and the PACS software were 10-bit compatible, the graphics cards in the PACS workstations supported only eight bits, thus converting everything to the 8-bit display mode! As a result, *the hospital radiologists kept doing their top-notch job on very basic monitor setups simply because they believed that their monitors could do much more.* An interesting case of viewing subjectivity and PACS vendor incompetence at the same time.

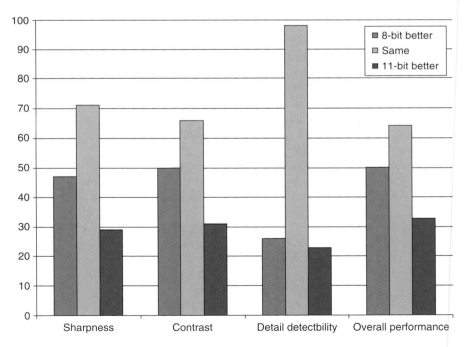

Fig. 6.14 Comparing 8-bit and 11-bit image display in (Bender et al. 2011) study: most radiologists did not see any difference, and many favored 8-bit monitors as providing sharper image display

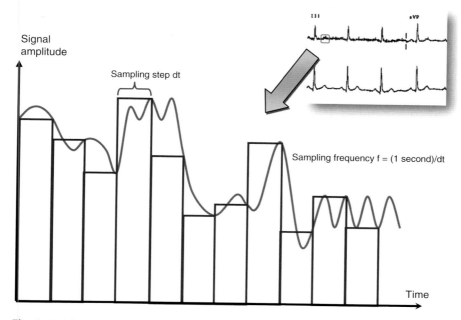

Fig. 6.15 Digitizing continuous (analog) signal into a sequence of discrete (digital) values

6.3.4 Waveforms

Waveforms are not images, but are close in many ways. As DICOM states:

> The Waveform information entity (IE) represents a multi-channel, time-based digitized waveform. The waveform consists of measurements of some physical qualities (for example, electrical voltage, pressure, gas concentration, or sound) sampled at constant time intervals. The measured qualities may originate, for example, in any of the following sources:
> - The anatomy of the patient,
> - Therapeutic equipment (for example, a cardiac pacing signal or a radio frequency ablation signal),
> - Equipment for diagnostic synchronization (for example, a clock or timing signal used between distinct devices),
> - The physician's voice (for example, a dictated report).

Digital sound is by far the most common waveform that we all know even before we get into any digital medicine business. ECG is another popular example. Arterial pulse and respiratory waveforms were added to DICOM last year. In each case, waveforms capture processes that evolve in time and can be represented with several signal channels (stereo sound, for example). In this respect, waveforms are very similar to images. But whereas images are characterized by two spatial coordinates (x and y), waveforms have one-dimensional amplitude changing in time t (see waveform screenshots on Fig. 12.3, left).

Consequently, just like images, analog waveforms must be converted to digital equivalents. This means that an analog signal is broken into discrete samples that are recorded as their amplitude values, thus forming a digitized waveform (Fig. 6.15).

Once digitized, this becomes a digital sequence of samples (amplitude values) that can be saved in DICOM the same way image pixels are saved. The terminology of bits allocated and bits stored applies to waveform representations.

In practice, DICOM waveforms are still rarely used compared to digital images, and are very poorly supported by DICOM vendors. Nevertheless, waveforms represent an excellent tool for storing one-dimensional, multichannel sequences; whatever they represent. If you are interested in learning more about waveform formats, check DICOM section A.34 in PS 3.3, and Supplement 30. As DICOM continues to embrace digital multimedia, the role of waveforms may only grow.

6.3.5 Overlays

Overlays (or overlay planes) are images that can be used to record graphics and bit-mapped text (such as annotations) on top of the regular DICOM images. This makes overlays very useful and widespread, although the long history of varying overlay formats in DICOM has contributed to poor overlay implementations.

Why do we need image overlays if we have images? Here is a simple use case: you want to draw an annotation on top of your CT image, tracing a tumor or some region of interest, and adding some measurement text. How would you do this? The first thing that comes into mind is "burning" (or "etching") the annotation into the image pixels – that is, making it a part of the original image. This is definitely the easiest approach; but unfortunately it is also the worst, and it won't work in most cases. First of all, it will destroy the original image data. Second, it will destroy the original image format. If you want to put a red circle on a monochrome CT image, you will have to convert the entire image from CT to SC screenshot; bye-bye, Hounsfield calibration! (Fig. 6.16).

Therefore, we need another image layer – that is, an overlay – to separately store additional graphics, and DICOM got busy with overlays quite a while ago. The original thought was to keep overlay pixels along with the original image pixel values in the (7FE0,0010) tag, as we discussed in 6.1. For example, if a CT image pixel usually takes 12 bits ("Bits stored"), it is rounded to 2 bytes = 16 bits ("bits allocated") of pixel memory; and we have $16-12=4$ unused bits to store something else such as overlay bits. This is what early DICOM used to practice; making a "pixel burger" with overlay bits on top. That approach was truly awful for many reasons, as you can easily imagine: different data always deserves separate storage. So the "burger" approach was eventually abandoned, and overlays (or "curves" before 2004 DICOM edition) were repackaged into separate DICOM elements: *repeating groups*[9] 60XX (Table 6.3).

The joy of moving overlay pixels from (7FE0,0010) to 60XX was spoiled by a few artificial limitations imposed by ever-creative DICOM authors. First of all,

---

[9]Repeating groups like 60XX are the leftovers of the pre-DICOM standards, which you can still find in a couple of places. They simply mean that XX can take different values in some range. DICOM wants to retire them eventually, using SQ sequences instead.

6.3 Working with Digital Medical Images

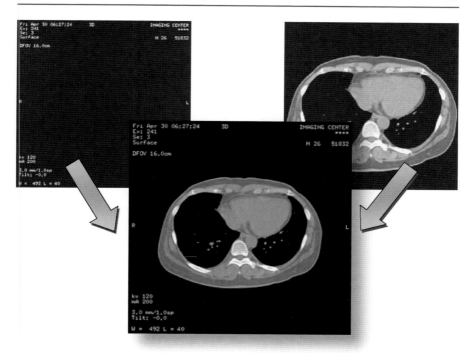

Fig. 6.16 Placing overlay (bitmapped text in this example) over CT image

overlays were reduced to only 1 bit/pixel "black-and-white" format. This left many users unhappy – grayscale or color overlays would be very appreciated in many cases. To make things worse, DICOM limited the span for hexadecimal XX from possible 00 to FF (decimal 0 to 255) to the even-numbered XX in the 00-1E range (decimal 0 to 30), which as you can easily count, produced only 16 possible group numbers.

As a result, you can have at most 16 overlays per image, each in 1 bit/pixel format. In theory, you can use them all – for example, displaying each in different color – but "there is no mechanism to specify with what color or intensity an overlay plane is to be displayed[10]," which means that your overlay coloring will be application-specific. As a result, nearly all DICOM companies default to a single overlay plane stored in the 6000 group (XX=00) as the most supported and cross-compatible solution. But even this should be regarded as a great step forward: many DICOM vendors, confused by the complex overlay history, do not support overlays at all, storing annotation and ROI data in their proprietary formats. No wonder that when their images are transferred to other systems, their overlays miraculously disappear from the PACS monitors as if they were written with invisible ink.

---

[10]See section C.9 in DICOM PS3.3.

Table 6.3 Overlay plane attributes

Attribute name	Tag	Type	Attribute description
Overlay Rows	(60xx,0010)	1	Number of Rows in Overlay (usually the same as image number of rows, that is, image height)
Overlay Columns	(60xx,0011)	1	Number of Columns in Overlay (usually the same as image number of columns, that is, image width)
Overlay Type	(60xx,0040)	1	Indicates whether this overlay represents a region of interest or other graphics. Enumerated values: G = Graphics R = ROI
Overlay Origin	(60xx,0050)	1	Location of first overlay point with respect to pixels in the image, given as row\column. The upper left pixel of the image has the coordinate 1\1 Column values greater than 1 indicate the overlay plane origin is to the right of the image origin. Row values greater than 1 indicate the overlay plane origin is below the image origin. Values less than 1 indicate the overlay plane origin is above or to the left of the image origin. Values of 0\0 indicate that the overlay pixels start 1 row above and one column to the left of the image pixels
Overlay Bits Allocated	(60xx,0100)	1	Number of Bits Allocated in the Overlay The value of this Attribute shall be 1
Overlay Bit Position	(60xx,0102)	1	The value of this Attribute shall be 0
Overlay Data	(60xx,3000)	1	Overlay pixel data, one bit per pixel The order of pixels sent for each overlay is left to right, top to bottom, that is, the upper left pixel is sent first followed by the remainder of the first row, followed by the first pixel of the 2nd row, then the remainder of the 2nd row and so on Overlay data shall be contained in this Attribute
Overlay Description	(60xx,0022)	3	User-defined comments about the overlay
Overlay Subtype	(60xx,0045)	3	USER (if created by user), or AUTOMATED (if created by software algorithm)
Overlay Label	(60xx,1500)	3	A user defined text string which may be used to label or name this overlay
ROI Area	(60xx,1301)	3	Number of pixels in ROI area
ROI Mean	(60xx,1302)	3	ROI Mean
ROI Standard Deviation	(60xx,1303)	3	ROI standard deviation

Therefore, please make sure that your DICOM software can handle overlay planes: just find some DICOM images with group 6000 and open them in your program – you should see the overlay. If you use overlays for annotations, keep in mind that any graphics or text you put in the overlay will be bitmapped – converted to overlay black-and-white pixels. It limits overlay use: once your text and graphics are bitmapped, you cannot edit them anymore. But it also makes overlays the simplest images on earth, impossible to get wrong.

6.3.6 Supporting True Video in DICOM

Want to store your favorite video in DICOM, and play it on PACS? Why not? Just imagine "House M.D." fans watching favorite episodes in the radiology department, straight from the PACS archive. I am almost tempted to start writing a business plan for a "PACS TV" startup. But before I digress into some hare-brained scheme for becoming an overnight Hollywood sensation, let's reel things back in and have a look at the basics.

The original DICOM had no support for digital video; all images were expected to be still frames. The need for the DICOM video, however, was soon realized with the earliest video modality: ultrasound. In ultrasound imaging, short video clips – called "cine loops" – are commonly used to record beating hearts, rolling babies, and blood flow to name just a few. Most of us have likely had some experience with them at least once in our lives. To accommodate these clips, DICOM applied the same idea that the first film inventors used from the early cinematographic times: a video is nothing more than a running sequence of still images. In other words, DICOM slightly extended its single image format to support multiframe images, storing each video as a sequence of its frames (still images as usual) packed into a single DICOM object (file).[11] Video parameters such as Frame Time (0018,1063) or Cine Rate (0018,0040) were recorded along with them, to indicate video format and to ensure correct playback.

Each DICOM workstation was expected to play the stored video accordingly; that is, to automatically scroll through the stored sequence of still images at a specified playback rate. To keep the data size small, lossy JPEG compression was applied to each stored frame (Fig. 6.17).

This "cinematic" approach worked for years, and still works pretty well for ultrasound images in particular. In fact, ultrasound imaging proved to be the ideal domain for the multiframe DICOM. Short cine loops (small numbers of video frames), inherently low ultrasound image resolution (ideally matching lossy JPEG compression), no need for audio, and the ability to extract and process individual image frames all transformed multiframe ultrasound images into a widely accepted and practically convenient standard, later adopted by the other video modalities. The only practical problem I ever ran into with multiframe images was their loading

---

[11] All frames are concatenated into the pixel buffer, (7FE0, 0010) attribute.

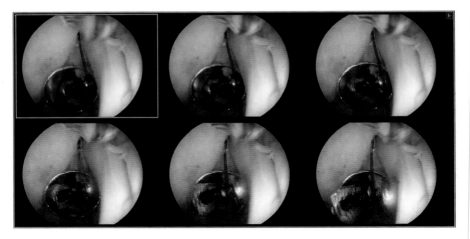

Fig. 6.17 Displaying multiple frames from DICOM multiframe image. The video – all 409 frames in this case – was stored in a single DICOM multiframe object, as a sequence of 409 JPEG-compressed color images, 480×640 frame size. Thanks to JPEG, the DICOM object size was reduced to 6 MB instead of the original 409×480×640×3 (*color bytes*) = 360 MB. Note that 60:1 JPEG compression had no negative effect on the naturally shaded image with a large black background

time: each image frame needs to be extracted from the data stream and uncompressed, thus taking substantial time and memory. But the ever-improving processing power of computers was able to keep this at bay.

During the past few years, however, the landscape of true video applications in DICOM has started to change rapidly. "Visible light" modalities (VL) – such as endoscopes, microscopes, and even plain video cameras – came into play, making their mark in DICOM (see Visible light IOD in PS 3.3). Users got really busy producing long-lasting videos with resolution and quality often surpassing that of good old ultrasound. Audio has become important to record physiological sounds and physician comments. The old multiframe format, although still applicable, soon started to reach its limits. The need for video-specific formats such as MPEG2 has become apparent.

We all are pretty accustomed to MPEG video in our everyday lives – playing it on iPods, digital cameras, and computers. MPEG does not cancel the fundamental "frames per second" principle; it still stores digital video as a sequence of frames. But instead of compressing and storing each frame independently, MPEG compresses and stores only the difference between the two consecutive frames, substantially minimizing the data volume: in most cases, only a few spots on the next video frame change, while the background remains largely the same and does not need to be encoded in each frame. Combined with more superior compression, MPEG definitely surpasses the quality of simple-minded multiframe images.

To make it work in digital medicine, the problem of MPEG support was solved in the typical DICOM way – by encapsulating MPEG2 video data into DICOM

6.3 Working with Digital Medical Images

Table 6.4 MPEG2 MP@ML video format attributes

Video type	Spatial resolution	Frame rate	Frame time (ms)	Maximum rows	Maximum columns
525-line NTSC	Full	30	33.33	480	720
625-line PAL	Full	25	40.0	576	720

objects. That is, MPEG-encoded video can be placed into the Pixel Data (7FE0,0010) attribute – the same attribute where still images used to be stored. In this way, DICOM support for digital video did not result in any new object types or definitions. Just like JPEG and PDF, MPEG has become yet another data (compression) format adopted by DICOM objects. First of all, this makes MPEG format negotiable at Association Establishment handshake; if it is refused, the video-sending device needs to use the default uncompressed multiframe image format.[12] Secondly, the use of MPEG is totally optional: one can still store long endoscopic video as a traditional DICOM multiframe. Moreover, this is still the most used approach. But when MPEG is used, the video will be stored in MPEG2 format, and its presence in the DICOM object will be indicated by MPEG2 transfer syntax – 1.2.840.10008.1.2.4.100 or 1.2.840.10008.1.2.4.101 (more on transfer syntaxes in 9.4).

Why two different MPEGs? The "MPEG2 Main Profile @ Main Level" was the one introduced originally. This is the same format used in most digital devices and videos, DVDs included. MPEG2 MP@ML supports the video types shown in Table 6.4 (DICOM PS3.5 and MPEG2-dedicated Supplement 137).

Video is always stored in RGB format (8 bytes per color channel, three color channels[13]), compressed with inherently lossy MPEG compression. Each DICOM object can contain a single video clip, limited by the 2 GB size (there are no "miltivideo" DICOMs yet). If the video does not fit into this size, it has to be cut into several fragments, each stored in its own DICOM object. Audio is supported just like with any video in general, being a part of the MPEG data stream.

In 2009, high-definition MPEG – "MPEG2 Main Profile @ High Level" – was added to support HD video.

As you can see from the format tables (Tables 6.5 and 6.6), the resolution and frame rates of the original "MPEG2 Main Profile @ Main Level" doubled in the newly added HD version.

Is it really needed? Only time will tell. Currently, the DICOM adaption of video codecs, like MPEG, was driven mainly by the need to store the videos from the VL modalities – digital video cameras of various kinds. Most of them recently went into the full HD video support, and DICOM merely followed this trend – no questions asked. On one hand, this opened the DICOM standard to the entire world of digital

---

[12]In theory. I wonder if video camera manufacturers ever considered providing this function.

[13]This makes it inapplicable to other types of medical images, such as 2-byte/pixel grayscale in CT, MR, or X-ray.

Table 6.5 MPEG2 MP@HL video format attributes

Video type (Hz HD)	Spatial resolution layer	Frame rate	Frame time = 1 s/rate (ms)
30	Single level, enhancement	30	33.33
25	Single level, enhancement	25	40.0
60	Single level, enhancement	60	16.17
50	Single level, enhancement	50	20.00

Table 6.6 MPEG2 MP@HL video frame sizes and rates

Rows	Columns	Frame rate	Video type (Hz HD)	Progressive or interlace
1080	1920	25	25	P
1080	1920	29.97, 30	30	P
1080	1920	25	25	I
1080	1920	29.97, 30	30	I
720	1280	25	25	P
720	1280	29.97, 30	30	P
720	1280	50	50	P
720	1280	59.94, 60	60	P

video. On the other, I have not seen a single major PACS workstation or hospital using DICOM MPEGs on a regular basis; the old multiframe image format remains dominant for the practical clinical needs. The use of MPEG-like video encoding calls for new image display, analysis, and processing tools; and they are not yet readily available.

In fact, following the same trend of being driven by the emergence of HD medical camera products, DICOM Supplement 149 (released in 2009 from the DICOM Visible Light workgroup) introduced into DICOM the MPEG2 successor: MPEG4, the "blue-ray" video format. And although we all know the advantages of blue-ray videos, their use in PACS has yet to be proven practically.

To conclude, it is worth mentioning that some older digital modalities relying on video display still lack adequate video storage. Let us consider digital angiography (DA) as one good example. DA involves sequences of grayscale X-ray images commonly taken to visualize blood flow. Unlike ultrasounds, these images have substantially higher resolution (averaging at 1000 × 1000 pixels), and 2-byte/pixel grayscale (unsupported by MPEG or "conventional" lossy JPEG). As a result, DA sequences cannot be efficiently encoded, and are still stored as multiframe DICOM, often with no compression of any kind. They produce DICOM objects of monstrous sizes, rivaling Hollywood epics (and I mean on the order of *several* gigabytes). From the users' perspectives, they are still video, and questions like "Why does my DA take so long to load, and forever to play?" are common – the users simply do not realize the scale of the data size.

Part III
DICOM Communications

DICOM SOPs: Basic

7

Anything complex is useless, anything useful is simple

– Mikhail Kalashnikov

Remember what the "C" in DICOM and PACS stands for? *Communications* of course; and DICOM networking is the glue that holds any medical imaging system together. While most of us used to think of DICOM as a simple medical image file format, it really is a much broader standard that directs all facets of the clinical workflow and goes far beyond the scope of managing formats for image files. The entire digital medical universe is created and populated by DICOM objects as they travel and interact through computer networks.

Interestingly enough, DICOM networking had been laid out in the standard well before computer networks came into existence. Part PS3.9 of the standard (Point-to-Point Communication Support for Message Exchange) used old-fashioned pin cables to interconnect DICOM devices. All this, including PS3.9 itself, has vanished with the introduction of modern networking hardware and protocols, which have become the foundation for contemporary DICOM data exchange.

In plain words, current DICOM uses the exact same underlying network protocol – Transmission Control Protocol (TCP) and the Internet Protocol (IP) – that you use for sending your email or watching online videos (Fig. 7.1). TCP/IP nicely accommodates all hardware and software variations, and delivers the most fundamental network functionality needed: sending information (as a sequence of bytes) from one port/IP address to another. DICOM only adds its own networking language (*application layer*), which we are about to explore.

This language consists of *high-level* services (DICOM DIMSE, the subject of this chapter) built on *low-level* DICOM association primitives (DICOM Upper Layer protocol, a more involved discussion reserved for Chap. 9).

Although sometimes technical, all concepts used in DICOM networking are quite intuitive – you really do not have to be an IT guru to understand them. Moreover, knowing the principles of DICOM networking will considerably improve your understanding of DICOM and PACS, and your ability to deal with related projects.

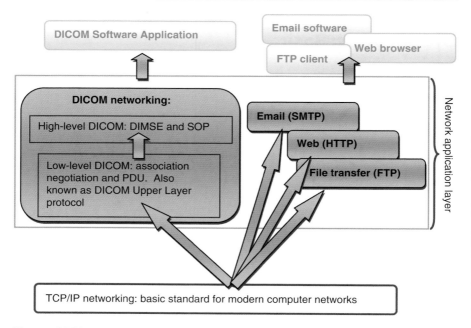

Fig. 7.1 DICOM and popular networking protocols. DICOM network application layer augments basic TCP/IP functionality with DICOM-specific protocols

7.1 Identifying Units on the DICOM Network

Each device residing on a TCP/IP network gets its own *IP address*, which is how the other networked devices find it. For instance, you can open www.whatismyip.com on your home PC, and it will show its IP address, assigned by your internet provider.

DICOM *Application Entity* (commonly abbreviated as AE, see Sect. 5.3.8) generally corresponds to any DICOM application on a networked DICOM device; for example, a DICOM server (archive), imaging workstation, film printer, or image acquisition device (modality). These four examples cover some 95% of all AEs that you will likely find in a clinical environment, so I will use them as our standard examples.

In addition to standard IP address, DICOM assigns to each AE its own DICOM name known as its *Application Entity Title* (AET). In DICOM, AET is encoded with the AE VR. As you might remember from the VR table in Sect. 5.3, the AE can have up to 16 characters. A practical approach for AET naming is to use either the application name (for example, PACSSERVER), or the computer name/location (DRBOBOFFICE); preferably without punctuation signs or spaces, and in uppercase to avoid ambiguity. This makes it simple to maintain and easy to identify.

7.1 Identifying Units on the DICOM Network

Unfortunately, certain PACS companies are infamous for using counterintuitive AE titles. When PACS software is installed at your site, make sure the AETs are assigned in a clear and consistent manner.

> **AEs as DICOM Applications**
>
> Important: As the name suggests, AE titles are used to label *applications*, not computers. Although in many cases you will have only one DICOM application running on each device, nothing prevents you from installing several of them on a single computer – server, workstation, DICOM printer server, and so on. In fact, this is a very common real-life situation. In this case, each DICOM application gets a different AE title and the other DICOM devices can talk to a particular application rather than to the whole computer.

All DICOM networking takes place between AEs when they exchange messages and data in DICOM format. If you are familiar with networking, you might know that TCP/IP always sends data to particular *ports* on each computer.[1] Ports are numbered from 0 to 65535. For example, your web browser (HTTP[2] protocol, based on TCP/IP) uses port 80 and your email (SMTP[3] protocol, also TCP/IP based) uses port 25. DICOM's default port is 104, but when you install your DICOM software, you can tune it to any other available port number, as long as:

1. You keep it consistent for all networked units; that is, as long as the receiving units use the same port as the sending units.
2. The port number is not already taken by another application. For example, using port 80 for DICOM would be a bit radical because it is traditionally used by web browsers, and won't be available for anything else. If you do not like the standard DICOM port 104, try using ports with high numbers (say, 10000 and up); their chances of being used are usually lower.

Port number comes in very handy when you have several DICOM applications on a single computer. While their different AE titles identify them as different DICOM applications, different port numbers separate them on the network. Even if they share the same IP address, each application gets called on its own port. Moreover, a single AE can have two ports: one to send data and another to receive data. Most current DICOM software provides this dual-port support for their AEs.

---

[1] If this is new to you, think about computer names as street names, ports as house numbers, and AEs as residents' names. You need to know all that to send a letter, right?

[2] HyperText Transfer Protocol.

[3] Simple Mail Transfer Protocol.

> **Connecting the Unconnectable**
> If you are shopping for DICOM software, make sure that it gives you complete freedom to configure AE parameters, both local and remote. Local corresponds with the application and remote corresponds with other AEs communicating with the software.
> Open the AE setup window in your DICOM software. You should not see any preset, read-only AE titles or impossible-to-modify port numbers.
> For example, in one recent project that required connecting a server from company X to a server from company Y, we discovered that:
> 1. X wanted to use *two different ports* – send port and receive port – where the send port *had to be* 104 and the receive port *had to be* anything but 104.
> 2. Y wanted to use *a single port* for send and receive.
>
> As a result, when X was asking for two different ports, Y was insisting on one; essentially making any connection between the two impossible. There is no rational explanation for this poor design on the parts of both X and Y. Likewise, there is no practical reason for insisting on using particular port numbers.

That's pretty much all you need to know about DICOM networking settings. Therefore, to configure your device on a DICOM network, you must assign to it a consistent:

1. *AET (AE title)* – Preferably alphanumeric, up to 16 characters. Think about easy-to-understand "CTWORKSTATION1", "ARCHIVE", or "PACS_SERVER".
2. *AE IP address* – Make sure it is reserved for this AE and will not change.
3. *AE port number* – Pick any (if not 104) and keep it consistent among all connected AEs. If you do not run multiple applications on the same computer, use a single port number throughout your entire DICOM network (Fig. 7.2).

AE properties need to be set for any DICOM application included in your network; all DICOM applications will have some menu or configuration utility to do so. Look for menu items such as "DICOM Properties," or "Add DICOM server (node)," and the like. AE setup is often performed by the device support personnel; and being a 5-min job, it ironically often takes several hours, if not days, to complete. Why? Because the support cannot be located or scheduled; because the configuration utility password was lost; because the entire PACS has to be rebooted; and for many, many other reasons you cannot imagine. Because of all these "becauses," device manufacturers like to charge for this service, often asking for a few thousand dollars for something a child can do. Therefore, plan any AE configuration ahead of time, and make sure you have all the pieces in place – this will really save you time and money.

7.2 Services and Data

Who are You?

Although it is not required by the DICOM standard, many DICOM manufacturers implement additional AE verification logic, requiring that connected AEs have complete knowledge of each other's configuration. In the DICOM standard, if AE *X* wants to connect to AE *Y*, *X* needs to know the AE configuration for *Y*. This makes sense because *X* has to know where to find *Y* on the network (name, IP, port). What is often required by some devices in addition to this is *Y* knowing what *X* is, even if *Y* never initiates any connections to *X*.

This mutual awareness could be presented by some as a coarse security feature (don't talk to strangers), but in reality it is a rather annoying hassle: you added archive settings to your CT scanner, the scanner attempts to send images to the archive, and nothing works – you have to spend another day chasing your archive support. To avoid it, always add AE configuration *symmetrically*: if you add *X*'s configuration to device *Y*, always add *Y*'s configuration to device *X*. In our example, don't forget to add CT scanner settings to the archive.

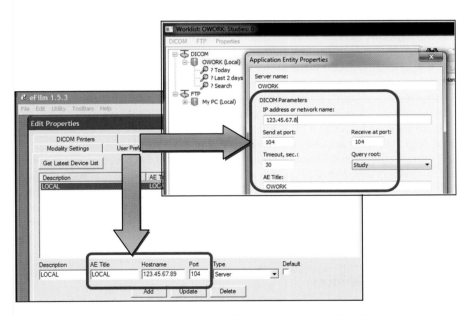

Fig. 7.2 Configuring AE specs in various DICOM software (AE title, IP address and port)

7.2 Services and Data

The model of data processing and exchange adopted by DICOM is classy and elegant – DICOM Application Entities *provide services* to each other. One DICOM entity can *request* a service from another, and that entity *provides* service to the first.

Fig. 7.3 SCU-SCP model

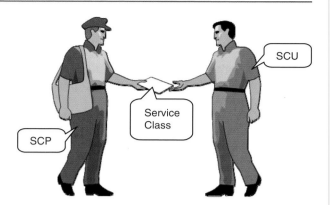

In DICOM lingo, a service-requesting AE is viewed as a *Service Class User* (SCU), and a service-providing AE is viewed as a *Service Class Provider* (SCP). In other words, AEs can play SCP or SCU *application roles* to communicate with each other (Fig. 7.3).

As the SCP and SCU names suggest, all DICOM services are rendered on the level of DICOM Service Classes. Service Classes in DICOM bind DICOM data with data-processing functions. In more strict terms, DICOM Service Class associates one or more DICOM Information Objects (IODs) with one or more commands. Consider printing digital images on film, for example. The DICOM Print Management Service Class is responsible for printing (command) various images (IODs, such as CT or MR images). Consequently, any DICOM printer can provide this service (that is, act as a Print Management SCP). Any DICOM device sending images to the printer requests the service – acting as a Print Management SCU.

In this section, you will become more acquainted with the structure and meaning of DICOM services. I need to say that while the DICOM standard is doing a particularly great job detailing the contents of its services, the overall relationships between them can often look extremely confusing because they are spread over multiple DICOM volumes and sometimes seasoned with inconsistent terminology. Reading this section should help.

7.2.1 DIMSE Services

I hope that by now you are becoming comfortable with the structure of DICOM IODs. So let's take a closer look at another part of any service class definition: IOD-processing commands. How do DICOM applications (AEs) ask each other for services? Essentially the same way we humans do.

DICOM AEs send *service messages* to each other, *requesting* or *providing* service information. This is why all service commands are known in DICOM as *DICOM Message Service Elements* (DIMSE*)*. DIMSE protocol sets the rules for DICOM service exchange – the backbone of DICOM networking. Consequently,

7.3 Storage

Table 7.8 C-Store-Rq

Message field	Tag	VR	Value/description
Command Group Length[a]	(0000,0000)	UL	The even number of bytes from the end of the (0000,0000) value field to the end of the C-Store-Rq message
Affected SOP Class UID	(0000,0002)	UI	Contains SOP UID for this image type – for example, 1.2.840.10008.5.1.4.1.1.2 for CT Image Store
Command Field	(0000,0100)	US	0001
Message ID	(0000,0110)	US	Unique numerical ID for this message
Priority	(0000,0700)	US	One of the following choices: 0002 (for low priority) 0000 (for medium priority) 0001 (for high priority)
Data Set Type	(0000,0800)	US	Anything *different* from 0101
Affected SOP Instance UID	(0000,1000)	UI	Contains the UID of the SOP Instance to be stored (that is, UID of the image to be stored).
Move Originator Application Entity Title	(0000,1030)	AE	Contains the DICOM AE Title of the DICOM AE which invoked the C-MOVE operation from which this C-STORE sub-operation is being performed
Move Originator Message ID	(0000,1031)	US	Contains the Message ID (0000,0110) of the C-MOVE-RQ Message from which this C-STORE sub-operations is being performed

[a]This item encodes the total length of all following items from 0000 group, as we learned in Sect. 5.5.2

- *Move Originator Title and Message ID* fields – As we will soon see in the C-Move SOP section, C-Store can be invoked by other DIMSE commands, such as C-Get or C-Move. In this case, the title of the invoking AE and the original message ID will be included in these fields.
- *Data set type* – You might remember that in C-Echo this field was set to 0101, which means NULL (no data attached) in DICOM. Consequently, a C-Store-Rq followed by data (the image to be stored) must have this field set to *anything but* 0101. What this is going to be is decided by each DICOM manufacturer and really does not matter. Some might use 0102 and some might use 0000 – ironically, in this context, 0000 indicates not-NULL (attached data) as opposed to the DICOM NULL, 0101.

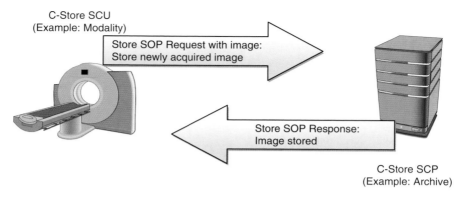

Fig. 7.9 DICOM C-Store

Table 7.9 C-Store-Rsp

Message field	Tag	VR	Value/description
Command Group Length	(0000,0000)	UL	The even number of bytes from the end of the (0000,0000) value field to the end of the C-Store-Rsp message
Affected SOP Class UID	(0000,0002)	UI	Contains SOP UID for this image type – for example, 1.2.840.10008.5.1.4.1.1.2 for CT Image Store
Command Field	(0000,0100)	US	8001
Message ID Being Responded To	(0000,0120)	US	Shall be set to the value of the Message ID (0000,0110) field used in associated C-Store-Rq Message
Data Set Type	(0000,0800)	US	0101 (meaning no data attached to C-Store-Rsp)
Affected SOP Instance UID	(0000,1000)	UI	Contains the UID of the SOP Instance to be stored (that is, UID of the image to be stored)
Status	(0000,0900)	US	0000 (if successful), FF00 (if pending), or other vendor-supported values for warnings and errors (see vendor's Conformance statement)

Because the Data Set Type field is not NULL, a C-Store-Rq message will be immediately followed by the image to be stored (one and only one image object). In other words, a C-Store-Rq always sends an image to its peer AE, asking for storage (Fig. 7.9).

The C-Store-Rsp returns from the data-receiving AE. It is shown in Table 7.9. Nearly everything in a C-Store-Rsp is derived from the original C-Store-Rq

Table 7.10 Query SOP

SOP class name	SOP class UID
Patient Root Q/R Find	1.2.840.10008.5.1.4.1.2.1.1
Study Root Q/R Find	1.2.840.10008.5.1.4.1.2.2.1
Patient-Study Root Q/R Find (Retired)	1.2.840.10008.5.1.4.1.2.3.1

message, except the ever-important Status field. Status tells you whether the image was stored (sent) successfully (Status = 0000), is still in the process of transmission (Status = FF00), or caused any warnings/errors (other values of Status).

The list of data-dependent C-Store SOPs keeps changing in every new DICOM revision; old data/image types are eventually retired while new types are added. If you are buying a new DICOM software or unit, always make sure that your data type is listed in the unit's DICOM Conformance Statement.

7.4 Query: Find

Now we can verify DICOM connectivity. We can even send images from one AE to another. But how can we find out *what* data needs to be sent?

One of the principal advantages of DICOM networking over simple file-sharing protocols is the ability to *search* for specific DICOM data, using DICOM C-Find messages. Three C-Find SOPs classes are provided to implement DICOM queries as shown in Table 7.10.

Searching for imaging data is not modality-specific, so C-Find does not use a multitude of C-Store-like, modality-based SOPs. In this respect, C-Find is very similar to C-Echo (Fig. 7.10). However, one thing about C-Find is still new to us; DICOM divides all C-Find data searches into three data levels: Patient, Study, and Patient-Study.

Those levels are called *roots* and C-Find has a separate SOP to implement data searches on each of them.

The need for DICOM query roots follows from the DICOM Patient-Study-Series-Image data hierarchy discussed in Sect. 5.6. DICOM organizes data into four hierarchical levels, and searching this data works best when limited to the same levels. For example, if the *Patient* Query/Retrieve root is supported, all searches will follow the Patient-Study-Series-Image hierarchy, starting from the Patient; with the *Study* Query/Retrieve root, they will be limited to Study-Series-Image levels only. In the latter case, all Patient attributes (such as patient name or ID) will be included in Study attributes to identify a study.

Because the current radiology's workflow is study-centric, the Study root is the most widely supported in DICOM applications and is usually always provided by

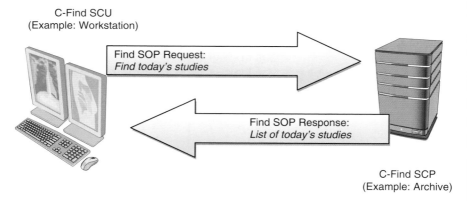

Fig. 7.10 DICOM C-Find example: retrieving a list of all today's studies from an archive

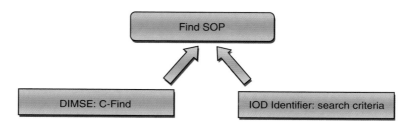

Fig. 7.11 Query SOP

default. Patient and Patient-Study SOPs for Query are rarely implemented. In fact, the Patient-Study root has been recently retired in the DICOM standard, meaning that it will not be supported in future editions of DICOM and it needs to be gradually excluded from DICOM implementations.

Needless to say, the C-Find SOP follows the same DIMSE+IOD structure, as shown in Fig. 7.11. The DIMSE object (encoded as a DICOM command object, group 0000) conveys the C-Find message parameters, and the attached IOD object (encoded as a DICOM data object) contains the search criteria to be matched on the C-Find SCP.

7.4.1 A Few Words on Data Matching in DICOM

When a C-Find SCU sends a find request, it includes a set of attributes to be matched. These attributes work as search fields that need to be compared against the data on

7.4 Query: Find

the target AE. Consequently, DICOM offers a few ways of specifying the search values:

- *Wildcard matching* – This one is already known to us. We first glanced at it in Sect. 5.3.2 when we talked about DICOM wildcards (* ?). Wildcard matches are commonly used to match strings, and not in DICOM only. For example, if we know that the patient name starts with "Smit", we can set the Patient Name (0010,0010) attribute in the C-Find request to "Smit*" using the asterisk (*) to indicate any sequence of symbols. *Smith, Smithson,* and even *Smit III the Great* will match this wildcard search. Another DICOM wildcard, the question mark (?), means a single unknown symbol, but it is rarely used for that reason; if we do not know the symbols, we more likely do not know how many there are.
- *List matching* – This technique uses the backslash (\ ) wildcard, which means "or." For example, "Smith\Graham" specified in the patient name will be used to find all Smith and Graham patients. You can definitely combine list and wildcard matches, with something like "Smit*\Grah*" especially when you deal with potentially mistyped data (and manually entered patient names do get mistyped more than we might like).
- *Universal matching* – This is the most general matching type. If the attribute to be matched has zero length, it will match everything. For example, if we provide a blank patient name in our C-Find query, all patient names in the target archive will be matched. Essentially, universal matching means *anything* and is identical to using the asterisk (*). However, there is a difference between *providing a zero-length matching attribute* in a C-Find request and *not providing it at all*. Including a zero-length attribute means that we want (or have to) use it for matching and we want to receive its matched values in a C-Find response. Not using an attribute means that we do not want it to be matched (it might not even be supported) and we don't care about retrieving its values. For example, if we do not want to retrieve patient names, we need not include a Patient Name attribute, empty or not, in the C-Find request.
- *Range matching* – This matching type is used for attributes that have ranges, such as date or time. In range matching, you can specify start and end attribute values, separated by a hyphen (-). Anything within this range will be matched. For example, range date match 20000201–20100202 means any date between February 1, 2000 and February 2, 2010. If either start or end is unknown, it can be omitted; so 20000201- means "February 1, 2000 and after."
- *Sequence matching* – Perhaps the most complex form of DICOM attribute matching, sequence matching is typically employed when an entire sequence of attributes (formed with the SQ VR, see Sect. 5.3.10) is used to match data. For example, to match a modality-scheduled patient study, DICOM uses a sequence of attributes such as patient ID, study date, and accession number. Each attribute in this sequence can have either exact values, or can use one of the above matching types. Grouping attributes into an SQ sequence works as a logical "and" (meaning that all attributes must match), as opposed to using the backslash (\ ) wildcard as a logical "or."

- *Single value matching* – This simply means using the exact attribute value as the matching parameter: using "Smith" for patient name, "20000201" for date, and so on. Naturally enough, single value matched attributes must not contain wildcards or ranges. Single value matching is commonly used for various IDs and UIDs, and in particular for hierarchical key attributes (see Sect. 5.6.3).

All attributes in DICOM data matching can be either *required* or *optional*. Required attributes, as the name suggests, must be present in the matching request. If we have no idea what their values might be, we simply insert them with blank values (universal matching). This also implies that we are guaranteed to receive the matched values. Optional attributes may be included if we are interested in using them. The DICOM standard usually specifies required and optional attributes for each query type (such as C-Find on Patient, Study, Series, or Image level), but you always need to check the DICOM Conformance Statements for the devices you are querying – they commonly override more generic DICOM specifications. This is understandable in part because attributes used on an ultrasound scanner will definitely differ from those used on a CT teaching archive. However, this always presents a certain implementation headache when you have to deal with different query attribute profiles for different devices.

Finally, nearly all matching in DICOM is case-sensitive. Case-insensitive matches are permitted for certain attributes such as names (PN VR), where they can also be space- and accent-insensitive. Personally, I doubt that case-sensitivity brings any advantages to DICOM whatsoever: first, case can be easily altered when typed; second, they almost never matter. Worse, some major PACS interfaces require users to enter certain data using a certain case: for example, typing patient names in uppercase only. This quickly turns into a major annoyance when patient Smith cannot be found unless you type him as SMITH. Practically, it often forces users to "Caps Lock" their PACS keyboards, which, as we can easily guess, inevitably creates an abundance of other typing problems, especially if other software is used on the same workstation. DICOM and DICOM applications should not be case-sensitive whenever possible.

Appendix A.4 gives you an idea of varying query attribute support from different DICOM manufacturers.

7.4.2 C-Find IOD

After our little voyage into the land of DICOM attribute matching, we can look at C-Find queries with a better level of understanding. C-Find IODs contain the search parameters to be matched on the C-Find service provider (digital archive, for example). Table 7.11 shows an example taken from a real Conformance Statement.[7]

As we discussed in Sect. 5.6.3, all data in DICOM follows the Patient-Study-Series-Image hierarchy, and C-Find queries are no exception; they must belong to one of those four levels. C-Find query level is reflected in the (0008,0052) attribute

---

[7] Because this C-Find IOD sample is taken from a particular DICOM application, yours could have a different list of optional items.

7.4 Query: Find

Table 7.11 Query parameters

(Group, Element)	Name	Required/ optional	Example	Matching (see Sect. 5.3.2)
(0008,0052)	Query Level	R	STUDY	Can be PATIENT, STUDY, SERIES, IMAGE. This element defines the level or hierarchical search
(0010,0010)	Patient's name	R	Smit*\ Grah*	Wildcard matching: * stands for any substring (empty included),? stands for any single symbol, and \ means "or"
(0010,0020)	Patient ID	R	12345	Typically, exact value is needed. Some systems support wildcard ID matches
(0008,0020)	Study date	R	20091231–20110201	Typically, range matching between two dates in YYYYMMDD format
(0008,0030)	Study time	R	015500–235559	Typically, range matching between two times in HHMMSS format. If study dates were given as a range, then the start time belongs to the start date, and the end time to the end date. In our example we are looping for all studies done between 01:55:00 on December 31, 2009, and 23:55:59 on February 1, 2011
(0008,0050)	Accession number	R	Abc789	Typically, exact match. Accession numbers are often imported from Radiology Information System
(0020,0010)	Study ID	R	1.234.567	Almost always exact match
(0008,1030)	Study description	O	*knee\ elbow*	Almost always wildcard matching, where keywords are used to locate studies with specific descriptions
(0008,0090)	Referring physician name	O	*Sinitsyn*	As for any names, wildcard matches are preferred
(0008,1060)	Reading physician name	O	*Bakhtin*	As for any names, wildcard matches are preferred
(0008,0061)	Modalities in study	O	MR\CT	Exact match or list match
(0010,0030)	Patient's birth date	O	19560101–19860101	Range match. Used to determine patient age

(required), and can be Patient, Study, Series, or Image. This also means that, in addition to SOP roots, the following should apply at any C-Find search level:

1. Key level attribute values[8] from all higher query levels must already be known. For example, before starting a Study-level search, we must know the Patient ID.

---

[8]The key level attribute values in Patient-Study-Series-Image hierarchy, as we learned in Sect. 5.6.3, are Patient ID (0010,0020), Study Instance UID (0020,000D), Series Instance UID (0020,000E), and Image, or SOP Instance UID (0008,0018), respectively.

2. Key level attribute values from the current level will be returned by the C-Find SCP. For example, in a Study-level search, "Study Instance UID" (0020,000E) will always be returned in response to any C-Find request. This enables us to proceed to the lower levels (Series, Image) according to rule 1 above.
3. In any C-Find request, we can search and match attributes only from the current C-Find level. For example, a Study-level search can search only the study attributes and cannot search individual series or images.

Look at the sample IOD in Table 7.11; what level is it on? The answer follows immediately from the (0008,0052) value: it is the Study level. But even if you did not know this value, you could have reasoned differently. The IOD seems to contain Patient ID (Patient level), but does not yet have a Study Instance UID (Study level). So according to rules 1 and 2 above, it is clearly on the Study query level. This logic is also useful for pinpointing DICOM problems. For example, if the level we determine from the key attributes does not match the one declared in (0008,0052) the C-Find query is destined to fail.

Certainly, you do not have to build your own level attribute tables. The DICOM Conformance Statement for each particular DICOM application lists all supported attributes for each supported level (and identifies them as required or optional). In fact, a particular device might not even support all four hierarchical levels – in which case, its Conformance Statement will contain only the levels supported.

Poor, Poor Modality

The most commonly level-misplaced attribute is imaging Modality (0008,0060). Knowing modality is important without question. However, most radiologists associate modality with a study and will likely be very disappointed if a study search (Study-level C-Find) does not return modality information.

But this is a well-anticipated result – nearly all DICOM Conformance Statements list Modality as a Series-level attribute. This means two things:

1. A DICOM study can be multimodality. Few people are used to this concept, so here is a simple example: a CT study with a few 3D-reconstructed images added to it. Those 3D reconstruction screenshots are more likely stored with the SC (Screen Capture) modality value and not with CT.
2. To find study modality, you should either search at the Series level with the (0008,0060) Modality attribute, or use (0008,0061) the "Modalities in Study" attribute, which belongs to the Study level. Searching a series is cumbersome. It requires stepping one level down from the Study level, and it might not even be supported on the target device. On the other hand, the (0008,0061) Modalities in Study attribute is not always supported.

This often makes retrieving a modality value problematic. But if we cannot fix our problems, we should at least understand them, right?

7.5 Modality Worklist

Table 7.14 Modality Worklist SOP

SOP class name	SOP class UID
Modality Worklist	1.2.840.10008.5.1.4.31

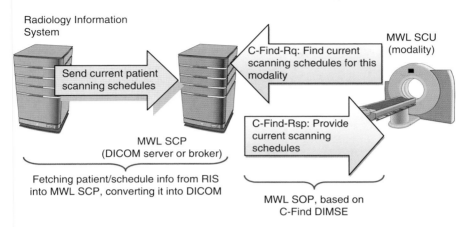

Fig. 7.13 DICOM Modality Worklist example: populating imaging modalities with basic patient data

most recent scheduling information. In addition to this standard workflow, modality operators can also use manual search interfaces, as shown in Fig. 7.14, for more specific schedule updates. When the patient is scanned, all MWL-transferred data (such as Patient Name or DOB) is embedded into DICOM images, leaving no room for errors.

What are the principal pros and cons of the MWL SOP? The main advantages are clear:

- MWL eliminates manual data entry on the modalities, reducing the main source for human errors and wasted time.
- Automatic fetching of MWL data directly from the RIS makes the entire process fast, clinically sound and robust.
- MWL parameters such as pregnancy status or allergies, commonly supported by modalities, are essential for many types of radiological exams.

The principal drawback of the MWL lies in its passive nature: modalities repetitively *pull* the MWL data from the MWL SCP server, and the latter has no ability to undo or delete retrospective transfers. Once patient/schedule information is passed to the modality, it is there, and it can be erased or edited only by the modality operator. In a busy clinic, patient/schedule information can change at a moment's notice, and manually editing it on the modality after the initial MWL fetch defeats the purpose of MWL.

How can you deal with this problem? Do not populate MWL lists days or weeks ahead of scanning time. I knew one clinic that tried to use MWL as their principal

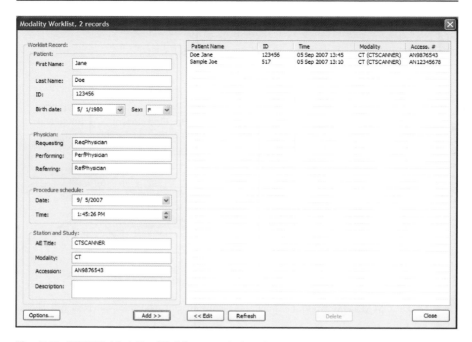

Fig. 7.14 DICOM Modality Worklist: sample interface (AlgoM server, www.algom.com) to retrieve MWL records from MWL SCP

patient scheduling engine, storing months of perspective scanning data into the modality worklists – *bad idea*! Instead, provide a "just-in-time" interface on the RIS side so MWL data can be sent to the MWL server right before the scan is needed. This approach minimizes the probability of cancelling or editing the scan information – and you will still benefit from the automatic, typo-free data flow.

7.5.1 MWL IOD

As you know, the Modality Worklist IOD contains information about the scheduled patient's study. In its minimum form,[9] it includes the most frequently used elements, as shown in Table 7.15.

Note that the (0040,0100) "Scheduled Procedure Step Sequence" element is encoded here with SQ VR (see Sect. 5.3.10), that is, it includes a subsequence of items (0040,0001), (0040,0002), and more. This sequence encapsulates the schedule for the patient scan. When retrieved from the MWL SCP, DICOM *sequence matching* couples it to a particular modality and time interval. The Accession Number in (0008,0050) is used to bind the original study record in the Radiology Information System (where the Accession Number is usually generated) with its DICOM images

---

[9] The complete Modality worklist attribute list can be found in PS3.4, Sect. K.6.1.2.2.

7.5 Modality Worklist

Table 7.15 MWL IOD

(Group, Element)	Name
(0010,0010)	Patient Name
(0010,0020)	Patient ID
(0010,0030)	Patients Birth Date
(0010,0040)	Patient's Sex
(0010,21C0)	Pregnancy Status
(0008,0050)	Accession Number
(0032,1032)	Requesting Physician
(0008,0090)	Referring Physician's Name
(0040,0100)	Scheduled Procedure Step Sequence
>(0040,0001)	Scheduled Station AE Title (name of the modality)
>(0040,0002)	Scheduled Procedure Step Start Date
>(0040,0003)	Scheduled Procedure Step Start Time
>(0008,0060)	Modality
>(0040,0006)	Scheduled Performing Physician's Name

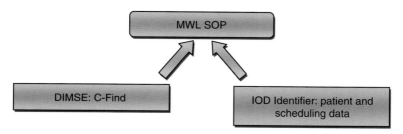

Fig. 7.15 Modality Worklist SOP

acquired on the modality. After the Accession Number is stored in its (0008,0050) DICOM image attribute, it uniquely links RIS and PACS study records.

As I mentioned, the list in Table 7.15 is minimal; more likely, a particular modality will require more data, which should be reflected in the modality's DICOM Conformance Statement. If some of those specific attributes are not provided to the modality, it will likely abort the MWL data transfer, insisting on a complete attributes list. In other words, if you are working on establishing MWL connectivity, always start by revising the modality's Conformance Statement. The list of attributes required for the modality should match those provided by the MWL SCP.

7.5.2 MWL DIMSE

The MWL DIMSE is nothing more than our good old friend C-Find DIMSE (see Sect. 7.4.3), which makes at least this part of the MWL implementation easy (Fig. 7.15). So no MWL-Rq and MWL-Rsp tables appear in this section – they are identical to the C-Find-Rq and C-Find-Rsp tables in 7.4.3. The only obvious change is in the (0000,0002) attribute value, which is now 1.2.840.10008.5.1.4.31 for the Modality Worklist SOP.

7.6 Basic DICOM Retrieval: C-Get

Let's drift back a couple of chapters and recall what we learned about C-Store. If you had carefully read the description of the DICOM Storage SOP (used to transfer DICOM images) you might have been puzzled by a simple question: "How do we know what to store?" Indeed, the C-Store SOP *transmits previously identified images* one-by-one, but provides no means to decide *what* these images should be.

Quite often, we do not need to think about image selection. For example, a CT scanner is usually set to transmit all newly acquired CT studies to the digital archive. Because the scanner will be producing those studies, it will know exactly what needs to be C-Stored. But what if we need to retrieve the most recent patient's images from a digital archive?

Basic DICOM image retrieval is accomplished with the C-Get SOP. Conceptually, *C-Get blends C-Find and C-Store into a single service class* where the required images can be identified based on a C-Find-like query, followed by a C-Store retrieval. Just like with C-Find, we form a C-Get request and we attach an IOD Identifier object with our image search criteria. When this request is sent to the C-Get SCP, the SCP first uses the search parameters to find the images then invokes C-Store to return them to the C-Get SCU, as illustrated in Fig. 7.16.

Thus, a C-Get SCU (such as our image retrieving workstation in Fig. 7.16) must also act as a C-Store SCP to accept the images returned to it. As you can see, each single image matched on the C-Get SCP is wrapped in a separate C-Store operation and sent to the C-Get SCU (C-Store SCP). During this sending process, the C-Get SCP can also send C-Get responses with status set to *pending* to acknowledge C-Store sub-operations in progress. In these pending replies, the C-Get IOD reply also includes the currently matched values of the C-Get search attributes. When all storage operations are executed, the C-Get SCP replies with the final C-Get-Rsp response containing no IOD and signaling the end of the C-Get operation.

If anything in this chain fails to comply, the entire C-Get operation is aborted with an appropriate error value entered in the C-Get status field.

C-Get inherits three retrieval roots from C-Find as we see in Table 7.16.

The most frequently used is the Study Root, meaning that we retrieve individual studies. As always, the C-Get SOP follows the same simple SOP layout with a DIMSE command and IOD data objects, as we show in Fig. 7.17.

7.6.1 C-Get IOD

The C-Get Information Object Identifier transmits the search attributes for the images to be retrieved. This makes it similar to the C-Find IOD; we provide attributes to be matched on the C-Get SCP end. Any image matching those attributes is

7.6 Basic DICOM Retrieval: C-Get

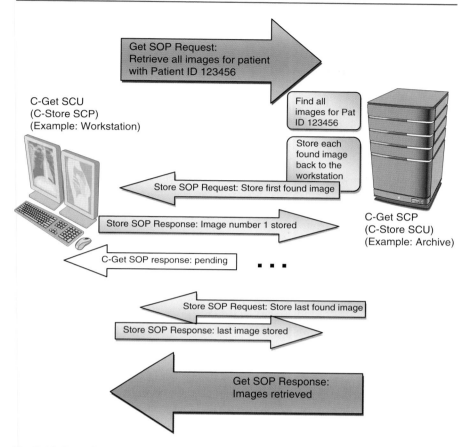

Fig. 7.16 Wrapping C-Store service in C-Get service

Table 7.16 C-Get SOP

SOP class name	SOP class UID
Patient Root Q/R Get	1.2.840.10008.5.1.4.1.2.1.3
Study Root Q/R Get	1.2.840.10008.5.1.4.1.2.2.3
Patient-Study Root Q/R Get (Retired)	1.2.840.10008.5.1.4.1.2.3.3

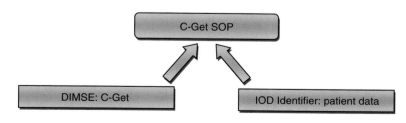

Fig. 7.17 C-Get SOP

Table 7.17 C-Get IOD example

(Group, Element)	Name	Example	Matching (see Sect. 5.3.2)
(0008,0052)	Retrieve Level	STUDY	Can be PATIENT, STUDY, SERIES, IMAGE. This element defines the level or hierarchical search
(0010,0020)	Patient ID	12345	Single value
(0020,000D)	Study Instance UID	1.2.840.1234567	Single value or list matching

returned to us. Consequently, the attributes for C-Get should also conform to the hierarchical DICOM Patient-Study-Series-Image search logic just as in the case of C-Find.

As you should glean from Table 7.17, one principal difference exists between the C-Find and C-Get IODs: the C-Get SCU must supply unique key values to identify an entity at the level of the retrieval. That is, instead of the *required/optional* key approach in C-Find, C-Get operates strictly on a hierarchical key level, using the unique keys for the current level and above to identify the images for retrieval.

Therefore, the C-Get Identifier IOD must contain:
1. *Query/Retrieve Level (0008,0052)* – Defines the level of the retrieval.
2. *Unique key attributes* – May include "Patient ID" (0010,0020), "Study Instance UID" (0020,000D), "Series Instance UID" (0020,000E), and "SOP Instance UID" (0008,0018).

The C-Get Identifier IOD *must not* contain any other optional key. *All unique key attributes in C-Get must have exact values*; that is, they will be matched with *single value matching*.[10] The C-Get SCP generates a C-Get response for each match with an identifier (DICOM data object) that contains the values of all key fields and all known attributes requested.[11]

C-Get performs the image query-and-retrieve job admirably, but the hierarchical *level-keys-only* model is clearly very restrictive – maybe too much so to be considered user-friendly. Only one of the four level key attributes, Patient ID, is commonly used in medical interfaces and known to PACS users. The other three (Study, Series, and SOP Instance UIDs) are usually automatically generated by the modalities. They contain up to 64 characters, are never displayed to the users, have no particular meaning, and consequently never get typed in interactive interfaces. This means that a PACS user willing to use pure C-Get interactively can do it only on the patient level, retrieving all images for a given Patient ID. However, Patient-level retrievals are rare in

---

[10] Study, Series, and Image levels may also support list matching, see Sect. 7.4.1. However, Patient ID must be unique.

[11] As usual, there is also a *relational* (extended) C-Get behavior, rarely needed or implemented, which is supposed to work with any nonhierarchical, relational retrieval. Most DICOM Conformance Statements will contain a phrase "C-Get Extended Negotiation will be NOT supported by the SCP," proving that any advanced features (relational searches included) are not very popular with DICOM manufacturers.

7.6 Basic DICOM Retrieval: C-Get

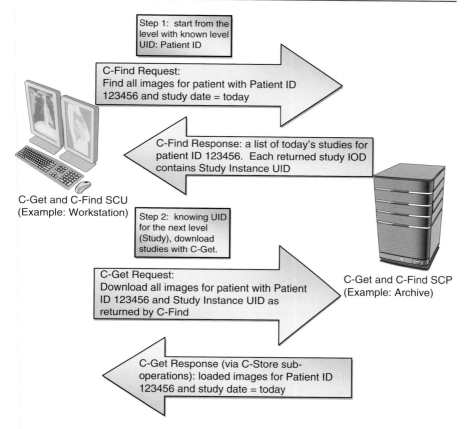

Fig. 7.18 Combining C-Find and C-Get example: retrieving today's images for a patient with known patient ID

radiology – we always start with the most recent studies and prefer to work on the study level. Besides, retrieving all images for a given patient might generate a huge data download.

So, can you use C-Get anyway? Yes, provided that you use C-Find *before* you use C-Get. C-Get does not really support optional key matching, but C-Find does. For example, any system can run C-Find by Patient ID and Study date to locate the most recent patient study. When the C-Find SCP replies to this search, it also returns with C-Find-Rsp IODs containing just what C-Get needs: the unique key UIDs for the next level. For example, C-Find on the Patient level returns the Study instance UID. When this UID is known, it can be used in C-Get to retrieve the images in question, as shown in Fig. 7.18.

Consequently, this approach is implemented in every single PACS. Users are first presented with a querying interface and always do a search (C-Find) first, before attempting to load anything. When search results are returned to the users, they also return those hidden hierarchical level UIDs that PACS software uses for subsequent

C-Get downloads. In other words, C-Get is used for retrieval of the images for which level key attributes are *already known*.

7.6.2 C-Get DIMSE

The C-Get DIMSE is quite similar to C-Find and C-Store. C-Get-Rq is shown in Table 7.18.

The (0000,0800) Data Set Type field is not NULL (0101) and the C-Get-Rq message is immediately followed by the C-Get IOD, conveying search attributes as we discussed. This DIMSE+IOD couple travels on the network from the C-Get SCU Application Entity to the C-Get SCP Application Entity. The latter receives the C-Get DIMSE first, identifies it as such, then takes the C-Get IOD and searches its local database for matches. When matches are found, the C-Get SCP replies with C-Get-Rsp messages; each complemented by a found C-Get IOD.

Because C-Get has a C-Store operation embedded in it, the last four attributes in Table 7.19 for C-Get-Rsp are used to return the current statistics on a C-Store execution. They tell you how many images (individual C-Store sub-operations) are still left to transmit, how many were already transmitted, how many have failed, and how many executed with warnings. For example, if a C-Get SCP returns *pending* messages during C-Store execution, those numbers (sub-operation counts) reflect the progress of the entire image retrieval.

C-Get warnings in most cases refer to some kind of acceptable deviations not leading to the entire C-Get failure (for example, if the C-Get SCP failed to support optional matching parameters). Failure to support any required parameter, on the other hand, would cause a C-Get error and failure. When all retrievals have been completed, the C-Get-Rsp delivers the final message. If everything goes okay, the message should have no data attached ((0000,0800) set to 0101; (0000,1020) set to zero; (0000,1021) containing the total count of all images transmitted; and (0000,1022) set to zero as well).

7.7 Advanced DICOM Retrieval: C-Move

C-Move is practically identical to C-Get, with just a little complexity twist: you can move to *third parties*. That is, where C-Get can be used to return images only to the requesting Application Entity, C-Move can send (C-Store) them to *any* other AE (Fig. 7.19).

Sure, in the simplest scenario an Application Entity can C-Move to itself, which means that it would do a C-Get-like download. For example, you can imagine that in Fig. 7.19 Workstation 2 is the same as Workstation 1. In reality, this is often the case: in most PACS, C-Move is used to do plain C-Get-like downloads, and this makes some sense. If Workstation 1 C-Moves Archive images to itself, we are at least sure that Workstation 1 is on, that it was able to issue a C-Move-Request, that it needs these images, and that it will more likely accept them. Moving to a real third party, such as another Workstation 2 located elsewhere, is a more daring endeavor.

7.7 Advanced DICOM Retrieval: C-Move

Table 7.22 C-Move-Rq

Message field	Tag	VR	Value/description
Command Group Length	(0000,0000)	UL	The even number of bytes from the end of the (0000,0000) value field to the end of the C-Move-Rq message
Affected SOP Class UID	(0000,0002)	UI	Contains SOP UID for this C-Move query root, that is, one of the following three: 1.2.840.10008.5.1.4.1.2.1.2 (Patient) 1.2.840.10008.5.1.4.1.2.2.2 (Study) 1.2.840.10008.5.1.4.1.2.3.2 (Patient-Study)
Command Field	(0000,0100)	US	0021
Message ID	(0000,0110)	US	Unique numerical ID for this message
Priority	(0000,0700)	US	One of the following choices: 0002 (for low priority) 0000 (for medium priority) 0001 (for high priority)
Data Set Type	(0000,0800)	US	Anything *different* from 0101
Move Destination	(0000,0600)	AE	Shall be set to the DICOM AE Title of the destination DICOM AE to which the C-Store sub-operations are being performed

how easy it can be to confuse these two, even for those writing the DICOM standard.

The new (compared to C-Get) Move Destination (0000,0600) attribute shown here specifies where the images need to be moved to by the C-Store sub-operation (Workstation 2 in our earlier example). When the C-Move SCP accepts this request, it will do the following:

1. Based on the unique level keys provided in the attached Identifier IOD, it will find the matching images in its own database.
2. For each of the images, it will issue a separate C-Store sub-operation request to store the images on the Move Destination AE. Note that only the AE title is provided for the C-Move-Rq destination. Based on this title, the C-Move SCP finds the remaining AE parameters (IP address, port number) in its configured C-Move destination list to open a second association with the destination AE (Workstation 2 in our Fig. 7.19 example).
3. As images are C-Stored on the destination AE, the C-Move SCP acknowledges the requesting AE (C-Move SCU) with the pending C-Move-Responses, just like we have seen with C-Get. In particular, those include the C-Store sub-operation counts (successful, failed, warnings, errors).
4. When the C-Store image transfer to the Move Destination AE is over, the C-Move SCP issues the final *success* C-Move-Rsp to the requesting C-Move SCU (or, if anything failed, an *error* C-Move-Rsp) – see Table 7.23.

As we will learn in a moment, C-Cancel command can be used by the C-Move SCU to cancel the C-Move operation in progress.

Table 7.23 C-Move-Rsp

Message field	Tag	VR	Value/description
Command Group Length	(0000,0000)	UL	The even number of bytes from the end of the (0000,0000) value field to the end of the C-Move-Rq message
Affected SOP Class UID	(0000,0002)	UI	Contains SOP UID for this C-Move query root, that is, one of the following three: 1.2.840.10008.5.1.4.1.2.1.3 (Patient) 1.2.840.10008.5.1.4.1.2.2.3 (Study) 1.2.840.10008.5.1.4.1.2.3.3 (Patient-Study)
Command Field	(0000,0100)	US	8021
Message ID Being Responded To	(0000,0120)	US	Shall be set to the value of the Message ID (0000,0110) field used in associated C-Move-Rq Message
Data Set Type	(0000,0800)	US	Anything *different* from 0101, if matched IOD is returned
Status	(0000,0900)	US	0000 (if successful), FF00 (if pending), or other values for warnings and errors
Number of Remaining Sub-operations	(0000,1020)	US	The number of remaining C-STORE sub-operations to be invoked for this C-MOVE operation
Number of Completed Sub-operations	(0000,1021)	US	The number of C-STORE sub-operations invoked by this C-MOVE operation which have completed successfully
Number of Failed Sub-operations	(0000,1022)	US	The number of C-STORE sub-operations invoked by this C-MOVE operation which have failed
Number of Warning Sub-operations	(0000,1023)	US	The number of C-STORE sub-operations invoked by this C-MOVE operation which generated warning responses

7.7.3 C-Move Versus C-Get

Because of the similar functionality of C-Get and C-Move, it is worth spending some time outlining their differences.

The need for C-Move to know its destination is often presented as an essential security feature. If some evil hacker attempts to steal a few images, he will fail miserably because his evil workstations are not in the C-Move destination list (C-Get *would* reply to any requestor). Sending images only to known destinations is definitely a nice C-Move feature; it can indeed be used for security – and often is.

Beyond the apparent practical security features, DICOM (in PS3.7) suggests that C-Get is practically archaic:

> It is expected that in most environments the C-Move is a simpler solution despite the fact that two associations are required. The use of the C-Get service may not be widely implemented. It may be implemented in special cases where a system does not support multiple associations. It was left in this version of the Standard for backward compatibility with previous versions of the Standard.

7.7 Advanced DICOM Retrieval: C-Move

So C-Get is supported only for the sake of backward compatibility? Can that really be? Calling C-Get archaic,[14] or considering a single-association model inferior to a more "advanced" dual-association model, seems like a very strange move on DICOM's part.

C-Get, with its single association model, relieves the user from one of the most severe DICOM problems: a statically configured communication setup (where each entity needs to know ahead of time the list of its peers). If you could expect phone calls only from the people in your phone book, life would get a little bit dull, wouldn't it? Plus, if anything changed, the phone book would need to be updated to make it work again.

These so-called "secure" features in the DICOM world translate into a lack of dynamic functionality in real life, where being dynamic is essential for survival.

With C-Get you can do teleradiology; you can connect to your DICOM devices from anywhere in the world; you can use mobile units; and you can rebuild your network any way you like without being concerned about updating the "phone books" on every C-Move SCP.

With C-Move, you are stuck in a very static world. Even a little disaster (such as your system administrator playfully changing a few IP addresses) can ruin the entire DICOM network. In the world of communications, any new link or association needs additional maintenance and creates additional overhead, which can potentially fail. PACS security should be based on functionality and on the ability to withstand hits; and not on the manual maintenance.

The single-association C-Get model adds another degree of freedom: it can work with firewalls (Fig. 7.21). Consider the following, very typical scenario: you need to read images from a remote unit or archive. You know their AE settings, you can connect to them, you can even query them, but when you try to retrieve data with C-Move, it fails. The reason is simple: C-Echo (for connectivity verifications), C-Find (for querying), C-Get (for retrievals) work on single associations. When you initiate a single-association connection from inside your firewalled environment (such as your hospital or even your firewalled computer), most firewalls would let this connection work – outbound requests are usually considered benign. However, C-Move response implies the remote system coming to you with another, inbound association – and this will be blocked by the firewall. Thus, C-Get can be even more secure than C-Move, because it does not require drilling firewall holes, and can coexist with your security policies.[15]

On the other hand, C-Move (as I have mentioned) is much more appropriate in complex, self-contained, multi-server PACS archives where image storage and processing loads are distributed between multiple archive computers on a local network. In those well-controlled, occluded environments changes are rare because

---

[14]The "It was left in this version of the Standard" mantra repeats itself in all recent DICOM revisions, year after year, without having any real effect on C-Get popularity. Maybe someone should update it finally.

[15]Sure, VPN would be even better, but they usually take more time to set up.

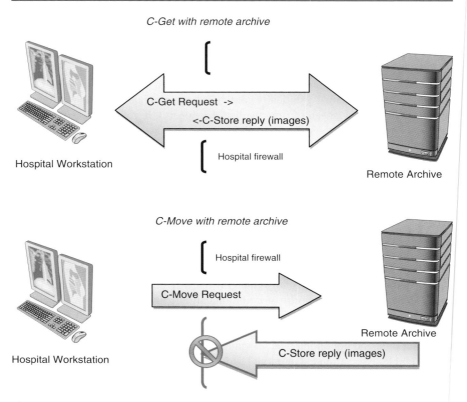

Fig. 7.21 C-Get from remote archive will use C-Store on the outgoing association, originally opened from the inside of the firewall (with the original C-Get request). C-Move will attempt to open an outside (inbound) C-Store association, which will be blocked

they are really supposed to work as a single, indivisible mechanism – they are meant to be static. In this case, C-Move becomes much more appropriate and brings substantial benefits to the internal PACS functionality. "C-Move inside, C-Get outside" really seems to be the most efficient combination, taking advantage of the two image transfer protocols to implement the most reliable and efficient DICOM solution.

> **50/50**
> The recent 2009 DICOM edition introduced some new language in C-Move SCP behavior. Now, when C-Move SCP responds to the request, it "shall either reuse an established and compatible association or establish a new Association for the C-STORE sub-operations." In plain words, when C-Move SCP does C-Store to return the images, it can grab some "established association" if possible, which makes it nearly identical to C-Get. It is still unclear how this can be implemented, which probably makes this provision completely useless; but it does look like a hidden tribute to C-Get single-association model.

Table 7.24 C-Cancel (C-Cancel-Find, aka C-Cancel-Get, aka C-Cancel-Move) DIMSE

Message field	Tag	VR	Value/description
Command Group Length	(0000,0000)	UL	The even number of bytes from the end of the (0000,0000) value field to the end of the C-Cancel message
Command Field	(0000,0100)	US	0FFF
Message ID Being Responded To	(0000,0120)	US	Shall be set to the value of the Message ID (0000,0110) field used in associated C-Find[Get/Move]-Rq Message
Data Set Type	(0000,0800)	US	0101

7.8 C-Cancel – Cancel Them All!

Let's say that you want to search (C-Find) a large PACS archive and you did not specify particular matching attribute values to limit your search. What would happen? A smart piece of DICOM software would recognize that your search is too broad and would either warn you about it or would artificially limit the number of returned matches to some threshold value (many systems use 500 or a similar number of maximum matches). A less smart system (and those, alas, prevail) would make you wait forever, retrieving tons of data that you will never need. "I wish I could cancel this!" you might say; and the first person who said this was definitely heard by the DICOM standards committee.

A C-Cancel-Find message allows you to cancel a C-Find search in progress. C-Cancel-Find needs no response, transmits no data (IOD Identifier), and has a very simple layout, shown in Table 7.24.

Now look closely: The only important element here is (0000,0120); it should contain the ID of the C-Find message that we want to cancel. All C-Cancel-Find is going to do is notify the C-Find SCP (processing the submitted C-Find) that the C-Find processing for message ID in (0000,0120) should be stopped. In other words, C-Cancel-Find bears no C-Find-specific semantics: *it simply cancels messages based on their Message IDs*. For that reason, C-Cancel-Find works with other messages such as C-Get and C-Move; therefore, the DICOM command dictionary (see Appendix A.1, (0000,0100) element values) knows only one C-Cancel flavor. Nevertheless, the DICOM guys added C-Cancel-Get and C-Cancel-Move names to call the same thing: C-Cancel-Get and C-Cancel-Move look and work just like C-Cancel-Find in Table 7.24.

Practically, one cannot really say how long the cancellation might take: C-Cancel exists only in the *request* (C-Cancel-Rq) version, it has no *response* counterpart. The C-Find (C-Get, C-Move) SCP application could spend considerable time interrupting its progress, which might prompt impatient users to keep pushing the *Cancel* button on their PACS interfaces. That's okay, it shouldn't break anything – you are only trying to kill a single message.

Part PS3.7 of the DICOM standard provides more details on C-Cancel behavior. Miraculously, Part PS3.4 uses the "C-Find-Cancel" name, and some other parts refer to *the same thing as* "C-Cancel." That's okay folks – we can understand it anyway. Besides, have I not mentioned the utmost complexity of the DICOM standard?

7.9 DICOM Ping, Push, and Pull

Practical DICOM jargon used by field engineers and PACS support specialists differs from that of the DICOM standard. You will not likely hear many references to C-Echo, C-Get/C-Move, or C-Store. Instead, they talk about DICOM ping, DICOM pull, and DICOM push. These are the same:

- *DICOM ping* – sending a signal to another AE using DICOM protocol to determine whether it is DICOM-connected. This is DICOM C-Echo (Verification SOP).
- *DICOM pull* – pulling (retrieving) images from another AE. Corresponds to sending either a C-Move or a C-Get request.
- *DICOM push* – sending (pushing) images to another AE (opposite of DICOM pull). Corresponds to C-Store.

DICOM push is designed for automated image routing (from modalities to archives, for example). DICOM pull is used predominantly in human interfaces when you select what you want to see, and then pull (retrieve) the images. From the DICOM point of view, *pull* (C-Move/C-Get) simply *initiates a push* (C-Store) to your computer (Application Entity). Essentially, *pull is a smart push* because you get to choose what will be pushed to you from a remote application.

The confusion comes when you open some DICOM software interface and see a *Ping* or *Test connection* button used to test connectivity between your AE and remote applications. Would it mean that it performs a simple TCP/IP connection test (checking whether two computers see each other on the network), or rather sends a true DICOM C-Echo (verifying that respective Application Entities can talk DICOM to each other)? The second always implies the first, but not vice versa; and you might have false expectations about your DICOM connectivity if only a TCP/IP ping was used.

Never underestimate the needs for correct DICOM connectivity verification (C-Echo). Always confirm with your manufacturer that you do in fact have true DICOM C-Echo functionality in your system interface.

7.10 Gentleman's Toolkit

C-Echo, C-Find, C-Store, and C-Get/C-Move protocols are by far the most commonly used in all DICOM implementations. In fact, most DICOM devices and software are completely based on these SOPs and do not implement anything else. This makes perfect sense. If you can verify DICOM connectivity, and you can find and transfer data between DICOM entities, you can consider your system DICOM-capable.

Also, if you are involved in DICOM software development, bear in mind that with proper SOP IODs and attributes you can squeeze a lot of functionality out of those few services. What immediately comes to mind as one of the most appreciated functions in any DICOM interface is the ability to do keyword searches in DICOM free-text fields. For example, searching for a Study Description (element (0008,1030)

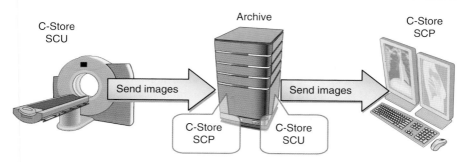

Fig. 7.22 DICOM application roles: digital archive acting as C-Store SCP and SCU at the same time

in the DICOM Data Dictionary), which is very commonly used in teaching archives as well as for clinical history.

Let's have a closer look at just such an example. Suppose you wanted to find all recent studies with the keywords "aneurism" or "endoleak" in their descriptions. If the list of your C-Find-supported attributes includes (0008,1030), then you can set the (0008,1030) value to "aneurism\endoleak" and use it in a C-Find-Rq message to find what you need. In fact, to include all potential word form variations, you can even specify "*aneurism**endoleak*" to ensure that all "aneurism*s*" and "*wejustdonottypespaces*endoleak*s*" will be found as well. As you know by now, if you can C-Find something, you should be able to retrieve it with C-Get or C-Move. In brief, with a few DICOM protocols and sufficient attribute support you can become extremely flexible in your DICOM data management, even if you are limited to hierarchical query/retrieve only.

7.11 Matching Application Roles

Before we conclude, let's take another look at the SCU-SCP concept of DICOM communications that was introduced at the beginning of 7.2. Folks with computer backgrounds tend to relate SCUs and SCPs to the well-known client–server view of computer networks and applications: SCPs are treated as servers and SCUs as clients. This is not exactly the case.

SCP-SCU is nothing but a *role* that any compatible AE can play depending on the current situation; the role is what this *particular application* is *doing* at this *particular moment* for another *particular application*. For example (Fig. 7.22), our digital archive SCP (typically considered a server) for a CT scanner plays the *role* of a CT image storage SCU (typically considered a client) *when it sends* images to another CT image storage SCP (such as workstation). As in nearly all DICOM SOPs, SCU initiates the communication and SCP replies to it – therefore, we cannot so easily assign the client/server labels as we might like.

For another example, think about a PACS archive application using DICOM as its internal language. To find an image in its database, it will issue a C-Find-Rq to itself and will reply to it with a C-Find-Rsp – thus being, with respect to itself, a C-Find SCU and SCP at the same time.

Another popular expectation is that SCP is somewhat *more advanced* than SCU and includes SCU as a sub-function. *This is not at all the case.* SCPs and SCUs can often rival in functional complexity, and being one does not imply being the other; once again, they are really two independent *roles* that any DICOM device can play. As a result, each DICOM unit can be SCU, SCP, both, or none with respect to any particular SOP Class. The DICOM Conformance Statement for the unit should provide exact specifications on this matter.

This brings us to our final observation. The concepts of *Service-Object Pairs* (SOPs), *Service Class User* (SCU), and *Service Class Provider* (SCP) are most essential for any practical implementation of DICOM. Only SOP SCUs and SCPs define exactly how any DICOM entity should interact, what it should process, and what information it should supply to other entities over the DICOM network. SOPs define the DICOM profile of any DICOM-compatible device – from the largest CT scanner to the smallest DICOM file viewer. Consequently, any DICOM Conformance Statement issued by a device manufacturer for its DICOM device or application is nothing but a list of supported SOPs defined as SCU/SCP roles. Traditionally, reading Conformance Statements is the point where many PACS administrators get really lost. In fact, most do not read them at all, and are overly trusting of DICOM manufacturers that *"it is gonna work okay for me, right?"*

Well, not necessarily, because:
- If you buy a unit that does not support the DICOM Verification SOP SCP, you will never be able to verify DICOM connectivity to that unit from another DICOM device. Verification messages sent to it will remain unanswered, as if the unit either does not exist or has a broken network connection.
- If you buy an archive that supports the MR storage SOP SCP, nothing implies that it should support the CT storage SOP SCP, and you might not be able to transfer your CT data to the same archive.
- If you have a workstation that supports the C-Find (Query) SCU, but does not support the C-Find (Query) SCP, you'll never be able to query that workstation from another workstation or archive. Only query SCPs can respond to queries, *serving* those responses to other units.
- If you buy a DICOM teleradiology server that does not support image compression for C-Store image transfers, you won't be able to send the images compressed; and you won't be able to run your teleradiology business.

This list can be continued indefinitely. Ignored, misunderstood, or misconfigured SOPs represent the bulk of DICOM and PACS problems.

Some units can be patched with additional software modules to add the required or missing SCU/SCP capabilities (the vendor will charge you for this, typically on a scale of several thousand dollars). But some units cannot be patched and need to be replaced (at your expense of course). If you are involved in any PACS administration or purchasing, always pay particular attention to the SCU/SCP support.

7.11 Matching Application Roles

Real Case: Printing to an Archive?

How well DICOM manufacturers adhere to those rules is, as usual, a totally different question. In one situation, we spent several hours trying to set up a CR unit to send its X-ray images to our digital archive. The CR unit had only two options: send images to an archive and send images to a printer. Despite all possible (and impossible) archive configuration settings, the thing just wouldn't work. So we resorted to our very last plan: calling onsite support from the CR manufacturer.

The guy came, looked at our desperate efforts, grinned, and informed us that all digital archives produced by third parties (including us) need to be added to this device as *printers*! That is, all we had to do was to enter our archive specifications into the CR "printer" section.

Certainly, the wisdom of those who designed this unit was highly questionable, but after a couple of minutes our "archive-printer" was receiving the images from the CR.

8 DICOM SOPs: Beyond Basic

The seemingly endless table in the Appendix (Sect. A.3) provides the list of all current SOP classes taken from PS3.6 of the DICOM standard, version 2009. The majority of SOPs in this table are included in the Storage SOP that we discussed earlier – they provide support for different image modality types. Regarding what remains, a few more SOPs deserve special mention because you just might find them in your DICOM Conformance Statements.

8.1 Storage Commitment

The *Storage Commitment SOP* was introduced in addition to the regular Storage SOP classes to ensure that the device receiving images for storage indeed *commits* to storing them – *explicitly taking responsibility for safekeeping the data*. For example, a simple workstation can implement a regular CT storage SOP Class just to be able to receive CT images for display, and delete them right after. Digital archives, on the other hand, are meant to support long-term (committed) storage and typically support the Storage Commitment SOP Class (DICOM UID 1.2.840.10008.1.20.1).

Nowadays, more and more DICOM devices offer Storage Commitment support; although the *real* commitment to store anything is strictly an administrative problem. In DICOM, Storage Commitment is merely another type of data transmitting protocol. If someone can log in to a storage device and delete certain studies, or worse, if a server's auto-delete function can purge the images when running out of disk space (a very common problem with many DICOM archives), then no DICOM Commitment SOP will help.

Various DICOM software packages implement different proprietary commitment strategies, often permitting the locking of certain studies (so that they cannot be deleted), marking them with no-delete flags, defining various storage rules, and so on. But clearly, none of this guarantees the safekeeping of data, and stays outside of the DICOM scope. Your best bet in any true storage commitment implementation would be backing up your DICOM archives daily and limiting any unauthorized access to them (placing them in isolated rooms, in particular). On an administrative level, this minimizes the chances of losing anything. For this very reason, the Storage Commitment SOP is commonly ignored in AE settings and is rarely enabled even when it is formally supported by the program.

8.2 Secondary Capture

Secondary capture storage SOPs (1.2.840.10008.5.1.4.1.1.7 and derived, as you will find them in Appendix A.3) were introduced into DICOM several years ago to recognize a simple fact that digital image data is collected not only from modalities, but from other sources as well. For example, digital images may be acquired when you scan (digitize) plain films, scan text reports, post-process[1] modality images (creating 3D images from the original slices, for example), or even if you simply make screenshots on a workstation and add them to the PACS database (Fig. 8.1).

Ironically, the most common problem with handling secondary capture (SC) images on PACS is identifying their modality.

Let me give you an example. Let's say that you scanned a patient on a CT scanner for a perfusion study and generated perfusion color maps, just like the one shown in Fig. 8.1 (right). Obviously, the best way to store those color maps would be to put them where they belong: added to the original CT study. But perfusion map images are clearly *not* CT images, and they do not match the CT image DICOM IOD: they are not monochrome, they are not associated with any CT scanning protocol, they do not have Hounsfield calibration, and so on. In brief, if you happen to label your perfusion maps with CT modality, you are in trouble; sooner or later some CT-processing function in your system (CT image storage, for example) will choke on using non-CT data.

The only way out is to label secondary capture images with SC modality, which would probably make perfect sense to most of us in the first place. But, unfortunately, you could now run into a different problem; for example, if you wanted to transfer your CT study (with some SC images included) to another workstation or digital archive. In most unsophisticated DICOM implementations, this will invoke a CT storage SOP, which will indeed transfer all your CT images – clearly *without* the SC maps! Because SC images in your CT study, as we just discussed, are not CT type, they will simply be ignored by the CT storage SOP. Radiologists reading the studies will also be puzzled seeing SC on their CT worklists.

Is there any solution to this? Yes. Make sure that your DICOM implementation can support SC Storage SOPs and, more importantly, make sure it will be checking for SC images when it transfers images for *any* specific modality. As we will see in Chap. 9, DICOM can negotiate several storage SOPs when transferring a digital study; if SC is always included in this negotiation, your SC images won't be forgotten. Practically, you should get a sample DICOM study with SC images included and use it to test any DICOM application you are about to purchase. If you are a radiologist, get used to seeing SC images in nearly any study, regardless of the original study modality.

---

[1]Post-processing creates what DICOM calls "derived images" – images in which the pixel data was constructed from pixel data of one or more original (source) images.

8.3 Structured Reports

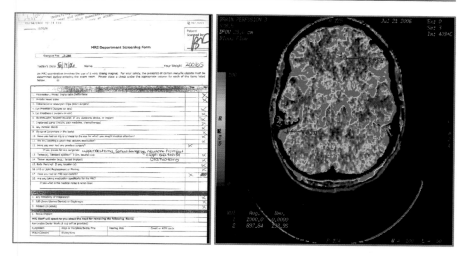

Fig. 8.1 Examples of secondary captures: scanned documents, screenshots of post-processed images

8.3 Structured Reports

For a long time, DICOM dealt only with digital images, strictly separating them by their modality types. If radiology always starts from the original digital images, complex post-processing, viewing, and analysis that follow produce much more diverse data types, which need to be handled with proper connection to each other. The most favorite (or should I say, the only) way of storing nonimage data such as text in earlier DICOM was to convert the data into images – just like secondary capture screenshots. Almost always, this would destroy the original data format and properties. For example, you can search text reports for keywords, but you cannot do the same with the scanned reports, stored as images.

The Structured Report (SR) SOPs are intended to create complex structured documents in which text, different images, and other data types can be mixed and organized together. They might have been meant for reporting, but they are capable of handling any complex multi-data document. SRs support basic usage of coded entries (titles, headings) and a hierarchical tree of headings under which text and subheadings may appear. Reference to SOP Instances (such as images, waveforms, or other SR Documents) is restricted to appearing at the leaf level (lowest subheadings) of this primarily textual tree. This structure simplifies the encoding of conventional textual reports as SR Documents; and it also simplifies their rendering.[2]

So, the easiest way to think about an SR object is to imagine a document that contains text and may also include referenced images, or even more complex data

---

[2]See section A.35, PS3.3-2009.

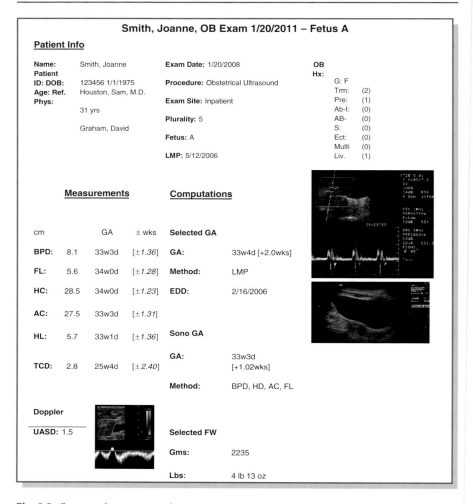

Fig. 8.2 Structured report example

such as sound recordings. The text can be structured into sections, subsections, and so on; the images can be original or reconstructed, as in our example in Fig. 8.2.

This book could be viewed as a DICOM structured report – in the most extreme form possible. In the simplest case, an SR can contain, for example, a single measurement performed on an ultrasound image (Hussein et al. 2004a, b). Moreover, SRs can be digitally encrypted and signed for security reasons.[3]

Structured reports are relatively new in the DICOM standard and older DICOM units/software might not be prepared to deal with them. For example, I have seen

---

[3] See section A.4, PS3.15-2009.

examples of PACS workstations attempting to open SR DICOM objects as digital images, which inevitably lead to failures and interrupted processes. Hopefully, as SR becomes more widespread, PACS manufacturers will become at least more aware of them.

On the other hand, structured reports have already experienced explosive popularity growth over the past few years. First of all, SRs can be used to transfer and manage valuable nonimage data, such as radiation exposure information for CT scans. Secondly, SRs provide *meta-modality* capabilities. If all DICOM IODs are modality-centric, SRs are not, and they allow you to mix and match unlimited numbers of various studies, scans, and documents. Consequently, in many cases SRs have become far more complex than conventional DICOM data, and certain radiological facilities have already made their workflows SR-based (instead of the traditional modality study approach). Balancing the benefits and the complexity of structured reporting is equally challenging and rewarding (Hussein et al. 2004a; Batchelor 2006).

The full overview of structured reports is beyond the scope of this book. If you are looking for in-depth structured report information, read an excellent "DICOM Structured Reporting" book by David Clunie (Clunie), or check out Supplement 23 of the DICOM standard.

8.4 Encapsulated PDFs

Just like the case with secondary storage images, it was soon recognized that DICOM needed to store more than just image data from the modalities. Portable Document Format (PDF), introduced by Adobe in 1993, has evolved into a universal and powerful document exchange tool, well-integrated into various applications.

Many medical practices use PDFs routinely because, just like with DICOM, almost anything can be put into a PDF file. Many documents (such as reports) are better scanned into PDFs than into plain images because PDF takes care of page order and scanned image compression. Typed (non-scanned) reports are often stored in PDFs as well. They are harder to modify compared to plain text, they can be digitally signed and secured (PDF supports a wide range of security features), they can have complex formatting, and they can include images – essentially acting as structured reports. Because such PDFs contain text, they can be searched for keywords, thus creating a searchable report database. In brief, if you have not yet enjoyed the benefits of PDFs in your document workflow, I suggest you investigate the rich feature set that this tool has to offer. Regardless of your adoption of DICOM, PDFs can make many of your documenting – and even imaging – tasks more solid.

For all these reasons, DICOM SOP 1.2.840.10008.5.1.4.1.1.104.1, Encapsulated PDF, allows you to store a PDF file as a DICOM object. To do so, a PDF document is complemented with a few DICOM-specific information modules, such as patient data, to provide all required DICOM attributes (Table 8.1).

Just like SRs, PDF SOPs are not yet widespread in DICOM/PACS systems. Complex data formats such as PDF need intricate software tools to display and

Table 8.1 Encapsulated PDF IOD Modules

IE	Module	Usage
Patient	Patient	M (mandatory)
	Specimen Identification	U (user-defined)
	Clinical Trial Subject	U
Study	General Study	M
	Patient Study	U
	Clinical Trial Study	U
Series	Encapsulated Document Series	M
	Clinical Trial Series	U
Equipment	General Equipment	M
	SC Equipment	M
Encapsulated Document	Encapsulated PDF Document	M
	SOP Common	M

manipulate them adequately. Essentially, you need to have the entire Adobe Acrobat Professional software integrated into your DICOM application. From the DICOM vendors' perspective, it is much easier to stay with the image-only DICOM systems; storing anything non-modality into plain secondary capture images. Besides, complex documents are meant to be used for complex tasks, and most radiology departments try to keep their DICOM and document workflow as straightforward as possible. The need for PDFs comes naturally only when you run into a multi-site, multi-practice document distribution; and then the ability to store PDFs in DICOM and PACS can come in very handy.

Nevertheless, a few commercial PDF plug-ins are capable of opening DICOM files and even sending them to/from PACS directly from Adobe Acrobat.

8.5 Hardcopy Printing

A wealth of *Print*, *Hardcopy*, and *Image Box SOPs* – retired and active – are dedicated to printing DICOM images on film. In many ways, those SOPs are meant to make you backward-compatible with the pre-PACS world (circa 1980) when film was the only medium used with medical images. In current PACS though, film has taken its proper niche: playing the role of reliable backup when nothing else is available. If your PACS network goes down; if you need to send a study to some disconnected rural location; if you have run into one of the few remaining retrogrades brandishing the "I just hate digital" motto, film will still save you. Having film printing SOPs on your archive and workstations will always be a good thing for these and other occasions.

Nevertheless, in the day-to-day radiology workflow, film is becoming increasingly rare – this was one of the main goals of the PACS revolution. Softcopy SOPs continue to infiltrate the traditional hardcopy domains. So if you want to add flexibility to your digital workflow, you'd better make sure that the PACS/DICOM prod-

9.1 Association Establishment Basics

Let's go back to our ARCHIVE-MR example. A new MR study has just been completed on the MR scanner and needs to be stored on the ARCHIVE server. An MR technologist pushes the *Send* button on her MR scanner interface to send the study to the ARCHIVE. If she could actually hear the AEs talk, she would hear something like this:

Act 1 – Association Establishment
MR scanner (to ARCHIVE): Hi, I am MR scanner and I speak DICOM. Do you?
ARCHIVE (to MR scanner): Hi, I am ARCHIVE and I speak DICOM, too.
MR: Are you an SCP for MR image storage? (Can you store MR images?)
ARCHIVE: I sure am.
MR: Listen, I have 100 new uncompressed MR images and I want to send them to you as is. I can also send them compressed with JPEG2000, or compressed with 12-bit lossless JPEG.
ARCHIVE: No problem, I can take MR images, but I prefer them uncompressed.
MR: OK, starting to send.
ARCHIVE: OK, ready to receive.

This dialog, which we translated from "Dicomean" into plain English, constitutes the association establishment part. In the very first lines, the devices introduce their functionality (Abstract Syntaxes), and then agree on image transfer format (Transfer Syntaxes). As images start to flow, the two units continue to communicate the image transfer part, verifying the process of image transaction:

Act 2 – Image Transfer
(Right after Act 1, same mise-en-scène, same actors)
MR (sending each image to ARCHIVE): Here is the first. Here is the second. Here is …
ARCHIVE: First received, OK. Second received, OK. Third…

Finally (yet still very importantly), when all images are transmitted, the AEs need to gracefully terminate their active association:

Act 3 – Association Termination
MR (after the last image is sent): All 100 images sent, 0 images failed, success, goodbye.
ARCHIVE (after the last image is received): All images received, goodbye.
(Association terminated)

As you can see, the association protocol is very simple and intuitive, and allows the communicating AEs to control the entire flow of the data exchange. You can also tell that the most important part is Act 1 – the actual *association establishment*. Now that we know the logic behind it, we can consider the technicalities.

9.2 Association Establishment

The contents of the DICOM association establishment are shown in Fig. 9.1. Do not try to grasp every detail immediately – we will learn everything step by step in the following sections. Instead, look at the entire structure and try to think how it fits into the "Act 1" logic.

To begin the process, the association-requesting (*calling*) AE builds and sends an *A-Associate-RQ* message (first part of the diagram in Fig. 9.1), requesting that the receiving (*called*) AE start an association. This message is packed with several Presentation Contexts (our *business cards*), and additional *user information data*, describing the capabilities of the Application Entity initiating the association (*user* refers to the requesting AE).

The receiving AE looks at all proposed communication parameters, picks the most appropriate, and replies with an *A-Associate-AC* message if the association is accepted, as shown in our diagram. If none of the proposed parameters matches the receiving AE profile (for example, you are trying to store an MR image to a CT scanner), it will reply with an *A-Associate-RJ* message, rejecting the association. It could also reply with a more general *A-Abort* message to abort associations at any time.

Straightforward, isn't it? So let's glance at the contents of the association establishment message first; then we can revisit the entire association messaging workflow.

9.3 Abstract Syntax

As I already explained, Abstract Syntaxes, present in A-Associate-RQ and A-Associate-AC messages, are very important for DICOM association establishment. They describe the services that DICOM applications can render to each other. In other words, Abstract Syntaxes encode SOPs (see Chaps. 7 and 8, and the table in Sect. A.3 of the Appendix) supported on the communicating AEs. We already learned that each DICOM SOP has its own Abstract Syntax Name such as "MR image storage," "CT image storage," "Modality Worklist," and so on, which DICOM encodes with an Abstract Syntax (SOP) UID. For example, 1.2.840.10008.5.1.4.1.1.4 is the UID for "MR image storage." Earlier (Sect. 5.5.8) we talked about UIDs and their importance for identifying object instances. DICOM networking uses UIDs richly to encode various transaction types; Abstract Syntax is just one such example.

DICOM offers dozens of Abstract Syntax UIDs – I sampled a few of the more important ones in Table 9.1.

9.3 Abstract Syntax

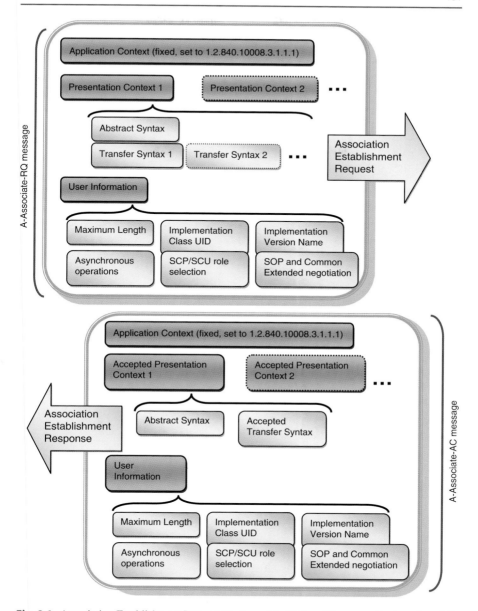

Fig. 9.1 Association Establishment Request (A-Associate-RQ) and Response (A-Associate-AC) Structures (optional items are *dashed*, subitems have *thin borders*)

As you can see from these examples, Abstract Syntaxes can be viewed as code names for DICOM networking functions. Let's consider the very first Abstract Syntax from our table: Verification (1.2.840.10008.1.1). If you have a DICOM

Table 9.1 Important abstract syntaxes

Abstract syntax name	Abstract syntax UID	Meaning
Verifying DICOM connectivity		
Verification	1.2.840.10008.1.1	Send to remote AE to verify its availability. Also known as "DICOM ping," this Abstract Syntax is used to confirm that the receiver AE is indeed working and available on the network.
Querying/Retrieving data from AEs		
Study Root Query/Retrieve Information Model – FIND	1.2.840.10008.5.1.4.1.2.2.1	Query AE for a list of studies (for example, query MR modality for the list of scanned studies)
Study Root Query/Retrieve Information Model – GET	1.2.840.10008.5.1.4.1.2.2.3	Ask AE to send study images to the requester AE
Study Root Query/Retrieve Information Model – MOVE	1.2.840.10008.5.1.4.1.2.2.2	Ask AE to send study images to another AE (requester or not)
Patient Root Query/Retrieve Information Model – FIND	1.2.840.10008.5.1.4.1.2.1.1	Query AE for a list of patients
Patient Root Query/Retrieve Information Model – GET	1.2.840.10008.5.1.4.1.2.1.3	Ask AE to send patient images to the requester AE
Patient Root Query/Retrieve Information Model – MOVE	1.2.840.10008.5.1.4.1.2.1.2	Ask AE to send patient images to another AE (requester or not)
Modality Worklist Information Model – FIND	1.2.840.10008.5.1.4.31	Retrieve from an AE its modality worklist (if supported)
Storing data on AEs		
CR Image Storage	1.2.840.10008.5.1.4.1.1.1	Storing images from various digital modalities on DICOM archive servers
CT Image Storage	1.2.840.10008.5.1.4.1.1.2	
MR Image Storage	1.2.840.10008.5.1.4.1.1.4	
Ultrasound Image Storage	1.2.840.10008.5.1.4.1.1.6.1	
Nuclear Medicine Image Storage	1.2.840.10008.5.1.4.1.1.20	
Positron Emission Tomography Image Storage	1.2.840.10008.5.1.4.1.1.128	
DICOM printing		
Basic Film Session Class	1.2.840.10008.5.1.1.1	Managing different parameters of DICOM printing (printing images on DICOM-compatible film printers)
Basic Film Box Class	1.2.840.10008.5.1.1.2	
Basic Grayscale Image Box Class	1.2.840.10008.5.1.1.4	
.....		

> MR: Listen, I have 100 new MR images, 1.2.840.10008.1.2, and I want to send them to you. I can also send them in 1.2.840.10008.1.2.4.90.
> ARCHIVE: No problem, I can take MR images and I prefer them 1.2.840.10008.1.2.

Using Transfer Syntaxes to encode image compression has one problem: all image compression algorithms, as you might know, depend on several important compression parameters (such as lossy compression quality or compression ratio). Transfer Syntax encodes only the name (and possibly the version) of the compression algorithm, but does not convey any information about the algorithm settings. Therefore, the values of compression parameters are not negotiable with Transfer Syntaxes and the DICOM handshake in general, and the receiving AE has to deal with whatever compression parameters the sending AE chooses to use.

This, and many similar problems, gave rise to the private (manufacturer-specific) Transfer Syntaxes used by various PACS manufacturers on their imaging networks. However, the private syntaxes by definition can be understood only by the devices from the same manufacturer and will be rejected by others (then defaulting, as we know, to 1.2.840.10008.1.2 transfer). This makes 1.2.840.10008.1.2 not only the default, but also the most preferred Transfer Syntax used in nearly all DICOM transactions. It ensures complete compatibility and keeps the system free of impossible-to-control compression artifacts.

9.5 Application Context

The Application Context item in Fig. 9.4 is also included in association establishment, although it adds nothing to parameter negotiation. Theoretically, the Application Context string represents the context of the association-requesting application (such as particular DICOM software running on the association-requesting AE). The association-responding AE can even abort the entire association if it finds the context unsupported.

For this purpose, NEMA (keeper of the DICOM standard) is also responsible for issuing unique Application Context names to various DICOM implementations and manufacturers (following UID encoding guidelines, see Sect. 5.5.8). In this way, various Application Contexts uniquely correspond to the DICOM capabilities of their respective applications, acting as Conformance Statement references.

Moreover, you can define your own private (unregistered with NEMA) Application Context and use it in your application. For example, if, during the negotiation process, your application receives an association request with an Application Context equal to yours, it will immediately know that an association is requested by another instance of the same software. In this case, you can enable advanced or proprietary data transfer protocols, which only your software supports – and you will know for sure that they will work.

Application Context item:

10H	00H (r)	Application Context length L	Application Context String
1 byte	1 byte	2 bytes	L bytes

Example:

10H	00H	0011H	1.2.840.10008.3.1.1.1
1 byte	1 byte	2 bytes	17 bytes (11H bytes)

Fig. 9.4 Application Context item, from PS 3.8, and its most typical example

Practically, however, DICOM offers a default Application Context name (1.2.840.10008.3.1.1.1) that many applications borrow. It would be impractical for any program to maintain a list of various Application Context names from other DICOM manufacturers and use them to negotiate additional DICOM capabilities during the Association Establishment process. Besides, all DICOM parameters needed for association (such as Abstract and Transfer Syntaxes) are explicitly included in association messages and can be used to capture any perceivable variety of communication options without the use of Application Context.

> **Application Context Wars**
> In essence, the Application Context item is meant to identify the application manufacturer. Consequently (as rumor has it), in the world of competing commercial PACS, where anything goes, it can be used to reject DICOM handshakes from competitors' applications – when they are recognized by their Application Contexts.
> It can also be used in a positive way: to enable manufacturer-dependent, proprietary DICOM Data Dictionary support (see Sect. 5.4.2) when the application manufacturer is recognized from its Application Context.

9.6 Presentation Context

A Presentation Context marries proposed functionality to format, and – easy to guess – comprises an Abstract Syntax plus a list of negotiable Transfer Syntaxes (Table 9.3). We already compared Presentation Context to a *business card* that any DICOM device will hand to its partner to initiate a network transaction.

9.6 Presentation Context

Table 9.3 Presentation context components

Abstract syntax		Transfer syntax		Role
Name	UID	Name List	UID List	see 9.7
Name	UID	Name1	UID1	SCP | SCU | BOTH
		Name2	UID2	
		...	...	

Table 9.4 DICOM AE, presenting itself to another AE for connection verification

Verification	1.2.840.10008.1.1	Implicit VR Little Endian	1.2.840.10008.1.2	SCU
		Explicit VR Big Endian	1.2.840.10008.1.2.2	

Table 9.5 MR scanner, presenting itself to DICOM archive for MR image transfer

MR Image Storage	1.2.840.10008.5.1.4.1.1.4	Implicit VR Little Endian	1.2.840.10008.1.2	SCU
		DICOM JPEG-LS Lossless compression	1.2.840.10008.1.2.4.80	
		DICOM JPEG-2000 Lossy compression	1.2.840.10008.1.2.4.91	

During this initiation, the Abstract Syntax establishes the subject of the *discussion*. The Transfer Syntaxes propose several *languages* in which the discussion can be carried out. Providing several Transfer Syntaxes is the essence of DICOM connectivity. This permits the receiving device to choose the Transfer Syntax it supports best.

In the Table 9.4 example, a generic Application Entity sends a simple verification request to another entity to confirm its availability on the DICOM network. Two Transfer Syntaxes are suggested: standard default Little Endian (1.2.840.10008.1.2) and the optionally supported Big Endian (1.2.840.10008.1.2.2). If the receiving device runs on a Little Endian system (such as Windows) it will likely prefer the Little Endian syntax; otherwise, it might choose Big Endian. In any event, the receiving device replies to the sending device with an Accepted Presentation Context message containing the same Abstract Syntax (Verification 1.2.840.10008.1.1) and the chosen Transfer Syntax. This completes the DICOM handshake: both devices agree on the communication format.

The second example, shown in Table 9.5, is similar to the first, but the request for MR image storage (1.2.840.10008.5.1.4.1.1.4) is accompanied by a choice of three Transfer Syntaxes. The first option, Implicit VR Little Endian, in this case also implies *uncompressed images* because it does not correspond to any compression algorithm. The other two Transfer Syntaxes offer two compression methods, which the MR scanner can apply to the images before sending them to the destination AE (such as an archive). The destination AE selects the most appropriate Transfer Syntax (for example, DICOM JPEG-LS Lossless compression, 1.2.840.10008.1.2.4.80) and communicates it back to the MR scanner with an Accepted Presentation Context

Presentation Context (PrC) item in A-Associate-RQ:

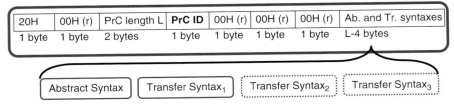

Fig. 9.5 Presentation Context (PrC) item in A-Associate-RQ. Bytes with (r) are reserved

Presentation Context (PrC) item in A-Associate-AC:

21H	00H (r)	PrC length L	**PrC ID**	00H (r)	Reason	00H (r)	Transfer Syntax
1 byte	1 byte	2 bytes	1 byte	1 byte	1 byte	1 byte	L-4 bytes

Fig. 9.6 Presentation Context (PrC) item in A-Associate-AC. Bytes with (r) are reserved. PrC ID must match the ID of the Proposed Context in A-Associate-RQ

message. As soon as MR scanner receives this message, it will start compressing the images with JPEG-LS, sending them to the destination.

Let's review this more carefully in the light of DICOM encoding. DICOM encodes the Presentation Context item similarly to what we have seen with Abstract and Transfer Syntaxes, but with one very important addition (which is often confusing to DICOM beginners). Presentation Contexts *exist in two different formats* used for requesting (A-Associate-RQ) and accepting (A-Associate-AC) a DICOM connection. Figure 9.5 shows this in more detail. The A-Associate-RQ Presentation Context (labeled in DICOM with the first byte as 20H) contains one Abstract Syntax and at least one Transfer Syntax. Its main goal is to suggest various Transfer Syntaxes to the peer AE so that it can choose the most appropriate one.

When the peer AE receives this Presentation Context in an A-Associate-RQ message, it does two things:

1. *Checks the proposed Abstract Syntax* – to see if the syntax matches its functionality. For example, if the imaging archive receives an A-Associate-RQ with an Abstract Syntax of 1.2.840.10008.5.1.4.1.1.4 (MR storage), it will agree to it if it can accept MR images for storage.
2. *Selects the Transfer Syntax* – If the Abstract Syntax is acceptable, the peer AE goes through the list of proposed Transfer Syntaxes and selects the one it can process best – for example, the most appropriate image compression format.

Now, assuming that the Abstract and Transfer Syntaxes were selected, peer AE needs to return this information to the association-requesting AE. So it constructs another Presentation Context message in a shorter format, which becomes a part of the A-Associate-AC, as shown in Fig. 9.6.

The *magic byte* is now set to 21H and the entire Abstract-Transfer Syntax sequence is reduced to a single Transfer Syntax item that the peer AE has selected

9.8 Protocol Data Unit (PDU)

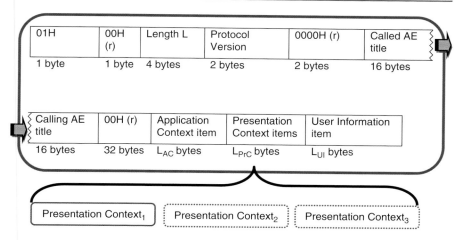

Fig. 9.9 A-Associate-RQ message structure, from PS 3.8

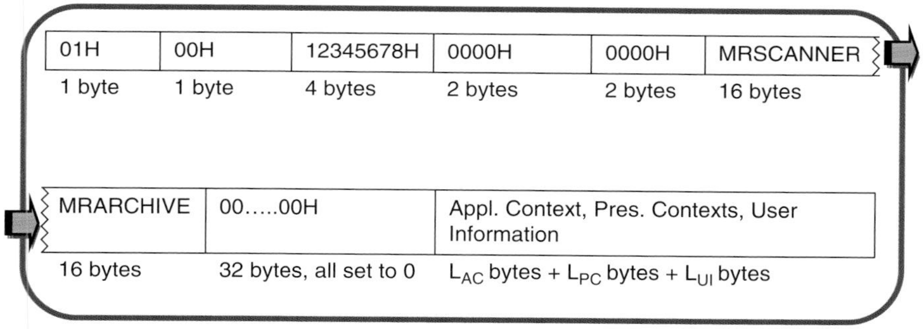

Fig. 9.10 A-Associate-RQ message structure example

To initiate a DICOM connection, the initiating AE proposes a message with certain connection parameters: an A-Associate-RQ. The receiving AE agrees on the most acceptable optional parameters (such as Transfer Syntaxes for each Abstract Syntax), and, if this agreement is possible, it accepts the connection with an A-Associate-AC message. Otherwise, if none of the proposed parameters satisfies the receiver AE, it rejects the connection with the A-Associate-RJ message.

9.8.1 A-Associate-RQ

As you can see in Figs. 9.9 and 9.10, A-Associate-RQ consists of several familiar structures, such as Application and Presentation Contexts. The A-Associate-RQ is the information that any *calling AE* hands out to its *called AEs*, proposing to establish a working DICOM association. Most importantly, the proposition includes one or more Presentation Context items (Abstract and Transfer Syntaxes) that reflect the DICOM functionality of the calling AE requesting the association.

Both *calling* and *called* AE titles must not be blank (undefined) and should correspond to the real, existing AEs on the given DICOM network. Because AE VR uses 16 characters (see table in Sect. 5.3), the A-Associate-RQ provides 16-character fields to hold calling and called AE titles. Shorter AE titles are padded with trailing blanks to ensure that all 16 bytes are used. Many PACS workstations and archives, acting as called AEs, first verify whether the calling AE title is present in their *white list* (list of permitted callers usually configured by the PACS administrator). If the calling AE is not in the white list, the A-Associate-RQ will likely be rejected as a *stranger*, with the A-Associate-RJ message. The message often contains the notorious "no reason given" reason for rejection, which we will see more of in the following sections. This archaic, primitive (and easy-to-bypass) security check nonetheless remains one of the most currently used in PACS networks: sometimes serving its purpose, and sometimes creating implementation problems.

The only new item in the A-Associate-RQ is the 2-byte Protocol Version. It is a constant with the first (zero) bit set to 0 to indicate Version 1 of the DICOM Upper Layer protocol. Because the values of the other bits are not used, you could simply set the entire Protocol Version field to 0 (0000H) treating it essentially as a reserved field – unless further editions of DICOM make changes.

Length L, the third item in the A-Associate-RQ, includes all the bytes from the fourth (Protocol Version) item to the very end of the A-Associate-RQ and can be computed as:

$$L = 2 \text{ (Protocol Version)} + 2 \text{ (r)} + 16 \text{ (Called AE title)} + 16 \text{ (Calling AE title)} + 32 \text{ (r)} + L_{AC} + L_{PrC} + L_{UI}$$

9.8.2 A-Associate-AC

A-Associate-AC (accept) is what we all hope to get from the called AE in reply to our A-Associate-RQ (request) message. Natural enough, right? After all, whether it is love or the DICOM Upper Layer protocol, no one likes to be rejected. If A-Associate-RQ *is* accepted, the called AE replies with an A-Associate-AC message of very similar structure, as shown in Figs. 9.11 and 9.12.

Can you spot all the differences from the A-Associate-RQ? Let's count them:
1. The first message byte is now set to 02H, corresponding to the A-Associate-AC.
2. Called and Calling AE items are now declared as Reserved, and "shall be sent with a value identical to the value received in the same field of the A-Associate-RQ, but its value shall not be tested when received." In plain words, these items contain the same Called/Calling AE titles.[4]
3. Presentation Context item (and this is important) slightly changes its format, as described in Sect. 9.1. Instead of Presentation Context for A-Associate-RQ, it becomes Presentation Context for A-Associate-AC. The most important part of this change is that the Presentation Context for A-Associate-AC retains *only one* Transfer Syntax (from several proposed in each A-Associate-RQ Presentation Context) – the one

---
[4]Do not be tempted to swap Called and Calling.

9.8 Protocol Data Unit (PDU)

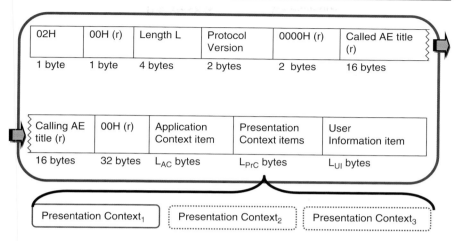

Fig. 9.11 A-Associate-AC message structure, from PS 3.8

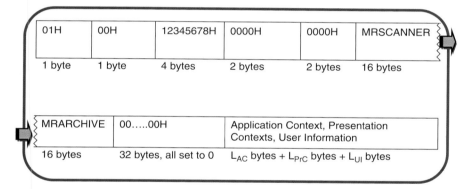

Fig. 9.12 A-Associate-AC message structure example

chosen as the best fit for the association based on the called AE capabilities. For example, the called AE might reject various image compressing syntaxes and default to uncompressed images only. Also, the Presentation Context for A-Associate-AC contains the "Reason" field, explaining why certain Presentation Contexts were rejected.

If at least one of the proposed contexts was accepted by the called AE, we have every reason to expect to receive the A-Associate-AC message – meaning that our DICOM association has been successfully established, and we can proceed with the actual data transfer.

9.8.3 A-Associate-RJ

The A-Associate-RJ message is used to reject a proposed association request (A-Associate-RQ). As we have already mentioned, reasons for rejections can be

A-Associate-RJ message structure:

03H	00H	00000004H	00H	Result	Source	Reason
1 byte	1 byte	4 bytes	1 byte	1 byte	1 byte	1 byte

Example:

03H	00H	00000004H	00H	01H	03H	01H
1 byte	1 byte	4 bytes	1 byte	1 byte	1 byte	1 byte

Fig. 9.13 A-Associate-RJ message structure, from PS 3.8, and its most typical example

many: incompatible devices, unsupported transfer protocols, invalid format, and so on. Unlike the A-Associate-RQ and the A-Associate-AC, which we have considered in all their complexity, the A-Associate-RJ message is really quite simple (Fig. 9.13).

The only parameters to be supplied here are:

1. *Result* – this field can be either 1 (rejected-permanent) or 2 (rejected-transient). Transient rejection can correspond to temporary problems (network congestion), but more common permanent rejection indicates mismatched association parameters, incompatible device profiles, and such.
2. *Source* – can be 1, 2, or 3 depending on the current provider and protocol type. The most typical code is 3, corresponding to service provider rejection.
3. *Reason* – can take a code value from 1 to 8. You can find them all in PS3.8, but the most typical reason code you will encounter in your practical experience will unfortunately be 1: "no reason given."

Because the choice of Result, Source, and Reason codes is left to the rejecting application, it really depends on how explicit it wants to be about the rejection cause. In other words, even if you set Reason, Source, and Result codes in the A-Associate-RJ to whatever codes you like, this will not change the outcome because none of these fields is meant for further processing. Simply, the association will be rejected, all association-related processing will stop, and (if we have a good piece of software) some error message will be written into the participating AEs error logs.

9.8.4 A-Abort

The A-Abort message does essentially the same job as the A-Associate-RJ, but at any time during the association processing. It reflects any insurmountable failure that leads to an abnormal association termination. Consequently, the A-Abort message has exactly the same structure as the A-Associate-RJ, except that the first message byte (PDU type) is set now to 07H (A-Abort type) and the Result field becomes unused, permanently set to 00H. This is shown in Fig. 9.14.

Source and Reason codes for A-Abort are different from those for A-Associate-RJ: the provider source code now corresponds to 2 (no reason given)

9.8 Protocol Data Unit (PDU)

A-Abort message structure:

07H (type)	00H	00000004H	00H	00H	Source	Reason
1 byte	1 byte	4 bytes	1 byte	1 byte	1 byte	1 byte

Example:

07H (type)	00H	00000004H	00H	00H	02H	00H
1 byte	1 byte	4 bytes	1 byte	1 byte	1 byte	1 byte

Fig. 9.14 A-Abort message structure, from PS 3.8, and its most typical example

A-Release-RQ message structure:

05H (type)	00H	00000004H	00000000H
1 byte	1 byte	4 bytes	4 bytes

A-Release-RP message structure:

06H (type)	00H	00000004H	00000000H
1 byte	1 byte	4 bytes	4 bytes

Fig. 9.15 A-Release-RQ and A-Release-RP messages

and reason corresponds to 0. Similar to A-Associate-RJ, no real processing is done with these Source and Reason fields. When an AE receives A-Abort from its peer, it will try to terminate the association as soon as possible; which, by the way, could still require a few long moments if the AE was busy processing.

9.8.5 A-Release-RQ, A-Release-RP

These two guys work just like A-Associate-RQ and A-Associate-AC. They are meant to gracefully terminate a successful association – everything that was neither rejected nor aborted. When data transfer is successfully completed, the data-sending AE issues a terminating A-Release-RQ message to its peer, inviting it to release the association. The peer replies with an A-Associate-RQ and the association between the two AEs ends at this point.

A-Release-RQ and A-Release-RP messages are the simplest in the PDU protocol.

As you can see in Fig. 9.15, the only difference between the two message types is in the first byte: hexadecimal 05H corresponds to A-Release-RQ and 06H encodes A-Release-RP. No reasons, sources, or results are communicated.

P-Data-TF message structure:

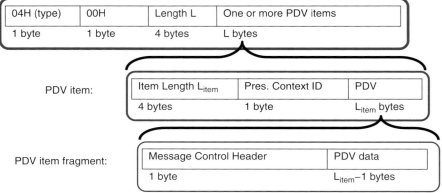

Fig. 9.16 P-Data-TF message, with PDV item

9.8.6 P-Data-TF

P-Data-TF is different from the other PDU types just considered; it is the only type responsible for transmitting the actual data. P-Data-TF sends DICOM objects cut into chunks known as Protocol Data Value (PDV) items[5] (Fig. 9.16).

As usual, P-Data-TF starts with the message type byte – this time it is 04H. It is followed by the 00H *reserved* byte then succeeded by the PDU-length field. The latter contains the length L of the remaining P-Data-TF message – the part of the message containing the actual PDV data block.

The PDV data block also starts with its own length value. Because one P-Data-TF can have multiple PDVs, we need to know the value of each one, which is the same logic applied to encoding DICOM VRs.

The Presentation Context ID byte, following the length, is nothing but the ID of the Presentation Context accepted during the A-Associate-RQ/A-Associate-AC handshake (see Sect. 9.1). This gives us the information on how to process the PDV data; for example, read it with Big or Little-Endian Transfer Syntax.

Each PDV data segment in the PDV item breaks into its Message Control Header and PDV data. Although the Message Control Header has a single byte, it encodes a couple of things:
1. If the first bit in the Message Control Header is set to 1, the following PDV fragment contains a DICOM Command Object (see Sect. 7.2.1). Otherwise, it is a DICOM Data Object.
2. If the second bit in the Message Control Header is set to 1, the following PDV fragment contains the last fragment of the DICOM Object. That is, when we receive this PDV chunk, we receive the last chunk in some DICOM Data/Command Object

---

[5]To meet the maximum PDU data length, as set by maximum length field in User Information item – see 9.7.

9.8 Protocol Data Unit (PDU)

and now we have the whole object to process. Otherwise, if the second bit is set to 0, this is *not* the last fragment and we have more to come.

From these bits and bytes of P-Data-TF you can tell exactly, at any time, what kind of data you are receiving, in what format, and how it needs to be processed. This makes P-Data-TF implementation very important on any DICOM software – the smallest mistake will make everything dysfunctional. If you are doing DICOM development, please read PS3.8 carefully; it will provide you with additional details on P-Data-TF implementation.

Keep in mind that the DICOM standard was developed by several groups of very creative people; the key word here being *several*. So, if in PS3.7 PDV stands for "Protocol Data Value" and in PS3.8 it becomes "Presentation Data Values" don't get your knickers in a twist – you do remember that old adage about "too many cooks" don't you?

9.8.7 How Associations Terminate

Associations start with the DICOM association establishment handshake (A-Associate-RQ). After they do their job (often with P-Data-TF data transfers) they need to be terminated. Moreover, many DICOM vendors license their software with limits on concurrent associations (10, for example), which makes exiting associations very important for remaining under the licensed limit. There are two possible ways to terminate associations:

- *By protocol* – A-Release-RQ for successful completion, and A-Abort to terminate incorrect associations on the spot.
- *By timing out* – Each AE is usually configured to wait a few seconds and, if nothing happens, simply close the association (without sending anything to its peer). This usually takes place after various connectivity problems: when the network goes down, when the peer AE freezes and becomes nonresponsive, when someone simply shuts down the peer AE, and so on. In such situations, the connected AE waits for T timeout seconds, and then picks up the trash by closing the nonresponding connection.

The second timeout mechanism is one of the nice freebies inherited by DICOM from TCP/IP. The timeout value T is usually configurable in the AE properties interface – the same interface you use to set up the AE title, port, and IP address (Fig. 9.17). For unreliable and slow networks, you might want to have a relatively high timeout (up to a minute); this will make your connection insensitive to the shorter interrupts. On the other hand, high timeout values can be inconvenient. Imagine that you are trying to C-Echo a workstation that someone has turned off. With a 1 min timeout you have to wait for a minute for C-Echo to stop expecting any response. In other words, if something does not work, it will take the entire *timeout* time to find out.

9.8.8 Communication Overhead?

It has become commonplace (especially on the part of PACS manufacturers) to blame DICOM for communication overhead. Every single time we exchange information

Fig. 9.17 Example of association timeout settings in commercial DICOM software

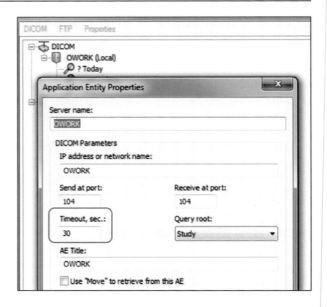

with another DICOM AE, A-Associate messages must be exchanged and an association must be established. In fact, most PACS companies often prefer to use their own proprietary data exchange protocols, at least between their own devices, to escape DICOM association complexities.

Indeed, encoding and decoding DICOM data and messages can introduce processing delays – at least, in theory. Moreover, on a slow network with frequent delays and interrupts, DICOM association establishment can take a second or two. If you have to transmit tons of small images, each one using its own C-Store handshake, these delays accumulate. However, nothing flows fast on a slow network. Let's not forget that the primary function of any DICOM network is image data transfer. Images (taking megabytes in size) are much larger than A-Associate messages (where every single byte counts). Even if you have to establish a new association for every image in a 1000-image study being transferred, 99% of the transfer time will be consumed by the image data. On the other hand, the DICOM association mechanism provides us with a universal and flexible data communication protocol, which is much more important than gaining a fraction of transfer time.

This can be seen in Fig. 9.18, showing network traffic for the same sample study download, performed in different formats and at different times. We used a sample CT study with 516 images (266 MB), downloading it from the same server over the same network as follows:

- D_1, D_2, and D_3 were DICOM downloads (C-Store), performed at different time intervals.
- S_1, S_2, and S_3 were downloads of the same data via shared folder copy, also taken at different time points. That is, the CT study folder on the server was copied to

9.8 Protocol Data Unit (PDU)

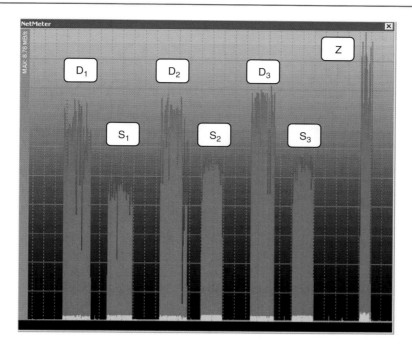

Fig. 9.18 Network traffic for various download types

the client "as is," in file explorer, using native operating system file-copying protocol.
- Z was similar to S, but the entire study (516 files) was written to a single ZIP file first (achieving roughly 50% compression), and the file was copied from the server to the client.

Looking at the widths of the red download regions (download time), you can see that DICOM download took the same time as native shared file transfer – a remarkable illustration of DICOM efficiency. Moreover, the average height of the red download segments indicates that DICOM used network bandwidth more efficiently. The yellow areas at the bottom of each transfer segment correspond to the upload traffic (communication overheads); as you can see, it was a minor fraction of the download volume regardless of the download format. In short, DICOM was not inferior to native file transfer protocol, and did not show higher overheads.

Zipped-file Z transfer, on the contrary, provided a much shorter download time (narrower red download zone, consistent with 50% data compression), which proves the most important point: the volume of data has much stronger impact on the download time, than the choice of data protocol.

In short, I do not believe in the "slow DICOM" theory – it typically sounds more like a cover up for poor DICOM implementations.

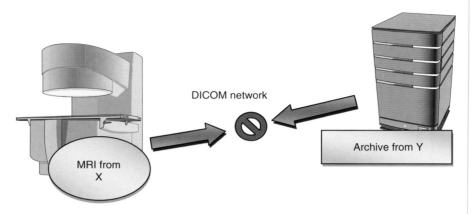

Fig. 9.19 DICOM failures – why?

9.9 What Do I Do When It Fails?

DICOM association failures definitely account for the vast majority of all DICOM networking problems, and I have not seen a single healthcare manager who has not run into some kind of DICOM association establishment problem. It *will* happen, sooner or later. What do you do when your DICOM association just won't work, and A-Abort gives you nothing but a "reason not specified" rejection? Let's take a look at some of the most reasonable DICOM connectivity *best practices*. Maybe they can help cheer you up from your DICOM blues.

First, *troubleshooting DICOM connectivity is the direct responsibility of your DICOM provider (manufacturer)*. They should be the ones to go through all the bits of the rejected association, trying to pinpoint the unknown reason. Your most typical DICOM connectivity problem will look like Fig. 9.19:

- You have one DICOM unit (or software) from manufacturer X,
- You bought another DICOM unit from manufacturer Y,
- You installed, connected, and configured both of them as instructed,
- And nothing worked.

Do not try to solve the problem yourself by talking to your DICOM providers X and Y independently. This will most likely start a long finger-pointing contest, loaded with countless confusing details that cloud the issues and make the real solution difficult to identify. Do not get in the middle. Instead, call both DICOM companies responsible for the noncommunicating units, put them in direct touch with each other (better still, make both of them come onsite on the same day), give them your deadline, and withdraw from the conversation until they produce a working solution. Remember, if either of them tells you that "it is not possible," the problem is definitely their fault. *Standard DICOM ensures that any two devices, which are supposed to talk to each other, will talk to each other.*

Second, *ensure that your DICOM software or device can generate a clear DICOM connection status and detailed error log in a format comprehensible by an average human being.* Ideally, you would take this precaution *before* you buy your software or device. Ask the salesperson to show how you can view this information. More likely, he won't know or care, so ask him to come back only when he finds out. If anything goes wrong with the association establishment a clear, understandable, and well-recorded error message is critical for any troubleshooting effort. You cannot troubleshoot a black box, and confusing error/transaction logs can make this work even more difficult. Logs saying nothing more than "invalid message received" without explaining exactly *why, where, and what* was invalid are useless.

> **Sprechen You English?**
> Here is a good example of what *should not* happen, but what *does* happen all the time. Once I worked on troubleshooting DICOM connectivity for a DICOM unit from a well-respected international manufacturer. The program interface contained no *view log* option. The log was hidden deep on a hard drive where it was broken into several files; and to complete the picture, half of it was in German and half in English. Making use of it was an adventure in itself and looked much more like reading the Rosetta Stone rather than DICOM. Make sure it won't happen to you.

The same issue applies to the connection status display. When your DICOM application sends or receives data on the network, it should provide a clear progress display for each transaction. It could be a graphical progress interface, or it could be a simple counter such as "Sending 85%... 95%... Completed successfully," but it should be there. Watching this progress is essential for identifying problems in real time, and not after every single radiologist in your department has complained about them. I have been in many situations where it took several hours – sometimes several *days* – just to realize that we *had* a problem because nothing in the interface was alerting the users. *Error-oblivious interfaces are something you cannot afford!*

> **Piling Studies**
> Many facilities configure their scanners (CT, MR, and so on) to send studies to their DICOM servers automatically. Many technologists working on those scanners become used to the automated workflow and do not check the status of sent studies. And many scanner manufacturers do not really display much of this status.
> What happens then if the DICOM server goes down? If nothing in the scanner interface warns the users, the error might not be noticed immediately, and it might not even be noticed for a long time. Quite often, the unsent studies will pile up on the scanners, and when the pile is finally discovered, its sheer size can easily reach the scale of a major problem.

Third, *understand what you are trying to achieve*. Let's re-visit the same example in which you have physically connected DICOM units X and Y, and you want to verify from X whether it can establish DICOM association with Y. Quite often, you will find a *Verify* button in X's interface, which is supposed to answer this question. You click this button and nothing happens. Failure?

Yes, but it may very well be an expected failure – a failure by design – as I explained earlier when talking about the Verification SCP. If unit Y does not support the DICOM Verification SCP, it won't be able to reply to verification requests from X. In DICOM parlance this means that the Verification Service-Object Pair (SOP) association establishment is not possible. However, this *does not mean* that other DICOM services will fail as well. For example, you could be perfectly able to send (store) images from X to Y, or to search for studies on X from Y. To verify the functionality, simply rely on our best friend; check the DICOM Conformance Statements for the units in question and match their SOPs to the functions they are supposed to provide.

Sure, DICOM was not meant to be learned in 24 h, but understanding even the simplest basics really pays off. Be patient and learn. At the very least, dealing with DICOM association establishment will be a good resource for both learning the issues and developing patience.

9.10 Point-to-Point Spell

I have already mentioned on several occasions that the DICOM standard once contained the PS3.9 part, "Point-To-Point Communication Support for Message Exchange". Remember, DICOM was first developed in the mid-1980s – a long time before TCP/IP networking broke onto the scene. Thirty years ago, one would have to use special pin cables to connect two computers together – this is what PS3.9 was all about.

The times have changed. PS3.9 was retired, pin-based connections were replaced by standard networking hardware and protocols, and the DICOM standard was updated to work over the same TCP/IP networks as your email or web browser – you do not need *another* network protocol or special hardware to put a PACS together. The galloping advances of wireless technologies can make network cables tomorrow's rarity. However, the very concept of point-to-point "pinned" connectivity was inherited in the most current DICOM editions. Nowadays, it means that any two Application Entities (AEs) on a DICOM network can be connected only directly and statically. That is, if AE_1 needs to connect to AE_2, both AE_1 and AE_2 have to know each other's network address and they must send messages to each other directly.

Consequently, when you connect any two DICOM units, you will always be required to do the same simple setup over and over again:
1. Typing the IP address, port, and DICOM title of AE_2 into the AE_1 configuration, and
2. Typing the IP address, port, and DICOM title of AE_1 into the AE_2 configuration.

As we all realize, this is not really different from the point-to-point concept of the venerable old 8-pin cables. The implication is immediate: should one of the units

9.10 Point-to-Point Spell

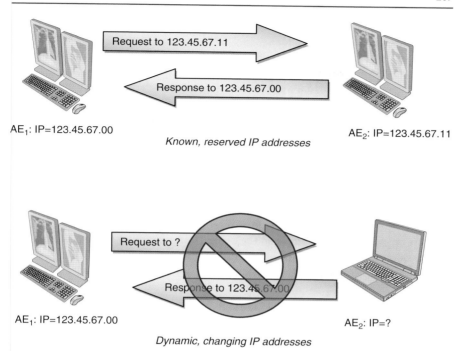

Fig. 9.20 DICOM point-to-point connectivity

change its network address or DICOM title, the DICOM network will break. The old hardware point-to-point has essentially become a new, virtual point-to-point requirement, severely limiting the application of standard DICOM networks.

The classic example of this limitation is shown in Fig. 9.20. If, for example, all your AEs reside on a local area network and have reserved (or static) IP addresses, you have a classic PACS layout where everything works nicely and is effectively point-to-point. However, if you decide to do teleradiology and check your PACS images from home – or from a cozy internet café, or from a conference hall – the communication will fail. The reason is clear: your home (internet café, conference hall, and so on) computer resides on a totally different network, and consequently will have a totally new IP address that is not recognized by your PACS. In fact, you do not even have to go far from your office to get into trouble. Just bring your laptop to work and plug it into your local network. Even if your laptop runs the PACS software, more likely than not you won't be able to load images on it because its IP address and AE title will be unknown to your PACS: for example, A-Associate-AC from your laptop will be rejected by PACS because of the unknown calling AE title. This leads to a sad paradox: you can be on a PACS network, but you won't be able to use PACS.

Real Case: Point-to-Point Failure

Point-to-point connections can often be blamed for DICOM network vulnerability. Soon after hurricane Katrina struck the U.S. Gulf Coast, one of my customers called me from there with a *really bad problem*. She was running an imaging center; they restored the power; they restarted all their PACS devices; but they just could not connect to their PACS server. Moreover, the server was used as a teleradiology backbone and they had to pay big money for couriers because they could not access the digital images on the server remotely. Losing time, money, and patience they seriously suspected that something had failed in the PACS server software we had provided.

The problem, however, was solved very fast with the help of the local network support engineer who visited their site. It was discovered that the local network router, after the hurricane power loss, reset itself to its factory defaults, essentially changing the IP address and network configuration of the PACS server. This address change made the server inaccessible and the entire PACS network dysfunctional – although it was still perfectly sound as a TCP/IP network. As soon as the IPs were restored, the entire PACS returned to normal.

Another direct consequence of the limited point-to-point design is a total lack of data forwarding in DICOM. Any data-receiving device always becomes the end point of the communication – it cannot be instructed, at least in DICOM terms, to relay the received data elsewhere. However, in a real medical workflow, forwarding is extremely important. For example, you might want to push a study to your PACS archive so that the archive would store the image and automatically forward a copy to a radiologist for review. Most current PACS/DICOM software vendors understand the demand and implement some sort of data forwarding on their devices – but only in their proprietary, non-DICOM ways.

As you can see from these examples, dealing with point-to-point limitations becomes a large and inevitable part of your PACS management. There are a few more considerations related to the point-to-point problem:

1. Certain DICOM manufacturers consider the point-to-point paradigm to be the quintessential security feature. It limits DICOM connection to known devices, thus naturally filtering out the *outsiders*. This may be true, but viewing security as limited functionality is wrong. The choice should be given to the PACS administrators and users. With the current multiplicity of other more efficient security solutions, the entire point-to-point approach looks quite ... Jurassic. It also impedes the growing number of the projects that cannot be done within point-to-point networks.
2. Some DICOM companies offer DICOM gateway software providing different, private extensions to the DICOM protocol, which remove the point-to-point restriction. If it does not affect their standard DICOM functionality, this is always a plus. When looking for PACS software, ask your PACS company whether they can provide this feature.

3. You could look into numerous teleradiology products, especially if you need to be *tele* (see Chap. 13). Teleradiology, as its name implies, mainly deals with remote access to medical images. In this case, the point-to-point technique is completely abandoned – it simply won't work. Bear in mind, however, that teleradiology often favors non-DICOM protocols to transfer DICOM data: for example, converting DICOM images to multimedia formats and sending them over the World Wide Web.
4. Some standard DICOM services also work beyond point-to-point networks, while others do not. For example, the Verification request does not really require the IP address of the receiver AE to be fixed, as long as it is known. Moving images on DICOM networks is implemented with two DICOM protocols: C-Get and C-Move. The first can work with changing IP addresses, at least theoretically (the practical outcome depends on the particular implementation of this protocol). C-Move, on the other hand, needs point-to-point. Unfortunately, for the *security* reasons mentioned, C-Move is also the most implemented image transfer protocol – only a few DICOM manufacturers support C-Get.

   I am giving you these examples to dispel false expectations that can sometimes arise when you plug your laptop into your PACS network, send a Verification request to the PACS server, and it works. This does not mean that your PACS is inherently better than others and somehow overcomes the point-to-point limitations. It simply means that the Verification service was not affected by them. Try to pull the study list and load some images from the PACS server; with a very high probability, you'll start seeing problems.
5. Make sure your security (firewalls in particular) does not block your point-to-point connections.

To conclude: know the limits of your DICOM point-to-point model, and do not expect DICOM devices to miraculously recover after failures or changes in your network. If you need more solid and dynamic connectivity, discuss it with your PACS vendor ahead of time to find a proper balance between limited DICOM-compliance and flexible proprietary solutions that they could offer.

> **Tip to the DICOM Committee**
> Please check the current DICOM standard. It still contains references to the retired PS3.9 and point-to-point connection architecture.

9.11 Networking: Standard and Beyond

As we conclude our review of DICOM networking, it is worth glancing at its practical implementations and possible deviations from the DICOM standard. DICOM vendors adore playing with the DICOM standard, and thanks to their creative thinking, they are always full of surprises.

Many DICOM modifications start at the DIMSE level as vendors try to *improve* DICOM services. For example, some DICOM programs will do C-Echo before they send any other command (C-Find, C-Move, C-Store, and so on). The rationale: use C-Echo to check DICOM connectivity before asking for data, or even to measure the current network speed. If you have read the previous sections carefully, you should realize that this check is totally useless. An A-Associate-RQ message will do the connectivity verification anyway, inside of each DICOM DIMSE command. Measuring network speed by using an extra C-Echo also sounds a bit strange, to say the least. With 68 bytes, which we counted in C-Echo in Sect. 7.2.2, you will never assess the network speed correctly because you need a much larger data sample. Besides, network speeds tend to fluctuate; even if your system measured something before sending an image, the speed could change by the time you start sending the data. With all this, there is hardly any need to add another C-Echo for an extra handshake. After all, would you shake hands twice with someone you just met to make sure the person is real?

I have seen cases in which the same approach was used with *dual* A-Associate-RQ requests – issued for C-Find or C-Store. The first A-Associate-RQ was simply meant to *verify* that everything was okay and the second was meant for the *real* processing. This gets even worse: instead of dealing with a *handshaking disorder*, we are now getting into *hearing problems* because we are asking for everything twice. The peer AE receiving these duplicate requests has no knowledge of our true intentions and will honestly try to process both. Consequently, our requests will either get lost (in case there is a limit on concurrent associations on the remote AE), or double-processed. Note that there is nothing DICOM-illegal in this behavior; but if your software does it, it invites serious problems and creates noticeable overhead.

The number of concurrent DICOM associations accepted by any AE is often also controlled by DICOM/PACS vendors. That is, the AE is programmed not to process more than a limited number of transactions at any given time. This has nothing to do with DICOM and is done mainly for software licensing purposes – the more concurrent associations supported, the more vendors charge. If you work in a complex environment with many interacting devices and you are faced with this licensing limit, I would recommend that you get at least 10 concurrent associations supported – if you can afford more, buy more. Dear DICOM vendors: Instead of charging for concurrent connections (with all the bookkeeping pain it entails, without adding *anything real* to the system), maybe you should charge for truly advanced functions?

Concurrent Users
Many vendors also set a limit for *concurrent users* who can work on their systems. This is particularly common for server architectures in which the same server (for image rendering or voice recognition) can be used simultaneously by multiple users.
The main issue here is how well your vendor controls the user concurrency. For example, ten users might be currently logged in, but only four are working

9.11 Networking: Standard and Beyond 211

> and the other six simply forgot to log off, or went to lunch, or switched to something else. In well-designed software, only the four currently active users should be counted as concurrent; that is, using the system at a given time. In real life unfortunately, most vendors would count all ten users as concurrent, even though no resources are allocated to six of them.
>
> Always ask your prospective vendors to define their interpretation of *concurrent*, whether for users or for associations – sometimes this might differ from what it should really be.

One of the best examples of both DICOM-compliant and proprietary tweaks would be the C-Store protocol (reviewed in Sect. 7.3). While other SOPs deal mostly with connectivity and searches, C-Store transmits the image data. Naturally, large volumes of digital images call for very efficient transmission techniques, and C-Store has become the most frequent target for enhancements.

Within the realm of DICOM, the major improvement to C-Store was the use of data compression. It was achieved with image compression Transfer Syntaxes, as we have already discussed in Sect. 6.2. Image compression does not change the overall structure of the DICOM data object containing the image. Instead, it simply compresses the contents of the "Pixel Data" buffer in (7FE0,0010), which holds image pixels. Because image pixels account for the bulk of the data transmission, and can usually be compressed even losslessly up to 3–4 times, C-Store with compressed images can significantly improve data transmission on a slow network. Therefore, various image compression techniques – public and proprietary – continuously contribute to improving DICOM network and storage efficiency (Fig. 9.21).

The next and less common extension to this is compressing the entire DICOM object, regardless of what it contains (images, large reports, and so on). This capability was added to DICOM as the "Deflated Explicit VR Little Endian" Transfer Syntax (1.2.840.10008.1.2.1.99). In simple terms, this corresponds to the well-known ZIP compression: DICOM can zip entire data objects, send them over the network, and unzip them on the receiver side.

Unfortunately, this DICOM-legal approach creates a major DICOM problem: *a zipped DICOM object is not a DICOM object anymore*, just like a zipped Word document is not a Word document. ZIP compression repacks object bytes into a ZIP-compatible representation. You cannot access the object's DICOM properties, and you cannot read and display it unless you unzip it first, in its entirety. In a way, this dilutes a nice VR-based structure of DICOM data and nearly contradicts the standard DICOM networking protocol. Possible gains from reduced data size are overshadowed by extra processing required to rebuild the DICOM object structure after it is unzipped. Practically speaking, this format is rarely supported in DICOM software.

Beyond DICOM, there is a wealth of proprietary data transmission protocols implemented by various PACS manufacturers to transmit data between their devices. Essentially, all of them either employ proprietary image compression algorithms

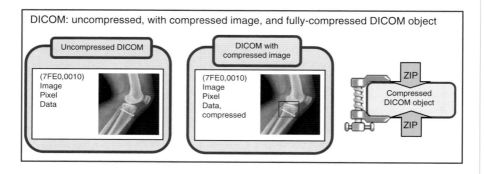

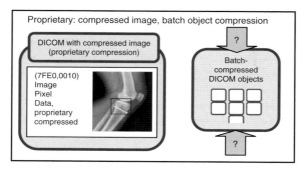

Fig. 9.21 Different compression methods (standard and proprietary) to reduce data size

(Transfer Syntaxes), or take data repackaging techniques to their ultimate extreme (Fig. 9.21, bottom part). For example, when a CT study with 1000 images needs to be transmitted, certain PACS will compress the images first, concatenate them into a huge single file, and transmit that file over the network in a single shot. This is meant to eliminate DICOM communications between separate images, and to ensure that the entire *package* arrives at its destination (Fig. 9.22). Another reason for proprietary batching lies in DICOM's inability to recover from interrupted transmissions. In standard DICOM, when C-Store is used to load a 1000-image CT study and the network connection breaks on image 1000, DICOM offers no means to identify and reload just the last, interrupted image – the entire 1000-image C-Store needs to be started again. This becomes extremely frustrating in many teleradiology projects when networks are often slow and occasionally go down.

The only way to make current DICOM transactions interruption-proof would be breaking each transaction into its smallest parts so that each one can be handled independently and recovered if needed. In our 1000-image study case, imagine breaking CGet requests for the whole study into 1000 CGet requests for each study image. In this case, if any image-level CGet fails, we can execute it again to retrieve only the failed image without affecting the rest. All you need to do is to use additional CFind requests to retrieve 1000 image SOP instances – first, using CFind to

9.11 Networking: Standard and Beyond

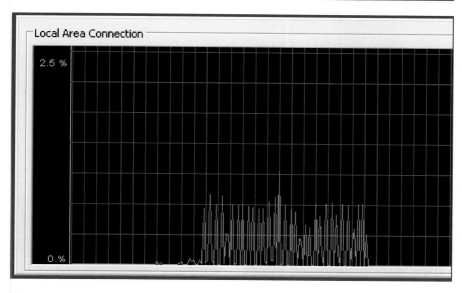

Fig. 9.22 Monitoring C-Store DICOM data download (a compressed study with 32 images) on a slow network. The peaks on this jigsaw pattern correspond to loading the images, and the gaps between them to C-Store association negotiations and to compressing each next image with lossy compression. Ideally, you would like the network to work at its highest rate; but with additional communications and processing, this may not be possible. In this case, concatenating all images might have worked faster

locate all study series and then using CFind to get a list of all images in the series. Then, you are ready to issue 1000 CGets (or CMoves) to load all the images (Fig. 9.23).

However, this DICOM-compliant robustness comes at a price to performance. Image-level retrievals (Fig. 9.23, left) requiring a CFind and association establishment handshake for each single-image download results in substantial overhead, dragging down the overall system performance.

Classic single-study DICOM CGet adds the risk of unrecoverable interruption, but it does the job much faster. This is why many vendors batch files or rely on other popular data transfer protocols, such as FTP, that are capable of autorecovering from interrupted transactions. But proprietary protocols work only between devices from the same vendor; they lead to self-isolation. And image batching, which may look like a great idea at first, has its own problems.

When images are transferred one by one (the DICOM way), the receiving application can take advantage of the transmission time: it can parse, load, and display the received images while still fetching the rest. In other words, DICOM's image-by-image transfer helps do several things concurrently, which ultimately speeds up the entire communication process. In comparison, when all the images are sent in a huge concatenated batch (the way many proprietary protocols do), the receiving

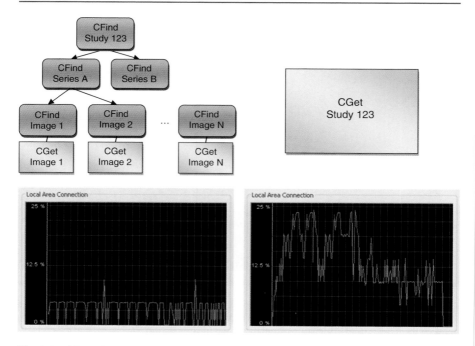

Fig. 9.23 Network performance for retrieving DICOM study image by image (*left*), and with single study CGet (*right*). While image-based CGet (*left*) took 20 min for a large sample case, study-based CGet was only 5 min

workstation has to sit idle until the entire batch is downloaded. The result: with smart multitasking, DICOM transfers can work considerably faster.

At the end of the day, nothing is ideal; but fixing DICOM networking issues still makes more sense than inviting problems by using obscure proprietary transmissions. I have already mentioned the lack of self-recovery and the point-to-point archaism that significantly limit the reach of DICOM connections. It's sad that DICOM – providing a complex association-establishing mechanism – does absolutely nothing to make these associations sturdy and self-healing. With some careful consideration, future revisions of DICOM will augment the functionality of existing DICOM networking with improved flexibility, error-recovery, and security.

Part IV
DICOM Media and Security

DICOM Media: Files, Folders, and DICOMDIRs

10

A substantial part of this book has been dedicated to DICOM networking, and transmitting data and messages between DICOM AEs over a TCP/IP connection. This is indeed the most common and efficient way to run any medical imaging project. Computer networks provide unsurpassed flexibility, reach, and throughput allowing you to collaborate with any partner, in any place, at any time.

Nevertheless, and quite frequently, we still need to export DICOM data from self-contained clinical networks into some media – be it a flash drive, CD/DVD, MOD, or another hard drive. We are not talking about the industrial-level PACS archive storage: PACS vendors do it in their own ways (which we will review a bit later in Sect. 10.5). DICOM Media Storage uses removable media to occasionally export DICOM data *from* PACS for external storage, viewing, and transfer into another DICOM application.

The classic example is using DICOM CDs (now more commonly replaced by DVDs due to ever-increasing data size). A patient can have his CT scan done in some imaging center. The center might not have a PACS and almost certainly does not have a PACS integrated into the hospital system that referred the patient. So the imaging center provides the patient with a CD containing his DICOM CT images, and the patient can take the disk to any other destination where he is being treated or accepted for health care.

This is more than a typical scenario; and, as you can see after reading Chap. 7, the patient essentially plays the role of the DICOM network (C-Store DIMSE), and the CD in his pocket plays the role of the attached DICOM Data Object.

DICOM email is another popular substitute for missing PACS networks. The original DICOM files can be attached to email messages and sent to another person (a referring physician, for example). Now, the email program acts as a DICOM network "C-Store" and the email attachment transmits DICOM data (which – behind the scenes – is encoded into email-compatible MIME[1] format).

---

[1]Multipurpose Internet Mail Extensions (MIME) is an internet standard that extends the format of email to support nontext attachments – DICOM binary objects (files) in this case.

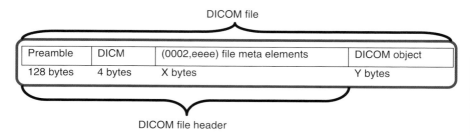

Fig. 10.1 DICOM file structure

As I have mentioned, none of these methods can even remotely compete with the power and throughput of DICOM networking in PACS, but for much smaller and infrequent projects, they quite capably play a vital role. Parts PS3.10, PS3.11, and PS3.12 of the DICOM standard deal with all the specifications of DICOM files and media, and I will review some of them in this chapter.

10.1 DICOM File Format

If we are talking about DICOM media, we are talking about DICOM files. DICOM files store DICOM data objects (also referred to as *Data Sets*) – most frequently, DICOM images. The data objects are written into the DICOM files with the exact same encoding rules as we used in DICOM networking: implicit or explicit VR encoding (see Sect. 5.5). The only difference is in the DICOM file header, which precedes the data object, as shown in Fig. 10.1.

The DICOM header plays the role of the missing DICOM Association Establishment: it explains to any file-reading application that the file stores DICOM data of a certain SOP type, and in certain Transfer Syntax format. The DICOM header includes a preamble, a DICM prefix, and a pinch of DICOM file attributes (file meta elements).

10.1.1 Preamble and DICM Prefix

The preamble is a string of 128 bytes, which opens any DICOM file. The use of a preamble is common in many imaging and data formats (consider TIFF images, for example), and DICOM adapted the same style. However, the DICOM standard does not define any particular preamble structure or content. It is up to each DICOM application to use the 128 preamble bytes to its advantage. Obviously, this makes preamble content application-dependent – different applications can use it differently. For that reason, the preamble in DICOM is generally ignored and filled with 0 bytes – in DICOM this simply means "unused preamble."

DICM prefix (indicating the DICOM file format) follows the 128-byte preamble verbatim – it simply consists of the four uppercase letters (D I C M) written into bytes 129–132. The use of a format prefix (often called the *magic number*) is also very common in many file formats (imaging included) and DICOM follows the same convention.

10.2 Special DICOM File Formats

File Indexing

File indexing – creating a special file that contains the information about the other files in a particular folder – is a very common task in many software applications. Operating systems, email, and multimedia software all try to index the files on your computer. File indexing speeds up the access to the file data, and improves searching the files with user-specified search keys (such as keywords). In particular, if file search key values are stored in the index file, only the index file needs to be searched.

The flip side is that creating and maintaining the index file takes processing power and the index file needs to be updated every time something changes in the indexed folder.

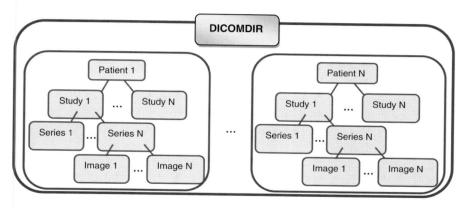

Fig. 10.3 DICOMDIR structure. Each image corresponds to a DICOM file in DICOMDIR directory

Consequently, just like any DICOM database (see more in Sect. 10.5), DICOMDIR organizes all directory data into four principal DICOM levels: Patient, Study, Series, and Image as shown in Fig. 10.3. Therefore, for each file in the DICOMDIR folder, DICOMDIR will record four entries – patient, study, series, and image information – corresponding to this file.

Table 10.2 (adapted from DICOM PS3.10) gives an example of the DICOMDIR file with sample data. It might appear lengthy, but look closer and you will see that the list of all DICOMDIR items (patients, studies, series, and images) is simply inserted into the DICOMDIR object as an SQ sequence element (0004,1220).

Table 10.2 DICOMDIR example

Entry type	Attribute tag	Attribute description	Value (example)
File Meta Information (must be present in any DICOM file)	128 bytes	DICOM File Preamble	All 128 bytes set to 0
	4 bytes	DICOM prefix	DICM (*required*)
	(0002,0000)	Group length	
	(00002,0001)	File Meta Information Version	0001 (*required*)
	(0002,0002)	Media Storage SOP Class UID	1.2.840.10008.1.3.10
	(0002,0003)	Media Storage SOP Instance UID	1.2.840.12345.6435.4
	(0002,0010)	Transfer Syntax UID	1.2.840.10008.1.1 (*required*)
	(0002,0012)	Implementation Class UID	1.2.840.4578.34.2345
	...	...	...
File Set ID	(0004,1130)	File Set ID	MYDICOMDIR01
	...	...	...
General Directory Information	(0004,1200)	Offset of the first record of root directory entity	1829
	(0004,1202)	Offset of the first record of root directory entity	6F18
	(0004,1212)	File Set consistency flag	0000
	...	...	...
Start of DICOMDIR record list	(0004,1220)	Directory record sequence. This SQ element contains the actual sequence of DICOMDIR elements, as follows	

10.2 Special DICOM File Formats

First DICOMDIR record (starts at byte 1829)	SQ item tag	(FFFE, E000)	SQ item data element (see Sect. 5.5.5) – start of the first DICOMDIR entry	
	Study 1	(0004,1400)	Offset of the next directory record	
		(0004,1410)	Record in use flag (set to FFFF for present files, and to 0000 for deleted files)	FFFF
		(0004,1420)	Offset of referenced lower level directory entity	2299
		...		...
		(0004,1430)	Directory record type	STUDY
		(0020,000D)	Study instance UID	1.2.840.1234.0125.5
	Study 1 selection keys	(0020,0010)	Study ID	MyStudyID01
	SQ item tag	(FFFE, E00D)	Item delimitation tag – end of the first DICOMDIR entry	
Second DICOMDIR record (starts at byte 2299)	SQ item tag	(FFFE, E000)	SQ item data element – start of the following DICOMDIR entry	
	Series 1	(0004,1400)	Offset of the next directory record	
		(0004,1410)	Record in use flag	FFFF
		(0004,1420)	Offset of referenced lower level directory entity	2681
		...		...
		(0004,1430)	Directory record type	SERIES
	Series 1 selection keys	(0008,0060)	Modality	NM
		(0020,0011)	Series number	2
	SQ item tag	(FFFE, E00D)	Item delimitation tag – end of the current DICOMDIR entry	

(continued)

Table 10.2 (continued)

Entry type		Attribute tag	Value (example)	Value (example)
Third DICOMDIR record (starts at byte 2681)	SQ item tag	(FFFE, E000)	SQ item data element – start of the following DICOMDIR entry	
	Image 1	(0004,1400)	Offset of the next directory record	3414
		(0004,1410)	Record in use flag	FFFF
		(0004,1420)	Offset of referenced lower level directory entity	00000000
		...	...	...
		(0004,1430)	Directory record type	IMAGE
		(0004,1500)	Referenced File ID	DIR\SUBDIR\ABC123
		(0004,1410)	Referenced SOP Class UID in file	1.2.840.10008.5.1.4.1.1.5
		(0004,1511)	Referenced SOP Instance UID in file	1.2.840.943.2345.54.778
		(0004,1512)	Referenced Transfer Syntax UID in file	1.2.840.10008.1.2.1
	Image 1 selection keys	(0008,0018)	Image SOP Instance UID	1.2.840.943.2345.54.778
		(0020,0013)	Image number	1
	SQ item tag	(FFFE, E00D)	Item delimitation tag – end of the current DICOMDIR entry	

10.3 DICOM File Services

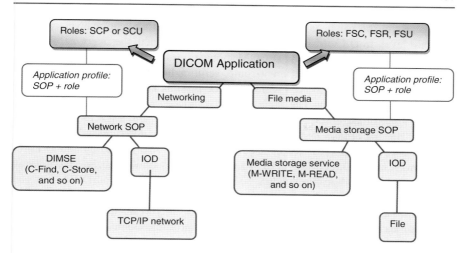

Fig. 10.4 DICOM media storage vs. DICOM networking – the big picture

its new version – even if the difference between the two was in a single character. The delete-write combination is conceptually simple, and it always works. Some file media will not let you modify the file content, so you really need to overwrite the file completely even for a minute change. This means that FSU often equals FSC + FSR, provided it can do M-DELETE to remove the old file version.

It is worthwhile to compare DICOM media storage services to DICOM networking because they follow the same framework. To begin the comparison, let's take a look at Fig. 10.4.

Both in networking and file management scenarios, DICOM applications communicate if they have matching *Application Profiles*:

- Application Entities on a DICOM network are communicating based on the supported SOP classes (such as Verification or Storage, which we studied in chap. 7). If two AEs support identical SOPs and their SCU-SCP roles match, then their profiles match and the AEs can talk to each other. For example, if two AEs could support Verification SOPs with one acting as the Verification SCU and the other as the Verification SCP, then their profiles match and the AEs can talk (see Sect. 7.11). In networking, application profiles are negotiated during the association establishment process: roles, SOPs, Transfer Syntaxes, and other options are compared by the communicating AEs, and the best match is selected when possible.
- File-processing Application Entities connect to each other in a similar manner. This means that the AEs should support the same type of Media Storage SOPs, and they should have matching roles; for example, one acting as FSC (creating files) and another acting as FSR (reading files). However, unlike networking, file-processing AEs cannot negotiate; the entire process of association establishment is lacking, at least in the current DICOM 3.0. Therefore, additional care must be taken to ensure that two Media Storage AEs can understand each other; if one is writing MR images, the other should not be expecting CTs.

Potentially, this can be done in one of two ways: on the application level, or on the standard level. In DICOM networking, as I have mentioned, the major application-profile matching work is done by DICOM applications. With file storage, the DICOM standard decided to take a different route, scrutinizing application profiles to the highest detail possible. So AEs with the same profiles *will have to match* without relying on any negotiation. This approach also produced a number of Media Storage Application Profiles, described in PS3.11. Let's have a look at a few examples.

The "Basic Cardiac X-ray Angiographic" profile handles only X-ray angiographic images up to 512×512 in size; another "1024 X-ray Angiographic CD-R" profile works with larger 1024×1024 images on CDs only; and the "1024 X-ray Angiographic DVD" profile handles 1024×1024 angio images on DVDs. As you can see, this is a very fine-grained approach compared to DICOM networking. To ensure application compatibility, every detail should be taken into account. Applications supporting certain Media Storage profiles should have them listed. Where? You got it: in their DICOM Conformance Statements.

This comparison with DICOM networking is a good place to conclude our review of standard DICOM Media Storage. If you are still interested in specific details, you can find them in parts 10, 11, and 12 of the DICOM standard. As I have mentioned, practical implementations of DICOM media exchange are still very diverse and often nonconformant, but this is the reality that cannot be ignored. Partially, in my opinion, this can be blamed on DICOM itself. The standard *can* be improved to become more media-forgiving and more efficient; and this is the subject of the next section.

10.4 Grains of Salt

Both DICOM networking and DICOM media serve the same purpose – accessing and manipulating DICOM data – but they have to play on very different stages.

DICOM networking is built on top of the standard TCP/IP networking protocol. When any two computers connect over a TCP/IP network, the human factor is almost totally excluded – no one messes with TCP/IP packets trying to modify or reorder them.

File media is just the opposite. We humans *like* manipulating files; and when we do so, we couldn't care less about what some silly old standard might require. What would be considered as audacious hacking in TCP/IP terms is commonplace and routine with file media. A good media-processing standard should take all this into account – DICOM does not.

10.4.1 DICOMDIR

I would consider myself an ardent opponent of DICOMDIRs. I do understand the rationale behind them, but I find them totally impractical, and for a few good reasons:

10.4 Grains of Salt

1. *DICOMDIRs are practically useless.* Any well-designed DICOM program should scan all the files in the given folder, identifying those in DICOM format and taking the required action. Certainly, for large folders DICOMDIR would save time, but just *how large* might these *large folders* be? Even a DVD filled with DICOM data can be scanned fairly quickly, and DICOMDIRs are not used for more industrial, PACS-level storage anyway (where they are replaced by databases). Most multimedia applications facing a similar task of identifying supported files on their respective media resolve the issue using the same scanning approach; this is how you play your videos and music, for example. And this approach produces the most complete and updated account of what *exactly is* stored on specific media instead of relying on some possibly wrong or outdated directory file.

   There are two major uses for DICOM media (files): they are either imported into a PACS, or they are viewed. In either case, all DICOM files from the media will be loaded and processed completely. In either case, DICOMDIR is not needed and adds negligible efficiency to the process.

   > **Developers' Tip: Indexing DICOM Files**
   > Indexing DICOM files in a folder can really be done *on the fly*, provided your application is smart enough to minimize file scanning overhead. For example, all essential DICOM information traditionally needed to index DICOM files (Patient name and ID, Study date and time, and so on) can be found in the first DICOM data groups (0008–0020), which usually take only the first kilobytes of a DICOM file.
   > To extract this data, your DICOM software *does not* need to read the entire file, and it certainly *does not* need to decode the image pixels – the most time-consuming task in DICOM file processing. Preloading data from the first DICOM data groups becomes a much faster task: hardly more complex than reading the DICOMDIR.

2. *DICOMDIRs are treacherous.* When we export DICOM data into DICOM files on removable media we open Pandora's Box. The media owner can copy these files somewhere else (for example, from a flash drive to another computer), rename some of them (for example, renaming the 8-character ABCD1234 DICOM-compliant folder, automatically generated by the software, into longer but more readable "MyInterestingMRCase"), delete some of them, and do whatever else is routinely done with the files. Well, any of these actions will invalidate the contents of the DICOMDIR file, but it still can be copied with the other batch and will eventually be delivered to another DICOM application for data import. If this application relies on DICOMDIR to import the files, it will produce anything but the correct outcome.

   From this point of view, DICOMDIRs remind me of the infamous DICOM point-to-point architecture – meaningful in the early PACS days, but obsolete now. DICOMDIR is based on the assumption that exported files will go straight into another file-importing application. This assumption is almost always wrong.

3. *DICOMDIRs are difficult.* DICOMDIR needs to be updated every time any DICOM file in the folder is updated or changed. This is not even always possible. If the media is update-protected, or you can write to it only once (CD-R, for example), then DICOMDIR should always be the last file recorded to provide the most accurate account.

To summarize, maintaining and updating DICOMDIR files introduces substantial overhead, rarely brings additional advantages, and has become something of a nuisance. For example, you can even find software dedicated to fixing invalid DICOMDIR files in case their file entries were deleted or renamed.

Of course, my vehement opposition to DICOMDIR does not mean anything for the DICOM standard, which requires DICOMDIR files to be present on any media containing DICOM data. Nevertheless, my observations on DICOMDIR come from practical experience with them. You can only improve your workflow if your DICOM software can import DICOM files based on their actual count and content, and not on the DICOMDIR data.

> **DICOM Committee Tip: Flexible Is Better**
> One practical way to avoid DICOMDIRs would be to add a new *M-INQUIRE-DICOM* FILE service. If present, the M-INQUIRE FILE can query only the file date and time, and an extended M-INQUIRE-DICOM FILE would be able to support a few DICOM search keys traditionally listed in DICOMDIRs (patient name, study date, and so on).
> As we have just observed, this would be easy to implement with a partial reading of DICOM data groups by looking for a few first-key elements instead of reading the files completely. In fact, a few years ago, I had to implement a *DICOM over FTP* protocol using the exact same idea of searching for DICOM data on any FTP-connected media, which enabled us to do DICOM searches on virtually anything – cross-platform and cross-space. Making DICOMDIRs virtual, and building them on demand at the application layer will substantially enhance the flexibility of DICOM software, and facilitate support for various types of local and remote media.
> Moreover, this approach could be taken even further if we extend DIMSE services (C-Find, C-Store, C-Move, and so on) to DICOM files. In essence, our hypothetical M-INQUIRE-DICOM FILE already implements C-Find, and the others would easily follow. This would lead to a very unified and consistent way of dealing with DICOM data, whether it is networked or read from DICOM files.

10.4.2 Media Storage

In many ways, the DICOM media storage model (and PS3.12 of the DICOM standard in particular) attempts to do what DICOM shouldn't be doing at all: giving

10.5 Storing DICOM Data in PACS

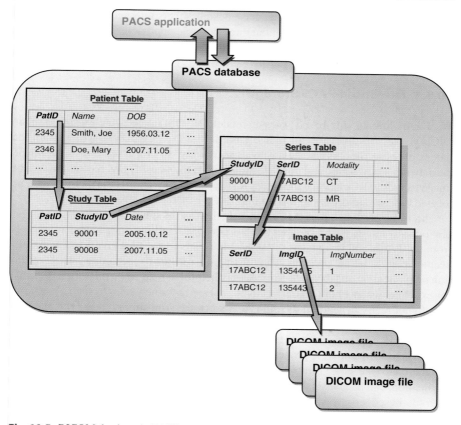

Fig. 10.5 DICOM database in PACS

Series will have Images in the *Image table*).[4] Figure 10.5 illustrates this basic PACS database layout.

Tables in this relational database will be related by certain common fields, such as PatID,[5] which uniquely identifies patients in the Patient table and, at the same time, identifies studies for these patients in the Study table. The breakdown into tables makes the entire database extremely efficient and well-organized. Instead of searching DICOM files or DICOMDIRs, the database can quickly locate the data in presorted tables, often limiting data searches to only a few affected tables to improve efficiency.

---

[4]Other tables in PACS databases will usually include the table of PACS users, Audit table (keeping track of who and how accessed the images), AE table (storing connected AE properties), and so on.

[5]In fact, PACS manufacturers rarely rely on the IDs extracted from DICOM data and implement their own identifiers (as table primary keys), to guarantee uniform format and uniqueness.

Consequently, this optimized database design affects internal DICOM data storage. PACS will usually take one of the three possible approaches to storing DICOM image data, and each of them deserves a little subsection.

10.5.1 File-Based PACS Storage

With a traditional, file-based storage model DICOM images are stored as plain DICOM files. In this case, an Image table in the PACS database will contain the names of those files. When PACS needs to retrieve an image for a certain patient, the patient's study, series, and image records will be found in the PACS database and the image records will include the file names for the patient's images. These files will then be located on the hard drive and loaded into PACS as DICOM objects.

The most obvious advantage of this method is its simplicity. The second, less obvious advantage lies in the fact that all DICOM data (files) are stored *separately* from the PACS and its database. PACS only points to the files and does the housekeeping part (deleting, updating, and relating file records to each other). This separation of application and data can be extremely helpful in many data migration projects; for example, when an old PACS has to be replaced by a new one. In such a scenario, you do not really depend on the old PACS software. You simply locate the place on the hard drive where it stores the DICOM files, and import these files into a new system. Data migration in this case becomes a data import task, which can be much easier if DICOM import is properly implemented in your new system.

One dark-side note: direct access to the application data (files), bypassing the application, can be abused. Files can be illegally copied, deleted, or modified. PACS with file-based storage should implement some security mechanism to prevent this from happening.

In-House Applications

Many institutions take advantage of this separate file storage to develop their in-house DICOM processing software. If, for example, you need to write an application to postprocess your nuclear images, and you know the folder where they can be found on the imaging server, your application may just read them from there, saving yourself from the trouble of DICOM networking development. Just limit your file access to read-only, and do not use this approach for any large projects.

10.5.2 Database-Based PACS Storage

Current databases allow storing large chunks of binary data directly in database tables – just like we store patient names or image IDs. Those large binary fields are known as *blobs* (binary large objects). Jim Starkey, a database architect who invented blobs, wittily describes them as "*the thing that ate Cincinnati, Cleveland, or whatever.*"

10.5 Storing DICOM Data in PACS

PACS blobs would then be *the things that ate DICOM objects* – whatever size these objects might be. A good, uncompressed ultrasound Cine loop stored as a single multiframe DICOM object/file could easily consume several hundreds of megabytes. Instead of storing DICOM objects in DICOM files, PACS would throw them all straight into the database – for example, in some Pixel Data column of that Image Table just mentioned.

The main advantage of this *all-in-one* approach is the ability to enjoy all the tools a current database can offer. For example, blobs with DICOM data can be encrypted with database encryption tools, immediately adding a strong layer of data security to your PACS application (while file-based DICOM security still remains in its infancy). Along with data encryption, all current databases offer you auditing tools to pinpoint when, how, and by whom any DICOM object is accessed or modified. In the same manner as data encryption, blobs can be compressed to optimize storage; that is, instead of relying on some DICOM image compression algorithm (compressing only image data), a database would usually offer its own built-in compression mechanism, which will losslessly compress the entire blob, whatever it contains.

Some database companies (such as Oracle) went even further, adding native DICOM support to their databases. That is, instead of managing rather amorphous blobs, these databases can:

- recognize DICOM objects,
- read and parse DICOM data,
- process the most common DICOM fields,
- anonymize DICOM data,
- map DICOM data to XML,
- and even convert DICOM images from the objects into nice preview thumbnails, which you can use in your PACS application (OracleDICOM).

Finally, keep in mind that current performance-optimized databases can access their blobs much faster than reading plain DICOM files. They can also run on different platforms and operating systems; they can do automated backups; and they can easily handle tons of DICOM images. In brief, on top of your database server you can get a nice set of tools that any PACS owner can only dream about. Nice! But what's the catch?

The main problem with "database PACS" is that it makes your PACS entirely dependent on that particular database product. You will have to rely on it for all DICOM storage-related tasks. With file-based PACS storage, should anything bad happen to the PACS or the PACS database, you will still be left with intact DICOM files – your sacred data that *everything* is about. With database-based storage, you put all your eggs in one basket – so you better make sure that your basket is 100% fail-proof.

10.5.3 Mixed PACS Storage Models

I have seen several mixed PACS storage models and have not really been impressed by any of them. As the word "mixed" suggests, the line between DICOM objects (files) and object housekeeping (database) is rather blurred – or even ill-positioned – often cutting through objects and records with little attention to the logic landscape. For example, one early version of a well-known PACS software would literally slice DICOM files into pieces. Only the database knew how these pieces were to be connected, and each piece was meaningless by itself. When this PACS aged to the point of falling apart and needing to be replaced by another system, the entire data-migration process turned into a long nightmare. Since then, I have worked with a couple of contemporary DICOM devices that store their DICOM data in a somewhat similar *piecewise* manner. Please remember that the DICOM standard is designed to store pretty much everything your digital device is acquiring as a well-structured DICOM object – there is no need to cut or redistribute anything.

Another example is somewhat opposite and is related to a well-known PACS company that chose to store certain DICOM data in the PACS database only; never updating the DICOM files (objects). In this case, these updates were annotations done by radiologists on the images. Although DICOM provides ample support for including annotations in DICOM objects, this was not implemented. Annotations were stored only in the PACS database, in a very obscure proprietary format. As a result, the radiologists had to do double work: first placing annotations on the images on PACS workstations, and then manually retyping these annotations into a separate hospital tool to track annotation measurements – just to record them in easily exportable text format. Needless to say, the process was time-consuming, annoying, and full of human errors. I have repeated this countless times, and I will keep repeating it: *when looking for any DICOM software, make sure that it can export all data it collects, in standard well-defined format.* This will make your life and projects so much easier!

10.5.4 Choice of Internal File Format

Especially if your PACS comes with file-based DICOM storage, the choice of the file format becomes essential for the efficiency and interoperability of your application. Ideally, this should be DICOM. Moreover, if you have to compress it (and with current volumes of digital data in radiology, you most certainly will), please rely on standard lossless DICOM compression (Sect. 6.2.1) such as 8-bit and 12-bit lossless JPEG. This will make your PACS-stored files compatible with nearly any other DICOM application.

Also, avoid *overstoring*. One popular medical imaging system, for example, decided to keep its imaging data in two formats – the original DICOM files (for compatibility), and the proprietary-formatted image files (for easier 3D processing). Needless to say, it doubled the size of the required storage, and added substantial processing overhead for continuously converting the data between the two formats. When this system was introduced in a busy hospital, its storage inefficiency was matched only by its slow and unreliable performance, both resulting from managing twice as much data when one copy would suffice. What started as a relatively small server soon took the entire server rack. PACS should be smart enough to work with a single internal data format – preferably DICOM.

DICOM Security 11

Ancient Romans used to shave their slaves' heads, write secret messages on them, and let the hair grow – an ingenious way of implementing data security. The papal scribes in the first crusades applied secret text-encoding tools and had to be executed after a year of active duty in order to maintain secrecy (share *this* with your system administrator). The whole history of human civilization is filled with attempts to encode secrets and, consequently, equal attempts to break the codes.

The main outcome of this quest was summarized by Mr. Sherlock Holmes: *"What is invented by one man, can be always understood be some other."* Applied to our subject of data encryption, this can be restated as: any security code can be broken. *It's just a matter of time*, and computer power, but this is exactly what makes a big difference. In the innocent era of the 1980s, when DICOM was first introduced, no one was really concerned with data protection: those playing Space Invaders at the time would never imagine that their own data and privacy could be invaded on a much more magnanimous scale. As a result, the sheer complexity of DICOM encoding methods has become the only DICOM data protection for nearly 20 years. It was believed to be complex, but it has never been. In fact, it was hardly enough to block even the least advanced threats.

11.1 DICOM Hacking

Let's look inside a DICOM file with some generic file viewer such as WordPad, Notepad, or Word. Sure enough, when you open a DICOM file in WordPad (Fig. 11.1), you do not expect to see any images or nicely formatted study information – WordPad has no idea what to do with the DICOM format. What you will see instead will be mostly unreadable gibberish corresponding to the binary (hexadecimal) contents of the file. However, look closely and you will see the valuable pieces of DICOM information and structure.

1. Symbols from 129–132 in a valid DICOM 3.0 file should read "DICM" (see Chap. 10). It means that you can open a file, and search it for DICM. If you find it somewhere in the beginning, it is a good indication that you are looking at a

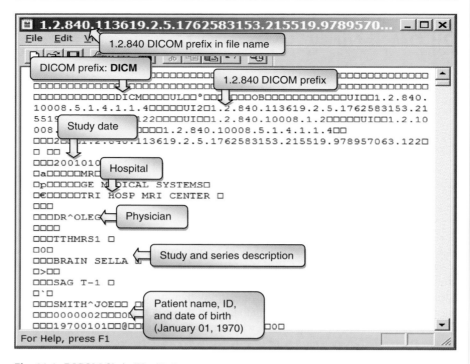

Fig. 11.1 DICOM file in WordPad

valid DICOM file. In fact, this is probably one of the best ways to recognize a valid DICOM file. Older ACR-NEMA versions might not have this, but they are becoming rarer.

2. The "1.2.840..." prefix is used in all standard DICOM identifier (UID) strings, and its presence in a file also confirms that we are dealing with DICOM. Often, DICOM files are named after their UIDs – in which case, DICOM file names begin with the same prefix.
3. DICOM dates follow the YYYYMMDD format and can be easily identified as such. Same is true for DICOM time strings in HHMMSS format (see Sect. 5.3.4).
4. Other readable strings such as patient and physician names, hospital, study, and series description can always be guessed based on their contents. In particular, the caret (^) character, used in DICOM as a name separator, helps locate names.

Thus, even without help from any DICOM software, one can easily interpret the textual part of a binary DICOM object.[1] The good news is that this often helps to identify the valid DICOM files and partially verify their contents. The bad news is that it also poses a serious security threat. Not only can we *read* the confidential clinical data, we can also *edit* it. This is possible provided our text strings remain at

---

[1]The same is true for the older ACR-NEMA files – see an example in section 5.2.

11.2 DICOM Anonymization

the same length (as you know, DICOM does keep track of each data element's size with VR lengths). For example, one can modify a patient's name by replacing "SMITH^JOE" with "GRAY^MARY". Worse, one can replace "NORMAL" by "CANCER" in the study description string. All DICOM dates, names, and other textual descriptions can be fiddled with in the same manner.

Consequences? *A devious person can easily alter and compromise your clinical data with the most primitive tools and you wouldn't even know it.*

What about the "bread-and-butter" pixel data, embedded in DICOM image object in binary format? Same story: extracting and viewing the image can be a bit trickier, but anyone with very little, if any, DICOM knowledge and very basic programming skills can do it. When I was starting my DICOM endeavors some 15 years ago, I came across a simple DICOM image viewer capable of displaying MR and CT images with no DICOM parsing whatsoever. The idea was simple and might provide a little entertainment for the IT-inclined readers of this book.

Most MR and CT images use either 256×256 or 512×512 pixel matrix with two bytes per pixel (16-bit) grayscale. Because image information takes the most space in a DICOM file, comparing file size to either $256 \times 256 \times 2 = 128$ KB or $512 \times 512 \times 2 = 512$ KB immediately reveals the actual size of the image matrix. Usually, image pixels come at the very end of the DICOM file. If we know, for example, that we are dealing with a 256×256 image, then we simply take the last $256 \times 256 \times 2 = 131,072$ bytes of the DICOM file and voilà – we end up with a *parsed* image, which with very little programming can be converted into a bitmap or any other conventional image type. And certainly one can easily modify the original image or even replace it with a different one – swapped from another patient, for example – without even bothering with any image conversion.

Good enough? Let's summarize our very basic yet fruitful DICOM hacking experience. With a little ingenuity and minimal skills, some socially deviant misanthrope can read and edit confidential DICOM information even without DICOM software. This poses two classic threats: unauthorized access to your data and tampering with your data contents. Common tactics used to combat these threats include permanently removing the confidential data (anonymization), or temporarily hiding it (encryption). Let's see how each works.

11.2 DICOM Anonymization

The main security breach in our DICOM hacking experiment was the readability of the textual part of the DICOM file content. As soon as we see "SMITH^JOE" in a DICOM file, we can easily realize that we are dealing with a person's name; probably followed by the person's ID and date of birth. If this data is so visible, can it somehow be removed or scrambled?

The simplest approach to hiding confidential DICOM data is *anonymization*. DICOM anonymization is the process of removing confidential entries from DICOM files. Anonymization is generally irreversible; that is, the original confidential data cannot be recovered from the anonymized file. This makes anonymization the most secure data protection: what is permanently removed cannot be recovered even by the most vicious hacker – it's gone. As a result, anonymized DICOM files can often be seen in public domains, and can be shared and exchanged with no risk of exposing confidential information.

This sounds like the ideal approach, but the flip side of irreversible anonymization is the permanent loss of important information that might be needed later. Moreover, you can easily run into other problems with complexity and consistency of the entire anonymization process. Therefore, let's have a closer look at the pitfalls of DICOM anonymization.

As you might remember, all standard DICOM data tags are listed in the standard DICOM Data Dictionary (part PS3.6 of the standard). Most of these tags such as "Image width," "Laterality," or "Echo time" reflect the material part of the image acquisition/display and are not confidential. Nevertheless, the dictionary also contains tags such as "Patient name," "Patient ID," "Reading physician phone number," and so on, which are clearly confidential and should not be open to the general public. The Health Insurance Portability and Accountability Act (HIPAA) of 1996, addressing the security and privacy of health data, defined the following list of 18 major identifier types, which have to be removed in Protected Health Information (PHI):

1. Names
2. Locations – all geographic subdivisions smaller than a state, including street address, city, county, precinct, zip code, and their equivalent geocodes.
3. Dates – all dates related to the subject of the information; for example: birth dates, admission dates, discharge dates, encounter dates, surgery dates, and so on.
4. Telephone numbers
5. Fax numbers
6. Electronic mail addresses
7. Social security numbers
8. Medical record numbers
9. Health plan beneficiary numbers
10. Account numbers
11. Certificate / license numbers
12. Vehicle identifiers and serial numbers, including license plate numbers
13. Device identifiers and serial numbers
14. Web Universal Resource Locators (URLs)
15. Internet Protocol (IP) address numbers
16. Biometric identifiers, including finger and voice prints
17. Full face photographic images and any comparable images
18. Any other unique identifying number, characteristic, or code

Some of these attribute types (such as license plate numbers) have nothing to do with DICOM and will hardly ever have; the others (patient IDs, study dates) are right on target and can be found as DICOM attributes in the DICOM Data Dictionary. Consequently, DICOM anonymization software should keep a list of these confidential attributes, and remove them from DICOM files. As a result, it would produce anonymized DICOM files still containing the image and nonconfidential data sufficient

11.2 DICOM Anonymization

for adequate image display, but lacking any confidential information. You can freely, publicly, and safely distribute anonymized DICOM files for any practical reason.

The early implementations of this approach produced a hodgepodge of DICOM anonymizers varying from simple delete-all-patient-information programs to intricate manual DICOM editors in which the user had total control over removing and editing DICOM file content (attributes). The latter choice, however, was already impractical; you do not want to manually edit some 500 files in your average MR study – it will take forever.[2] Therefore, automatic anonymization has become the most popular; but it soon ran into its own problems.

The biggest mistake made by many DICOM anonymizers was the automated *removal* of confidential fields from the files. Consider, for example, an attribute such as "Patient ID" (element (0010,0020) in the DICOM Data Dictionary, see also Sect. 5.6.1). This attribute is clearly confidential because it uniquely points to the patient. Moreover, many DICOM systems use patient name, social security number, or date of birth for Patient ID. However, one cannot simply wipe the Patient ID out of a DICOM file. This attribute is *required*, and its removal would make the file or DICOM object invalid. Therefore, the attribute has to be present, but it needs to be changed into something meaningless and absolutely unrelated to the original ID value (anonymization with pseudo values is sometimes referred to as *pseudonimization*).

OK, let's say that the original Patient ID value was "1234567", and our DICOM pseudonimization software automatically replaced it with "wo4_ejF9h". Mission accomplished? Not so fast! Not only should this replacement *hide* the original data, but it should also *consistently* reproduce the result regardless of how and when it was done. And combining *hidden* and *consistent*, as you might guess, becomes the most intricate part of the process. For example, all entries with the same 1234567 ID that we might encounter later on (say, 2 years later, when this patent comes for another exam), or all ID entries in a 2000-image CT study for this patient must be consistently replaced with the same "wo4_ejF9h" string. Otherwise, we would break a single patient into a mix of unrelated pieces, destroying the original image-and-data relationship. Thus, our anonymizing software should replace the confidential tag value with its meaningless placeholder in a unique way, which already begins to sound like data encryption.

Furthermore, no two different patients should receive the same anonymized ID: if we anonymize another one with the same "wo4_ejF9h", we would *merge* two totally unrelated people into a single Siamese twin with all the unpleasant consequences. In the extreme case, if we simply replace any patient ID with a blank (like many anonymizers do), we would essentially merge all patients into one big Mr. Unknown; because only patient ID (and not the name or anything else) is used in DICOM as the unique patient identifier.

Suddenly, all this makes DICOM anonymization quite a complex procedure, rarely implemented with sufficient thought. Just recently, I saw another popular anonymizer that was almost doing the required job except that it was still keeping

---

[2]Also, remember, that some attributes may depend on the others (see Sect. 5.5.6), so you cannot edit them freely.

the original confidential information. The trick was simple: to remove the original data from public display, the anonymizer would move it into proprietary DICOM tags in the same DICOM object (file). Unfortunately, what is simple to hide is usually simple to find. For example, opening such files in WordPad, as I showed in Sect. 11.1, will expose all this confidential data no matter where and with which tags it is stored in the data file. Nice try!

And this is only the beginning. Consider the "Patient's age" attribute; it is confidential, but knowing the age is often important for the clinical interpretation of the image. Study date can definitely be used to identify a patient, but would you like to remove it? Not really, because study date is essential for time-ordering of the studies and for making observations about the dynamics of the disease. So, although we listed study date as item three of our HIPAA confidentiality list, I would strongly recommend that you do not hide this information – at least from the reading radiologist. The same thing can be said about tags such as "Study description," "Patient comments," "Patient's weight," and many others in the 2000-tag DICOM Data Dictionary; albeit confidential, they are important for the correct image interpretation, and should not be anonymized.

Finally, did we forget about certain image types (such as ultrasound or secondary capture images) where proprietary information (patient name, ID, birth date) is not only stored in easy-to-remove DICOM tags, but also included in the images themselves – *burned* into their pixels, as in Fig. 11.2?

The only way to remove the confidential data from the image itself is to somehow erase it manually – blurring it or blanking the confidential image regions. But wiping these image regions automatically is definitely a challenge. You can probably teach your anonymizer to recognize text in the image (using some kind of OCR[3]), but how would you automatically distinguish which text fragments are confidential and need to be removed, and which have to stay (such as important measurements and annotations)?

Recently, I was involved in a large ultrasound anonymization project. The best automatic anonymization we came up with was to blank the upper section of any ultrasound image, and to completely remove the ultrasound header screenshots. Patient names were usually written in the upper section, and the header screenshots had no ultrasound data, but were filled with patient information. Fortunately, it worked for us because we never would have had time and resources to clean those images manually; but the same solution might fail for ultrasound images with different layouts. Scanned reports with less structured layouts present even larger problem (see example on SC images in Sect. 8.2); cleaning them up would require herculean patience.

In brief, anonymization provides the most bullet-proof security, but anonymizing confidential and semiconfidential DICOM data is not an easy task, and can

---

[3]Optical Character Recognition, used to recognize text on scanned images.

11.2 DICOM Anonymization

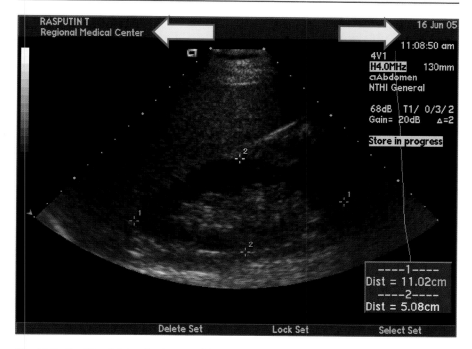

Fig. 11.2 Confidential data in ultrasound images: patient name, hospital, study date and time

inevitably reduce the clinical value of the subject DICOM file or image. I hope, dear reader, that after these few examples you will be more careful in selecting your DICOM anonymizer. Modifying the complex structure of DICOM data without making it incomplete and invalid is quite possible, but only when done with extreme care.

HIPAA and DICOM

Have no HIPAA illusions either: HIPAA security guidelines cannot be 100% compatible with DICOM. Consider, for example, item 17 on the HIPAA list above – full face images. It does not take much to reconstruct the head and the face of the patient from MR or CT head scan. Any current 3D medical imaging workstation can do this. Radiology is all about images, and about confidential images. Little things like piercing can uniquely identify a person.

Hopefully, this will prompt for better security methods than brute-force anonymization. Overdosed data cleanup, even with the best intentions, leads to informational gaps and inconsistencies. This can be more dangerous for a patient than the loss of confidentiality.

11.3 Understanding Encryption

Permanent data loss in anonymization calls for better approaches, and this is where digital data encryption comes into picture. Modern data security is shrouded by thick layers of myth, misunderstanding, and conspiracy theories,[4] so it is worth taking a little time to understand its principles. You are welcome to skip to Sect. 11.4 if you're not interested in encryption internals.

In brief, encryption is the process of changing the format of the data to protect its original content. Encryption can be viewed as translating your data into another language (code) that cannot be understood without a special key. Unlike anonymization, encryption has to be reversible; that is, you can always translate your data back to the original form without any loss or distortion. The reversibility of encryption eliminates the entire problem of data loss that we faced with anonymization. If you carefully read the previous section, you should realize that our attempt to encode confidential Patient ID tags in a unique and consistent way was, in fact, an initial approach to encryption.

Part PS3.15 of the DICOM standard, released a few of years ago, adopted the existing data encryption techniques to be used with DICOM data. These techniques pursue three important goals: *encrypting the data, verifying the data origin, and verifying the data integrity*. The DICOM standard still needs to do a good deal of explaining how this can be brought into practice; meanwhile, we can review the most important concepts.

11.3.1 The Main Idea Behind Encryption

Encryption of digital data can be compared to lossless image compression (see Sect. 6.2.1): you reversibly transform the original data into another format that is impossible to read unless you decrypt it to its original form. Consider something as simple as patient name, "SMITH^JOE". If left as is, it can easily be spotted in a DICOM file or DICOM object (see Sect. 11.1) without any particular DICOM software or skills.

Even if you merely replaced each letter in the patient's name with the following letter in the alphabet, you would get something more secure: "TNJUI^KPF". This is already a huge progress; the real name of the patient is completely hidden. You can show this to anyone and they won't be able to read it, but you (or your business partner, knowing the *"next letter"* encryption rule) can always decrypt the original name. This is the essence of data encryption, and the only problem with our *"next letter"* code is that it is too easy to break. There is another problem: the information about your *"next letter"* method may eventually leak into the public domain, which will immediately expose all your encrypted data. You will have to start over and encrypt everything using another method.

---

[4]Some believe that data encryption algorithms such as DES have intentional backdoors by their inventors. I do not.

11.4 Encrypting DICOM Data

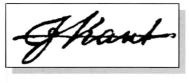

Digitized signature

```
KfJe98fdKel9jejKsdfjer498KasdfJ905Md
sbGK5N33nggJMGg45tG54kgrkgKg4gk
3tRkeg45Ggkwekg4ggwegjbKgwr6Kgw
Mvwrwknbn899did874jjhd9jskj84nnf983
928hlkd989jyg5lnbi3bzvmsjs640wjshg1
254ey9samag45HqfnaFl6ns52nd9tnhg
mabv215azkf85ls8sH8Umq9zms63bs8x
znxc73ndn6T7akz873Eydb3673fgks8wn
58fmsj580284e5d2c4840S0D00610a8c
aa8F96b192bbB550efb356972ecewcwc
23c23V==
```

Digital signature

Fig. 11.5 Digital signature

Digital or Digitized?
If you ask your software provider "Do you support digital signatures?" the answer will likely be "Yes!" As exciting as it sounds, it may rarely correspond to the true digital signatures. Many – sometimes inadvertently, sometimes intentionally – will confuse digital signatures with more naïve ways of signing your data on computers: typing your name or initials, inserting an image of your scanned signature, clicking on some "Signed" checkbox, and so on (Fig. 11.5). Clearly, none of these are secure. What was typed can easily be retyped; signature bitmaps can be replaced and manipulated; dates can be changed; and so on. Only the true electronic digital signature makes any of these manipulations impossible. Many popular software formats, such as Adobe PDF, become more and more proficient with the use of true digital signatures, and you can always take advantage of this in your workflow.

11.4 Encrypting DICOM Data

Data encryption was originally introduced into DICOM with PS3.15 in rather declarative form; therefore DICOM Supplement 142 was added in 2008 to sort out many PS3.15 mysteries. Some of them were mentioned in our Sect. 11.2 on anonymization. Therefore, it is interesting to consider both documents.

11.4.1 De- and Re-Identification: PS3.15

DICOM defines *de-identification* as protecting confidential attributes by either removing or encrypting them. DICOM defines *re-identification* as the inverse process of "removing the protection." Note that this definition is not without flaws: re-identification may not always be possible if the original data was cleaned or removed.

Table 11.1 Basic application level confidentiality profile attributes (PS3.15, Table E.1-1)

Attribute name	Tag	Attribute name	Tag
Instance Creator UID	(0008,0014)	Other Patient Ids	(0010,1000)
SOP Instance UID	(0008,0018)	Other Patient Names	(0010,1001)
Accession Number	(0008,0050)	Patient's Age	(0010,1010)
Institution Name	(0008,0080)	Patient's Size	(0010,1020)
Institution Address	(0008,0081)	Patient's Weight	(0010,1030)
Referring Physician's Name	(0008,0090)	Medical Record Locator	(0010,1090)
Referring Physician's Address	(0008,0092)	Ethnic Group	(0010,2160)
Referring Physician's Telephone Numbers	(0008,0094)	Occupation	(0010,2180)
Station Name	(0008,1010)	Additional Patient's History	(0010,21B0)
Study Description	(0008,1030)	Patient Comments	(0010,4000)
Series Description	(0008,103E)	Device Serial Number	(0018,1000)
Institutional Department Name	(0008,1040)	Protocol Name	(0018,1030)
Physician(s) of Record	(0008,1048)	Study Instance UID	(0020,000D)
Performing Physicians' Name	(0008,1050)	Series Instance UID	(0020,000E)
Name of Physician(s) Reading Study	(0008,1060)	Study ID	(0020,0010)
Operators' Name	(0008,1070)	Frame of Reference UID	(0020,0052)
Admitting Diagnoses Description	(0008,1080)	Synchronization Frame of Reference UID	(0020,0200)
Referenced SOP Instance UID	(0008,1155)	Image Comments	(0020,4000)
Derivation Description	(0008,2111)	Request Attributes Sequence	(0040,0275)
Patient's Name	(0010,0010)	UID	(0040,A124)
Patient ID	(0010,0020)	Content Sequence	(0040,A730)
Patient's Birth Date	(0010,0030)	Storage Media File-set UID	(0088,0140)
Patient's Birth Time	(0010,0032)	Referenced Frame of Reference UID	(3006,0024)
Patient's Sex	(0010,0040)	Related Frame of Reference UID	(3006,00C2)

Nonetheless, DICOM often uses re-identification as a metaphor for decryption, which implies that de-identification was rather reversible encryption. I hope further DICOM editions will make it solid.

To address multiple questions raised in our anonymization review, DICOM gurus suggested breaking the de-identification process into several Attribute Confidentiality Profiles. Each profile is meant to address certain parts of security and to target certain types of attributes.

DICOM PS3.15 defines the *Basic Application Level Confidentiality Profile* as the most conservative and crude way to hide confidential data. An application conforming to this profile should take at least all attributes listed in PS3.15 Table E.1-1 (we reproduce it here in Table 11.1), encrypt their original (true) values with a standard encryption algorithm (such as AES or Triple-DES), and store the encryption result in

11.4 Encrypting DICOM Data

(0400, 0550) Modified Attributes Sequence, while replacing the values in the original locations with dummy ones. In other words, we anonymize confidential attributes just like we would do with any anonymization, but we also store their original values in the (0400, 0550) "vault," locked by a digital key. This is where we can find them for re-identification (decryption) when needed. To flag DICOM objects as de-identified, we insert a special Patient Identity Removed attribute (0012,0062) in it with a value of YES.

Note that it is the responsibility of the application to replace these attributes at their original location with *consistent* dummy values, preserving the validity of the data – one of the trickiest parts of the anonymization process. That is, if one chooses to rename patient into SMITH^JOE into STROKE^CASE123 (I strongly urge you to use meaningful dummies), all instances of SMITH^JOE should become STROKE^CASE123. In this case, the dummy yet consistent STROKE^CASE123 would be stored in the patient name (0010, 0010) attribute, while the original SMITH^JOE value from there will be AES-encrypted and placed into the (0400, 0550) sequence.

Unfortunately, the rest of the specs in PS3.15 look rather suggestive. First of all, re-identifier application is supposed to decrypt the de-identified data, but without any guarantee of getting the original data set. This guarantee becomes impossible because Basic Application Level Confidentiality Profile does not store the original image (pixel data is not mentioned in Table E.1-1). Instead, it irreversibly wipes out the parts of the image containing confidential data (such as patient name, see Fig. 11.2). In this sense, as was mentioned above, we already violate the key principle of encryption: the decrypted data should be identical to the original.

Second, PS3.15 does not explain any further what and how to remove: "It is the responsibility of the de-identifier to ensure that all identifying information is removed." This raises many questions. What about study date and time attributes? They are not in Table E.1-1, but they can be considered confidential according to HIPAA and common sense. On the other side, what about potentially important items such as patient's birth data (0010,0030) or sex (0010,0040), which might be needed to correctly process the de-identified record? Not clear. We have to hide them on one side, but the de-identified record without them might become meaningless. What dummy value can one suggest for patient's sex? Either you keep it or you change it to the opposite value. The first option contradicts security; the second, common sense. In brief, all implementation decisions are left to the application designers, and should be documented in their application DICOM Conformance Statement. But as our experience suggests, leaving critical logic to the application developers paves a smooth road to chaos.

As a result, the Basic Application Level Confidentiality Profile merely projects the HIPAA requirements onto DICOM attribute sets by identifying the "most confidential" DICOM attributes and suggesting the generic approach to their hiding in the encrypted (0400, 0550) sequence. But the devil is in details, and from this point of view PS3.15 remains too sketchy for any practical use. "Just clean this mess, somehow, and don't ask too many questions."

DICOM Supplement 142 comes to the rescue.

11.4.2 De- and Re-Identification: Supplement 142

DICOM Supplement 142, a short 37-page document entitled "Clinical Trial De-identification Profiles," provides a much deeper insight into DICOM de-identification. The Supplement approaches the de-identification task from the most common practical angle: de-identification of the data used for clinical research, teaching files, and presentations. As it often happens, having practical use cases helps with making practical recommendations. Also, in its own way Supplement 142 makes a nearly perfect list of all roadblocks that DICOM de-identification has yet to overcome. I really recommend it to anyone interested in the current state of DICOM security implementation.

First of all, Supplement 142 makes several important enhancements in the suggestive model from PS3.15. It subdivides the Basic Application Level Confidentiality Profile into several independent options:

- *Clean Pixel Data Option*: delete confidential data (such as patient name or ID) burned into image pixels (see example in Fig. 11.2).
- *Clean Recognizable Visual Features Option*: clean image fragments that can be used to recognize the patient (photographs, facial features in high-resolution CT series, etc.)[7]
- *Clean Graphics Option*: remove confidential graphics from the images, such as annotations and overlays
- *Clean Structured Content Option*: remove confidential data from the structured reports (see Sect. 8.3)
- *Clean Descriptors Option*: clean data items such as Study Description (0008, 1030) or Series Description (0008,103E); free text fields, where confidential information can be entered.

In addition to this, Supplement 142 addresses the need to retain certain data (such as patient age or study date), which can be viewed as confidential, but may be required for adequate data processing. The options include:

- *Retain Longitudinal Option*: dates and times. For example, patient date of birth (DOB, attribute (0010,0030), see Table 11.1) may be needed for the clinical trial, but may also point to the patient identity. To resolve this conflict, Supplement 142 offers two choices: preserving longitudinal data as is, or modifying just enough to hide the patient identity, but to be still useful for analysis. Example: shifting all dates by a fixed amount of days.[8]
- *Retain Patient Characteristics Option*: when this option is chosen, patient characteristics such as sex, weight, and height will be preserved (not de-identified).

---

[7] There are amazing examples of CT surface reconstruction algorithms combined with forensic applications, such as enabling us to see the faces of ancient Egyptian mummies (Cesarani). It is also a nice illustration of how the old "data encryption" techniques (trapped pyramids, massive sarcophagi, complex mummification, and all the chants from the "Book of the Dead") can be "broken" with current technology.

[8] Ironically, this looks just like our "next letter" encryption, doesn't it?

11.4 Encrypting DICOM Data

- *Retain Device Information Option*: as its name suggests, retains the information about the data acquisition device.
- *Retain UIDs*: retains UIDs (unique identifiers associated with the original data, such as image UID, which is supposed to uniquely identify the image). Possible reason for retention: auditing.
- *Retain Safe Private Option*: retaining the private (proprietary) data elements created by various DICOM vendors.

Note that these items tackle the majority of our earlier questions about the "security vs. completeness" compromise. Given all these options, one can use them with PS3.15 Table E.1-1 (Table 11.1 in this book) to achieve different levels of de-identification. For example, with longitudinal attributes retained or modified. To make the process even more straightforward, Supplement 142 specifies the removal type for each attribute, depending on the removal option: replace (with a nonzero length dummy value), clean (replace by a zero-length attribute), remove (completely remove from the DICOM object), keep unchanged, and so on. This results in the "improved" Table E.1-1, conditioned on the removal types and reaching some 17 pages in Supplement 142. But at least for the most basic and conservative Basic Application Level Confidentiality Profile, this provides a sufficient level of detail for practical implementation, and a logical choice of data removal options to support.

11.4.3 Security and DICOM Images

Images are the Holy Grail of DICOM objects. Their countless pixels relay the most precious information about the patient, and image data can be processed and analyzed into an infinite number of ways. What security risks can one face with DICOM image data? Let's just name a few to sketch the entire spectrum of this problem. Imagine that you need to de-identify a set of DICOM images for a pharmaceutical company interested in their analysis.

First of all, images can be down-right personal. What if one of them contains a photograph of the patient? Worse, what if you have a CT scan of the head, and any 3D rendering software would be able to reconstruct patient's face from the sequence of CT images? There is no easy answer to this; and quite a few people write smart programs just to dilute the individual facial features in CT or MR head slices. There are well-established masking techniques to blur eyes or entire faces, but even those methods are not automatic and require human guidance. Moreover, a patient's face is not the only unique feature that can identify the patient. Any obvious abnormality, any visible pathology, any piercing or implant can be used to recognize the subject, especially when the range of candidates is small. Can one feasibly write software to "fix" all of them? Certainly not, so we have a problem; and the Clean Recognizable Visual Features Option in Supplement 142 meets a serious practical challenge.

Second, extensive image editing can render the image "unusable for the purpose for which it has been collected," as Supplement 142 recognizes. As an example of this case, consider removing dental image fragments from dental images. In essence, we apply a far-from-ideal anonymization approach to the image pixels, trying to modify only the confidential ones – out of billions of pixels. The approach is clearly counterproductive, at least to be used on a serious scale.

Third, there are more complex data types, such as structured reports or embedded video, for which image editing would require special software and unique skills. How would one edit individual frames in DICOM-encapsulated MPEG4 video? What about sound, which may be included and contain confidential information as well?

But the item that really tops my list of image security problems is intentional image modification. With any good image editor, one can cut a liver tumor from one DICOM image and paste it onto another patient's image, making it look totally natural and in place. One can edit anatomy features to completely alter the diagnostic result. In the present DICOM standard, there is no way to detect intentional image modifications, and there is no means to sort "benign" modifications (cropping, noise-filtering) from the "malignant" (intentional alterations of the diagnostic results). Clearly, we can see that the DICOM committee has its work cut out for it.

> **Next Level of Image Security**
>
> If you want to fortify your image protection, you will need to consider more complex techniques such as digital watermarking (Tan). Digital watermarking works similar to conventional watermarks seen on currency and passports: it embeds secret messages into the image. But in the case of digital images, the secret messages are invisible binary codewords and integrity checksums that are added to the least-important bits of each image pixel. Technically, they alter the image; practically, the alteration is so minute that it cannot be seen and it cannot affect diagnostic image quality. In this case, instead of applying encryption to the image as a whole, you apply it to a multitude of small image regions. If one of them gets altered (with a fake tumor, for example), you will be able to pinpoint its location.
>
> Keep in mind though, that increasing your defenses always comes at a price. Advanced techniques such as watermarking require substantial processing time, which can bottleneck your image workflow. Also, digital watermarks cannot differentiate between legitimate image modifications (QA cropping or rotation, lossy compression, denoising filtering) and illegal ones (fake tumors). As a result, you will always have to balance the pros and cons of augmenting security to find the model that fits your interests best.

11.5 Concluding Remarks on Security

As you should realize by now, blending DICOM and security is not an easy task; "it may be extremely burdensome," as Supplement 142 reminds. Largely, it is due to balancing on the thin edge of "preserving the diagnostic value while removing the confidential;" but a few other aspects contribute to this complexity as well.

The main problem of the DICOM format is that it does not easily blend with data encryption. When you encrypt a file with WinRar, you get an encrypted file: an

11.5 Concluding Remarks on Security

object of the same "file" type that you can store, delete, FTP, or email just like the original. But if you take a DICOM object – with all its VRs organized in a complex internal structure – and encrypt it in its entirety, the result won't be a DICOM object anymore. Instead, it will be a binary blob that no DICOM application would ever recognize or process. This creates a fundamental problem, and the only way to bypass it without rewriting the bulk of the DICOM standard would be embedding the *encrypted* DICOM object into a *regular* one, to be carried through the regular protocol traffic much in the way that DICOM embeds video or PDF documents (8.4). But then, someone has to decide how much of the original data can still "leak" into the embedding "carrier" object. From a security standpoint, we want it to be as dummy and impersonal as possible; but for all practical reasons, we want it to make sense and somehow correspond to the original (encrypted) data. The problem is that this *correspondence* still has no practical answer.

In addition to pure encryption, there is a wealth of related problems making secure DICOM a much harder nut to crack. Consider long-term archiving; can one store de-identified (encrypted) images for years? The answer is not obvious. First of all, the advances in computer processing power can make old encryption techniques too weak to be adequate. Second, some 10 years from now you might not even find that old decryption software and the private keys to decrypt (re-identify) those encrypted DICOMs (think about VHS tapes in your closet). *Memento mori*: all current encryption methods are designed to protect the data at the given moment (bank transactions, online data transfers, etc.) with no guarantee of long-time persistence. Where would one keep the private RSA key for 10 years anyway? Carve it in Rosetta stone?

However – and I cannot overstate this – none of this is meant to disenchanter you from building a secure clinical practice. Above the application-specific realm of DICOM security, there is a wide spectrum of tools – VPNs, digital signatures, access logs, and policies – already available to you and designed to near-perfection. Securing the entire workflow still remains your best bet in securing DICOM as a part of it. Therefore, work with your IT and always ask your potential PACS/RIS/HIS provider about their security options. Make sure you have an accurate account of what is *really* supported by your software. In this case, you should be concerned with DICOM de-identification only when DICOM files leave your secured environment, such as when you send them to the third parties for teaching, trials, and demos. But in this case, retaining the original data would be your least concern. The most basic DICOM anonymization will solve the problem and will protect your data forever. Anonymize!

Long Way to Go!
This year one of my friends, the CIO of a large hospital, decided to buy a new CR for mammography. As scrupulous as he was, he first identified the leading CR manufacturers and contacted them to get a few DICOM CR image samples to be evaluated by his radiology team.
The samples arrived from *three reputed CR companies*.
We opened them in a PACS workstation.

We looked at the patient data and saw what appeared to be real patient names, DOBs, IDs, *everything – on the images with breast tumors*. Two out of three companies sent us the real patient data! Moreover, it was not even data they acquired (they had no patients of their own). It would have had to be real patient data from their affiliated hospitals, beta sites, and wherever else their CRs were used.

It wouldn't take a genious to grab a few names and DOBs from these images, type them into Facebook, and find the matches. These very *real* people did not have a clue that their personal data and health problems had become common knowledge, exposed to the entire planet.

No standard – and certainly no encryption algorithm – can protect from sheer human ignorance and neglect.

11.6   What Else?

Anonymization (pseudonymization) and encryption secure DICOM data, but they will be of little help if you do not implement the entire scope of safe work practices. What's the point of encrypting DICOM tags if anyone can log into your computer, or if a virus can ravage your entire image database? Securing and safeguarding the *entire medical imaging workflow* is the most solid approach to digital health. Not only will this protect the DICOM files, but all other pieces of confidential information in the bargain. You should recognize this practice by now as the familiar HIPAA (Health Insurance Portability and Accountability Act) approach, which provides you with a strong grip over when, how, and who had access to the confidential information. Based on my own experience, let me offer a few practical tidbits on keeping your operation secure:

1. All medical images (as well as other confidential data) should reside on a separate, dedicated server. The banality of this statement, unfortunately, often becomes obvious only after something has already been compromised or deleted. Your medical imaging enterprise should function pretty much like a bank, where even the best customer does not have access to other accounts. The server should be placed in a secure location, its password should be available only to a closed circle of administrators (but more than one), and it should be changed on a regular basis. No other programs or users should be hosted on this server.[9]
2. The critical data on the server should be backed up regularly (at least daily) to another external disk, server, or remote backup provider (depending on your budget and network).
3. Despite any financial or technical reason you might have, *never* share servers with other medical enterprises. Medical imaging startups tend to do this to split costs

---

[9] I cannot tell you how many times I have seen folders like "MyWeddingPics/" on clinical server desktops!

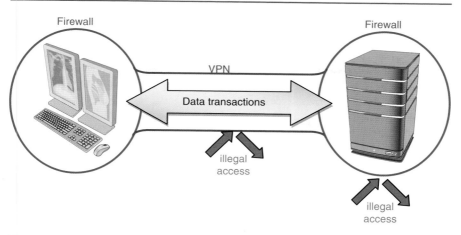

Fig. 11.6 VPNs and firewalls

and often run into serious security problems later. If you absolutely need it, set up a separate server for your sharing needs, but do not compromise the main one.

4. Be in charge of your defense. I have seen many hospitals fall prey to (often outsourced) IT groups with change-adverse authoritarian mentality. When the time comes to do a minor security update – such as creating a VPN tunnel to another partner – the entire task degrades into a never-ending saga with documents, committees, meetings, and managers gnawing on the simplest problem. As a result, nothing gets done and radiologists often hang their heads in despair: it is easier to drive to the new partner with a flash drive in a pocket than to network with their servers. Out-of-control security simply compromises the entire security model, and invites hacking as the only way to get the job done.[10]
5. All internal users in your enterprise should have access to only their data. Their passwords should also be changed regularly.
6. Consider dividing your hospital network into two separate parts: clinical use (where all confidential data resides) and general use (for email, web-browsing, and so on). This segregation makes your clinical traffic more secure (you can isolate the clinical network from the Internet, for example), and it alleviates the bandwidth problem. Large medical image transfers would not bog down your Internet traffic, and the usual lunch-time email peak pattern would not slow down your PACS.
7. All external connections to your network should go via Virtual Private Network (VPN) or a similar data-encrypting channel. Your computers should be located behind a firewall. In case you are not familiar with the difference between a VPN and a firewall, here it is in a nutshell in Fig. 11.6. A firewall only protects each

---

[10] For that reason, out-of-control security promotes the use of firewall-independent DICOM applications relying on web-browsers, emails (see Sect. 13.5) and other indirect channels to break free from authoritarian IT management. However, this does not justify mismanaged security.

computer from prohibited external access (hacking), while a VPN protects the entire communication between two computers (network). If you rely on a firewall only (which is often the case), data sent from your computer to another over a public network is still unsecured, and can be intercepted and compromised. VPN will encrypt the data when it is being transmitted, thus protecting it from any unauthorized access.

8. There is a wealth of administrative software that can monitor your server performance and automatically notify you of critical issues. I have seen cases where PACS servers lost data because their disks became full and they could not store or send anything else; but no one discovered the problem for days.

9. Do not rely on user guides; test any new protocol or function that you plan to implement. In the case of PACS, this can be automated image prefetching, automated deletion, and more. Test every feature and function before assuming that they will run correctly. I was working with one hospital in which the radiologists were sending reports by email client, embedded into PACS interface before they realized – *7 months later* – that the client was not properly configured.

10. Avoid overloading your system. For example, do not run several important tasks at once. First of all, this can result in freezing, or crashing. Second, this can produce unpredictable results. Think about running image import and auto delete at the same time – partially deleting the newly imported files. Use task scheduling to spread the load.

Just Log into My Server
A popular way of sharing imaging data, especially for small teleradiology projects, is letting your business partner or offsite radiologist log into your imaging server remotely to view images. Do not do this! It is indeed the easiest way to view your images remotely. It is also the easiest way to compromise your security and to kill your entire business with a couple of misplaced mouse clicks.
Please invest in a well-structured teleradiology system from the start. If you're sharing needs are low, use a secure file-sharing provider.

Did I forget to mention power backups, access logs, and antivirus software? Computers automatically locking screens after some 15-minute timeout? I do not want to go into the depths of network security in this medical imaging book, so here comes the most important advice of all: *There is no way a contemporary medical imaging enterprise of any size can function without a cautious, well-trained system administrator.* The sooner you hire one, the better.

Finally, I would like to say a few passionate words to lay bare the most common fallacy of achieving computer security – eliminating computers. How many times have we been through hospitals, research institutions, and imaging centers where the mantra *"the fewer computers and networks the better"* was recited as the quintessential approach to clinical security? How many old, DOS-era systems have we seen around long after their time, maintained under the pretext that *"they are more secure than the new ones?"* Sure, current hackers do not mess with Windows 3.1 anymore. Why should they if these systems do not even implement basic user and file security? Anyone walking by can do whatever they please with them. Can you imagine a bank with wide-open bamboo doors, simply because they believe that *"no locks attract no thieves?"*

> **"I'm Kinda Busy"**
> Bradley Manning, the principal contributor of a major U.S. military documents leak to WikiLeaks, achieved his goal with the most primitive tools: downloading classified cables to his pop-music CDs. "Listened and lip-synced to Lady Gaga's *Telephone* while exfiltratrating [sic] possibly the largest data spillage in American history.[11]" Not exactly the stuff of 007 movies!
> While we may have different opinions on his motives, his remark on "weak servers, weak logging, weak physical security" is worth keeping in mind. Wide-open honey pots attract bees, sooner or later.

The "fewer computers, better security" approach is nothing but a fanciful attempt to justify stone-age management, disguise ignorance, and quite often, conceal financial abuse at the site. This becomes painfully obvious when the inevitable lightning strikes; and with Jurassic mentality and hardware, one has no means of recovering or protecting permanently lost data. Having a well-developed, well-structured, contemporary network with adequate hardware/software and a qualified IT staff is the only foundation for building sane and pragmatic clinical security.

---

[11]http://en.wikipedia.org/wiki/Bradley_Manning

This brings us back to the absolute importance of pure DICOM standardization. There is no *our DICOM* vs. *their DICOM*. If company X's claims that its device can store its images on another DICOM server, then it becomes company X's responsibility to make it work with *any* server – the one from company Y included. Your knowledge of your DICOM provider's Conformance Statement becomes your main line of defense in any DICOM compatibility argument; it is their documented claim to what the device does, and how it conforms to the standard.

12.4 DICOM from a Black Box

Have you ever wondered why, when you buy a DICOM unit and you see on your bill a list of items for things related to DICOM output (DICOM compatibility, DICOM connectivity, and so on)? Shouldn't these items be included in the unit cost? Not really, and for several reasons.

First of all, while DICOM meticulously explains the required *external* functionality of any DICOM device, it's really up to the manufacturer to decide what happens *inside* the device. DICOM only describes the exterior, and not the interior. In fact, most manufacturers design proprietary standards to run their DICOM units and software. Then, only when they are required to talk to DICOM devices from other DICOM providers will the internal proprietary format be converted into external DICOM output. When you pay for DICOM on the outside, you are paying for that proprietary internal-format-to-DICOM translator that the manufacturer has to add to the unit to make it truly DICOM-compliant.

Second, the use of internal proprietary standards certainly brings several important advantages to medical device manufacturers. Mainly, it gives them the freedom to do whatever they like without being bound by standard requirements. Indirectly, this may affect the results and the performance of your clinical projects (we have already seen a few examples in Sect. 9.11). Take our favorite company X and company Y case: let's say that company X has developed its own proprietary medical standard, XCOM, which is used to connect all X devices. You might come to a clinical site and hear a story like this:

> At first, we tried to use company Y's server with our company X's MRI, but image transfer was so sloooow, and we could not get some important information out! So we bought a DICOM server from X, and now it works like a charm!

Does this mean that X implements DICOM better? Certainly not. Simply, in addition to DICOM, all devices from company X speak XCOM, which provides richer internal information and substantially facilitates the X-to-X workflow. When you interface two DICOM devices from X, they might recognize each other as such, and switch to XCOM. If it seems to work better on the outside, do not rush to blame it on Y (Fig. 12.1).

Add to this scenario the wealth of DICOM providers, multiply by the never-ending company merging and outsourcing, and you will see a large, boiling mix of X, Y, and Z "DICOMs" floating around. Eventually, every large DICOM

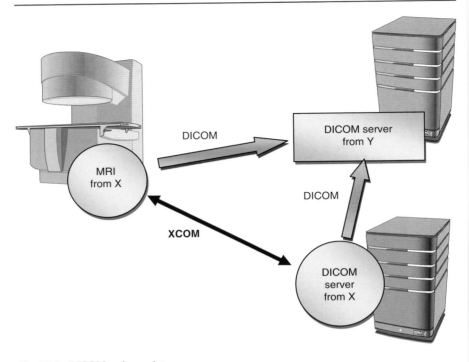

Fig. 12.1 DICOM and proprietary

market player promotes its proprietary standards as universally adopted. When this is done for marketing reasons, it certainly dilutes the fundamentality of pure DICOM. It confuses end-users and downgrades the efficiency of any medical enterprise. Compared to many proprietary protocols, DICOM is neither *slower* nor *less-efficient*. More often than not, pure DICOM is simply neglected and not implemented properly. Enforcing DICOM compatibility and requiring clean DICOM support from all your DICOM providers still remains your main tool in building an efficient and manufacturer-independent medical imaging network.

12.5 "Home-Made" DICOMs

This little section is meant for IT gurus and their administrators. Whereas knowledge of DICOM helps you deal with compatibility problems, lack of such knowledge often lures one into creating dysfunctional medical islands running on their own protocols. Why deal with DICOM if it is so complex and even expensive?

Here are a few scenarios we have dealt with many, many times:
1. A clinic buys a medical device but does not pay for its DICOM compatibility – just to save some money. As is often believed, a DICOM device is a DICOM

device anyway, and with a little help from a local computer science student, the missing compatibility part can easily be *enabled*. We should all realize by now how far this belief is from reality. Not only won't you be able to hack into a complex (and totally foreign) internal proprietary standard of your medical device, but also you will also void the manufacturer's warranty – that is, if you manage not to break the unit completely. If you find yourself in this unfortunate situation of missing DICOM on a DICOM-capable unit, do not try to get creative. Contact your device manufacturer and try to acquire all the necessary DICOM upgrades.

2. A clinic, puzzled by the infernal intricacies of 16 DICOM volumes, decides to develop *its own* medical system. To *standardize* the process, the new system is based on some MS Access database with a couple of Visual Basic forms, possibly accompanied by an A3 flatbed scanner to scan the films. Wrong, wrong, wrong move! This *solution* is nothing but a primitive patchwork: nonstandard, nonscalable and, in the long run, very expensive. In addition to this, keep in mind that any nonstandard software dies the very next day after its developer quits. Finally, you are reinventing the wheel; throwing away 20-plus years of solid DICOM experience and trying to develop a system that would never even approach ACR-NEMA 1.0. Your time, money, and effort will simply be wasted on creating some isolationist software that no other device understands.

3. A hospital with existing Hospital Information System (HIS, we will see more of it in Chap. 14) decides to add medical images to its digital HIS records. But instead of buying a fully functional PACS system as they should, they implement some simple DICOM-to-BMP software, converting DICOM data from the modalities into HIS-compatible multimedia formats (bitmaps, PDFs, JPEGs, … – pick anything). Now they have digital imaging integrated into HIS! What a feast! And who needs these DICOM troubles anyway? Well, if you care about your patients and diagnostic image quality – *you* do!

4. A small clinic decides to implement teleradiology, so they use a remote desktop access application (such as LogMeIn or WebEx – your choice again) on their imaging computers to view the images from outside of their network. Sure, it does something, but what exactly? The answer: it wastes your time, network traffic, and once again downgrades the image display quality. You cannot treat your DICOM data as screenshots or video feeds. Remember one thing: all teleconferencing tools are great: for teleconferencing – as they should be. They are not substitutes for DICOM display or networking. Don't eat your soup with a fork.

Stick to the standard! Use DICOM!

12.6 Open-Source DICOM

When commercial solutions become too expensive and home-made solutions too primitive, many institutions and departments take chances using open-source DICOM software. Open-source software is typically distributed free to the general public along with the complete software source code, which the public can modify to its liking. In essence, open-source attempts to blend the flexibility of home-made (you can modify it any way you like) and the reliability of commercially distributed (what is written, tested, and used by many is more likely to be bug-free and more standard-compliant). Many open-source applications originate from academic institutions or research groups that took the effort to transform the scientifically viable into the practically applicable.

Open-source has become a religion for many of us, opposed to the Big Corporate Brother who sells us underdeveloped, proprietary, and expensive products while having no interest in human creativity or software efficiency. I am not an advocate of commercial proprietary monopolies either, but let's put our personal views aside and consider the problems from a practical point of view. Open-source offers certain advantages to be sure, but do not ignore the potential problems:

Advantages of Open-Source:
1. Often comes free – at least for noncommercial use.
2. Tends to be pretty standard and is not influenced by any particular proprietary format or manufacturer.
3. Because of the above, it tends to be reasonably popular within a diverse audience, which ensures that it is constantly used and tested, and problems are being fixed.
4. If you are really into coding, it provides a nice foundation for adding your own functionality on the fly simply by adding your own source code.
5. Sometimes, it just makes you feel good.

Problems with Open-Source:
1. *Free*, unfortunately, means no contractual responsibilities, and no dedicated support/maintenance. If anything happens, you are on your own.
2. Rarely have sufficient medical clearances and certifications (they are expensive to begin with).
3. Originally developed for limited problem scope; does not scale well to complex projects and diverse clinical environments.
4. Having the software source open to you can rarely buy you anything. Implementations of complex things such as DICOM take thousands and thousands of code lines. If you want to modify something in there, you will need a set of very skilled and professional developers (and *that* will cost you).
5. Because of problem 1 above, software bugs still exist, even in the most popular open-source software.

As a result, open-source products usually fit best with audiences similar to those where open-source usually comes from: relatively small, well-confined, research-oriented groups – such as clinical scientists. Those groups are not facing industrial data loads, pressures of real-life healthcare, or even liability problems. Nor are they burdened by huge budgets, which makes open-source an even better match. In a real hospital where problems need to be resolved immediately while complying with a defined chain of responsibilities, open-source will quickly become a challenge.

Open-source often blends into commercial products. On one hand, commercial developers might *borrow* things from the open-source – sometimes without giving enough credit to the open-source developers. On the other hand, commercial developers sometimes *contribute* commercial source code to the open-source domain, without getting appropriate permissions from their companies. All this keeps pouring gas on

12.6 Open-Source DICOM

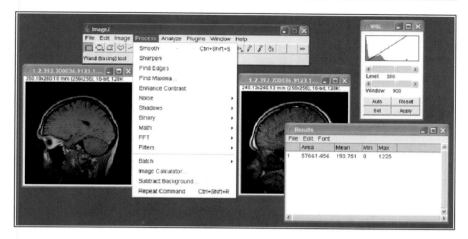

Fig. 12.2 Running Image J. Note manual controls (such as window/level window in the top right corner), separate windows per each tool/image, filters and mathematical functions – typical attributes of scientific software, rarely found in PACS

the flames of never-ending legal battles between the open-source community and commercial, closed-source companies – battles that rarely benefit any side.

The best known open-source DICOM software is probably Osirix (http://osirix-viewer.com). At the time this book was written, Osirix[3] was running on Apple computers only, but since Apple started adopting Intel processors, it widened the range of its potential users. (A lighter Osirix app has even been made available for the iPhone.)

On one recent occasion, we attempted connecting Osirix to another PACS at our radiology department. Osirix worked nicely for relatively small studies (below 200 images), but couldn't extend to larger loads. At the same time, Osirix offers excellent 3D rendering that otherwise would cost thousands of dollars. This example nicely illustrates the pros and cons listed above: the product may not be fit for the industrial use, but it does provide excellent complementary functionality. In fact, I would like to thank the Osirix R&D group for their outstanding efforts. They proved that many great things can still be developed by a few bright individuals, simply knowing what they are doing (Fig. 12.2).

Another popular open-source project is the ImageJ DICOM viewer (http://rsbweb.nih.gov/ij/). Programmed in the platform-independent Java language, it can run on virtually any system, offering a blend of most basic and rather scientific DICOM tools (consider image math like square roots). If you want to have a DICOM image viewer that is not restricted by your computer operating system (Windows, Mac OS, or Linux), this is a good choice. On the other hand, viewers such as ImageJ were clearly designed for imaging scientists, do not provide PACS functionality, and will likely get many clinical radiologists lost in layers of unknown image processing options.

---

[3]Version 3.8.1.

Want to Go Commercial?

It has become a trend over the past few years for research-minded, open-source-oriented groups to go commercial. If you decide to do the same, do not forget to bridge the gap between your research product and what is expected in a demanding clinical workflow. Designing a simple straightforward interface, using clear and accurate terminology, optimizing performance, implementing load balancing, and considering tolerance to data and input diversity are just a few items on the most essential list defining "research-to-commercial" software conversion.

If proper software does not happen, it becomes extremely visible to the clinical guys. Using one practical example, I have seen PACS software asking "Use recursion?" in reference to opening multiple images. Just think about how many doctors would answer this prompt right. In another case, the buttons on the software interface were overlapping – literally (as crazy as it may sound), only because no one from the "post-research" vendor company bothered to test it on different monitors, and it did not matter for the research guys anyway.

My fellow research colleagues, if you decided to commercialize your inventions, please do not embarrass yourselves and do not invite problems for your customers. Hire professional developers to clean your products before selling them to the medical community.

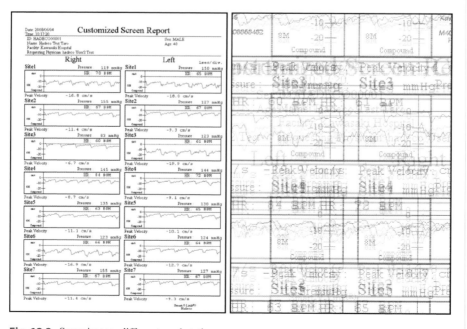

Fig. 12.3 Same image, different workstations

12.7 DICOM Validation Tools

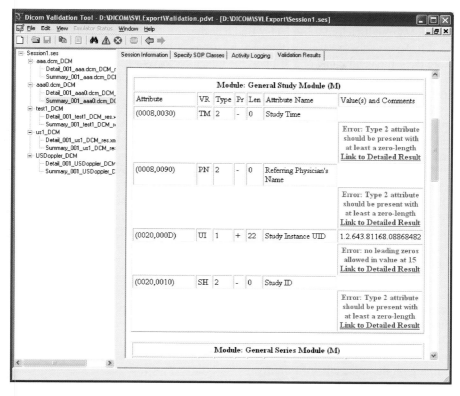

Fig. 12.4 The above DICOM image, analyzed in DICOM Validation Toolkit. You can clearly see DICOM format errors – missing tags, errors in data formats

If you are interested in exploring DICOM development further, take a look at Chap. 17 of this book.

12.7 DICOM Validation Tools

Being a complex and ever-changing standard, some DICOM guidelines, rules, and formats can be understood (or misunderstood) in many different ways. Moreover, as we already know, there are rules and formats that can be required, optional, conditional, and entirely dependent on the particular modality. As a result, making a correct DICOM object takes some time and effort – not always wisely invested. Creating semivalid DICOM objects, files, or images are commonplace.

Here is a very typical scenario. Your PACS application makes an image, and it looks like the one in Fig. 12.3 (left). Then the same application sends this image to another DICOM workstation, and it displays there as Fig. 12.3 (right). What is wrong? You start pulling your hair out, calling your DICOM engineers, then they start pulling their hair out, but the image is not getting any better. Different color format? Wrong byte order in pixels? Bad hair day?

What makes these cases particularly hilarious is when both workstations come from the same vendor and one displays the image correctly while the other does not. In fact, this is how I made Fig. 12.3; I used a PACS terminal and a standalone workstation from the same well-reputed vendor.

You would never imagine that this could happen because some "Referring Physician Name" tag was missing. That is, you could spend hours troubleshooting the image settings when in fact the origin of your problem might be in a totally different place that would never enter your mind.

This is when DICOM validation tools come in very handy. While it might require a little time to get used to, the DICOM Validation Toolkit (DVT) from DICOM@OFFICE group (http://dicom.offis.de) is one of the most popular and liberally licensed applications that you can use to help troubleshoot such problems. Figure 12.4 shows how the DICOM Validation Toolkit dissects the DICOM object shown in Fig. 12.3. You can take this hard evidence to your PACS vendor, making a much more solid argument about your DICOM problems.

It's hard to develop DICOM validation software without implementing DICOM – I'd say, it is plain impossible. Therefore, all DICOM validation providers – DVT being the best example – are also known for their DICOM implementations used in third-party products. I have seen DICOM@OFFICE library in virtually any free DICOM viewer, and some commercial products as well. This is another reason for using this validation tool – it makes you compliant with countless DICOM software, running on the same DICOM library.

Part V
Advanced Topics

Wouldn't it be excruciatingly boring to deal with some 20-year-old standard without being able to apply it to the most interesting things in today's digital imaging? When DICOM was born, surrounded by Stone Age computers of the 1980s, it was very much ahead of its time. Today, DICOM is constantly at risk of falling behind. Expanding clinical networks, increasingly complex hardware, and the advancement of the entire radiology workflow challenge not only the standard, but any current tools and abilities – human included. DICOM is forced to evolve daily, struggling to adapt to technological progress and new realities.

In this part of the book, we will entertain ourselves with an overview of the most dynamic areas of digital medicine, and the challenges they present.

DICOM and Teleradiology 13

When PACS started gaining popularity in the late 1990s, they instantly proved a very important concept: there is no limit on how far computer networks can transfer digital data. Surprisingly, it took several years to realize that this concept could become a powerful tool in rebuilding the entire medical workflow. For too long, PACS users, developers, and administrators were much more preoccupied with imaging rather than networking. As a result, the road to making medicine truly *tele*, or distance-independent, took a few interesting turns before returning to the PACS domain. Its history is worth a quick review.

13.1 Can I See the Image?

As we learned in Sect. 9.10, to make PACS work, DICOM has always relied upon point-to-point connections between any two units. This artificial constraint inherently limited PACS to a few neighboring offices in the same radiology department. The classical PACS or DICOM implementations were not really any more *remote* or *tele* than a stethoscope; rather, they were multimonitor extensions of their digital modalities. Besides, even though the need for remote clinical data transfer was realized a long time ago, it was hampered by DICOM imperfections that were accompanied by the inadequate hardware of the time – mostly networks. The inertia and conservatism of traditional clinical practitioners also contributed to keeping PACS *locally minded*.

> **Nota Bene**
> Theoretically, nothing prevents one from connecting two very remote computers in a point-to-point pair; provided that they are networked and have static IP addresses. However, this would link two remote networks, raising many potential security and workflow concerns. This is why point-to-point connections between remote devices or PACS were judged very unsafe and were rarely used in practice. The problem was exacerbated by the lack of security protocols in previous DICOM editions.

On the other hand, mankind has been experimenting with telemedicine applications for at least a century before the proliferation of PACS. In 1905, Dutch physician Willem Einthoven (invented the electrocardiogram – ECG) started transmitting ECGs from the hospital to his laboratory 1.5 km away via telephone cable. I greatly respect and admire his vision; but a century later, many hospitals are still fighting with the same "1.5 km" problem: they are unable to efficiently transmit their data anywhere beyond a couple of reading rooms.

It's no wonder then that, while PACS were battling with those technical and logistical problems, similar and somewhat *lighter* approaches were explored. These approaches were easy to implement, often did not require any special or expensive equipment, and more importantly, could easily be done by the doctors without relying on slow-moving administrative or technical resources.

In the early 1960s, a classic and widespread example of transmitting medical data remotely was achieved by sending electrocardiograms over phone lines (just like Dr. Einthoven prescribed). It worked well even then. First, because ECGs were much smaller in data size compared to digital images, they matched the low bandwidth of the phone lines. Second, even half a century ago, phone lines were already in place, thus providing a ready-to-use infrastructure. Finally, ECGs were conveniently transmitted in their original analog format, which was very handy before the entire spectrum of data digitizing techniques had been worked out.

By the 1990s, these and similar experiments gave rise to a new innovation called *telemedicine*, which addressed all possible ways of providing clinical services remotely. Back then, the most typical features of telemedicine projects included:
1. Using standard (often analog) networks and equipment to transfer data remotely: ISDN,[1] TCP/IP, analog lines.
2. Using standard multimedia formats for clinical data: for example, converting images to JPEGs, AVIs, or word-processing documents.
3. Using standard teleconferencing software and hardware (online meetings, internet chat-like applications, web-cameras, faxes, and so on) for remote consultations.
4. Lack of any serious PACS interface or DICOM support.

In brief, at that time the word "medicine" in "telemedicine" was reflecting only a particular choice of *data*, but not the choice of *tools*. The same systems could have been used for telematchmaking, telecooking, tele-practically-anything-else. In one respect, this generality made many early telemedicine projects popular and easy to use – no learning curves, no complex installations.

Unfortunately, the same generality that contributed to the spread of telemedicine applications has also become its main limitation. While telemedicine systems proved to be important and efficient in areas such as remote education, they never really made it to the heart of medical imaging: radiology (here they were sarcastically nicknamed *talking heads*[2]). The main reason for this failure was the lack of sophistication and relevant radiology-specific imaging tools, crucial for remote image reading.

---

[1] Integrated Services Digital Network.
[2] Referring to the videoconferencing.

> **Stealth Teleradiology**
> There is another important reason for web-based teleradiology clients. For pure convenience, reading radiologists in many hospitals would like to run their teleradiology projects on the same viewing workstations they use for their local hospital PACS. However, PACS vendors would definitely oppose installing third-party teleradiology software on their workstations. Light web-based clients do not require installation, and therefore can be run on any computer without violating local PACS policies.

When teleradiology started to flourish some 10 years ago, nearly all major PACS providers offered some variety of their own *light* teleradiology solutions. In almost all cases, those solutions were the same old heavy PACS workstations reprogrammed to run in web browser interfaces – definitely, a quick-and-dirty fix that hardly solved any teleradiology problem. Running a 20-megabyte PACS plug-in in a web browser is no different from simply installing a full-blown PACS workstation on your computer. You still need certain software libraries, certain very restrictive system requirements, high network bandwidth, often static IP addresses, and many more things to make it work – just as you needed all this in conventional PACS. A serious teleradiology system should solve all these problems rather than put them on the users' shoulders. Let's emphasize this once again: a true mobile teleradiology system should work with virtually any contemporary client computer and network, and should not require any heavyweight installations. Asking your remote expert to go out and buy another computer just to be compatible with your teleradiology system does not make any sense (Fig. 13.3).

> **Personal Experience**
> Many of these lessons were learned the hard way when my friends and I started one of the first teleradiology companies in the late 1990s. We knew what we were trying to achieve, but even in the late 1990s the state of computer technology was very diverse and far from sitting on common ground. Microsoft, Sun, and a few others were fighting to promote their solutions to building web projects (the essence of the teleradiology user interface). DICOM was still not addressing this problem (as it does now partially with PS3.18). PACS provided no universal interface for exporting data outside of PACS networks. Eventually, we managed to solve all these problems, but it took several years for us and for the technology to mature. When I read DICOM PS3.18 now, I see many things that we designed back then for our product, and I can confess that building a true teleradiology application is not easy.

There is no way one can satisfy the above teleradiology requirements without mobilizing the entire set of modern programming, data-sharing, and image-processing

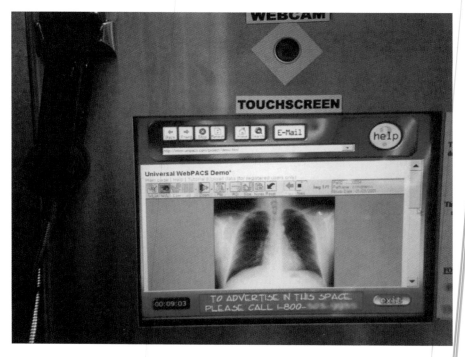

Fig. 13.3 Behold, smartphone addicts: here is what we did some 10 years ago. Conceptually, this is lightweight teleradiology at its best. With a system we developed, we were able to pull and display full-quality DICOM images even from other, third-party PACS. Our system would run on virtually any internet-enabled device, such as this antiquated pay phone at an airport. You can laugh at the phone, but can you do the same now?

techniques. In fact, as we have outlined, teleradiology cannot rely on any assumptions about the client computer. In order to survive, teleradiology applications must be software-smart. In particular:

1. There is no teleradiology without advanced image compression algorithms. If a teleradiology system relies only on good old JPEG, it is pitiful and won't serve the purpose. It should take full advantage of the much more appropriate and diagnostically safe compression methods such as JPEG2000 and JPEG-LS (see Sect. 6.2). Compression is also the only way to overcome slow network bandwidth.
2. DICOM implementation for teleradiology systems must be much more flexible and stable, compared to what we see in contemporary PACS. First, DICOM in a teleradiology system will have to work with a variety of other PACS and DICOM clients – absolutely no place for playing *proprietary games* here. Second, a teleradiology DICOM implementation must be much more forgiving for potential problems – such as broken network connections – automatically recovering from them whenever possible.

13.3 Teleradiology

3. Teleradiology must rely on security and data-encryption protocols such as RSA, Triple-DES, and SHA. Because external security setups (VPNs for example) are not always available, teleradiology solutions must be fully capable of securing their data themselves.
4. Teleradiology applications should inevitably comprise two major parts: server and client. Designing their interaction and carefully balancing the computational load between server and client is essential. The client should run on any computer, be small in size, and intuitive in interface. The server should be the processing brain and the data warehouse. These very uneven parts should connect seamlessly and spare users from any extra work or decision making.
5. The teleradiology client should support dynamic image manipulations (window/level, zooming, panning, certain reconstructions, and so on). Delegating all these functions to the server will make the teleradiology solution extremely network-dependent. The need for a smart, data-processing client immediately rules out simple static HTML-based web pages and calls for advanced web client technology such as JavaScript and AJAX, or even more powerful Java.[6]
6. Teleradiology apps should have versions tailored to run on the most popular multimedia devices: iPhones, Androids, and tablet PCs for example. This enormously increases the reach of teleradiology projects, allowing the participants to remain productive at any time.

It takes time to teach the clinical community not to fall for simple and cheap teleradiology substitutes. For example, we have noted that teleradiology succeeded *email radiology* and, in fact, the first teleradiology systems did not look much different. They had the ability to retrieve DICOM images from PACS, but then the images were converted into static JPEGs and posted online as static HTML pages – very much like email attachments or your online photo album. First, those images were impossible to manipulate: essential radiology tools such as window/level were not available. Second, to minimize image size, the exported JPEG images were often compressed with shockingly high lossy compression, annihilating any diagnostic quality of the original images. *Pretty* and *easy* often do not mean *clinically adequate*.

However, when properly implemented, teleradiology turns into a revolutionary tool, appreciably improving any clinical project. In remote areas, in small hospitals, in imaging centers, and simply in many places where an expert opinion cannot be available on a 24/7 basis, teleradiology systems have proven to be extremely efficient and productive (Fig. 13.4). At the same time, many large hospitals were able to survive through crises by providing teleradiology outsourcing to others – which often was the only way to maintain large radiology staff. Besides, in large well-staffed hospitals where clinical personnel can often be dispersed and dedicated to many different tasks, teleradiology added the ability to instantly check images on any networked computer (PACS or not), work from home, and respond to emergencies – thus eliminating many PACS bottlenecks. Teleradiology brought images to many PACS-neglected areas, such as the OR and ED rooms. I have seen many radiologists who became advocates of teleradiology systems simply because they would save an

---

[6]ActiveX, supported by Internet Explorer browser, becomes increasingly marginal technology.

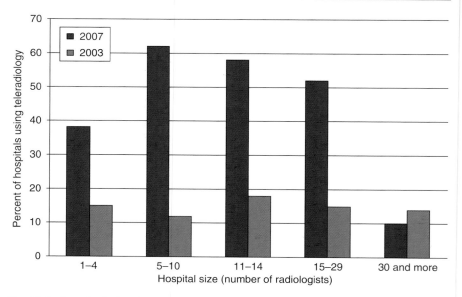

Fig. 13.4 Growth of teleradiology in US hospitals – year 2007 vs. 2003 (Lewis et al. 2009)

extra hour of commuting in a traffic jam – an hour that could make the difference when trying to save someone's life.

In the end, we have every reason to hope that gradually teleradiology gateways will become an integral part of any PACS solution, transforming the latter into mobile and easy-to-reach systems.

13.4 DICOM and WWW

We have to admit that DICOM, at least in its classical incarnation, was probably the least-suited tool for teleradiology solutions. The reasons are well-known:
1. The rigid, point-to-point logic of DICOM connectivity makes a connection to a dynamically changing remote client (such as a web user) impossible. The approach lacks the ability to relay data transfers.
2. Lack of integration with multimedia and WWW software such as web browsers.
3. Lack of control over the exported image quality (such as lossy compression ratio, impossible to negotiate at DICOM handshake).
4. Lack of download status controls. In standard DICOM, it is almost impossible to tell when the requested study will be downloaded and how large it is.
5. Lack of delayed and interrupted download support.[7]
6. Lack of user account management.

---

[7] As opposed to, for example, many FTP download clients that can resume interrupted downloads.

13.4 DICOM and WWW

As a result, many teleradiology companies had to develop their own, nonstandard DICOM extensions, eventually sliding into the same chasm of self-occlusion and incompatibility that made telemedicine applications so hard to manage. Several years ago, I was also involved in a similar process for the teleradiology company we founded. Although it was extremely interesting technically, the feeling that we were fixing an outdated standard – inadequate for the task – often loomed, contributing to the doldrums in the development team. And the disquieting feeling of diluting the standard with nonstandard solutions was even worse; we were merely putting lipstick on a pig.

The DICOM committee realized the need for standardized teleradiology extensions and released part 18 (PS3.18) proudly named "Web Access to DICOM Persistent Objects (WADO)." It is currently the smallest of all the DICOM parts (not counting the PS3.1 brief introduction) and contains things that are often more declarative than complete. Nevertheless, it does create a sense of direction and it does provide several standardized mechanisms for implementing web-based DICOM – the key to any teleradiology or remote-access imaging system.

What are the main highlights of the PS3.18 approach to providing DICOM on the web?

First, PS3.18 introduces the idea of the *DICOM persistent object* – a securely allocated instance of a standard DICOM object that can be stored for some period of time. The most important types of DICOM persistent objects include text and images (single or multiframe, encoded in JPEG, GIF, PNG, and JPEG2000). These object instances, no surprise, have their own unique identifiers (UID, see Sect. 5.5.8) and are meant to be transmitted to web clients (web users, viewing images in their web browsers). Because web browsers are based on the HyperText Transfer Protocol (HTTP), and have no idea of what DICOM is, this transmission needs to be done in HTTP format – the same format used to load any web page.

Part PS3.18 proposes an HTTP-compatible version of the classic DICOM query and retrieval requests. All basic elements such as annotations, regions of interest, anonymization, window/level, and more are supported and can be provided as parameters in web requests, using URL syntax. For example, a task of retrieving a region of a DICOM image that has been converted to JPEG2000, rescaled, and contains the patient and technical annotations produces the following HTTP request (as one large URL string with parameters):

```
https://YourHospitalServer/imageaccess.js?requestType=WADO
&studyUID=1.2.250.1.59.40211.12345678.678910
&seriesUID=1.2.250.1.59.40211.789001276.14556172.67789
&objectUID=1.2.250.1.59.40211.2678810.87991027.899772.2
&contentType=image%2Fjp2;level=1,image%2Fjpeg;q=0.5
&annotation=patient,technique
&columns=400
&rows=300
&region=0.3,0.4,0.5,0.5
&windowCenter=-1000
&windowWidth=2500
```

This can be typed into a web browser address window to display the resulting image. You do not need to be a DICOM or HTTP guru to read this request: parameters such as *objectUID* specify the image identifiers to be retrieved[8]; *region* defines the region of interest (ROI, measured in fractions of the images sizes); *windowCenter/ windowWidth* specify the window/level settings; and so on. A web-compatible DICOM server (that is, a DICOM server complying with PS3.18) that receives this request should retrieve the requested DICOM image, format it to the provided specifications (convert it to JPEG2000 with given resolution, ROI, and window/level) and return it to the web client browser application. Because all image formatting is done on the server side, the web client only has to display the result. It's really that simple and straightforward.

Formatting all transactions as HTTP requests serves another important purpose. These transactions can easily be inserted into various documents (such as emails) as web links, which is what they are anyway. These links can be also embedded into other hospital software – such as Hospital Information System (HIS, see Sect. 14.1) – pointing to the most critical images and binding different hospital application together. Single studies, as well as entire worklists and databases, can easily be shared in this form. A user can simply click on the transaction link to launch a browser with the requested image – a very convenient mechanism for image distribution and teleradiology in general.

In essence, PS3.18 delivers a brief yet solid standardization of *email radiology* and similar web-based systems. Nevertheless, it still provides a very limited set of tools and leaves many questions unanswered. For example, while it provides a standard web-compatible extension to classic DICOM, it makes no argument on its efficiency or applicability. Consider, for example, the suggested use of static HTTP pages. When a radiologist reviews an image, she often needs to change many image parameters (such as window/level, ROI, zoom) on the fly. Unfortunately, with the proposed model, any change of this kind would produce another request to the web-enabled DICOM server which, in turn, would have to retrieve the image, reformat it to the new specifications, and download it to the user. This constant back-and-forth server-side reformatting, even on the fastest network connection, will certainly take its toll on time, making any real-time image manipulations impossible. We have discussed this problem before. Building a functional teleradiology system requires more than simple static HTTP. Most radiology tasks need very dynamic, real-time image rendering.

Another critical functionality still missing in PS3.18 is the ability to manage remote user accounts and bind them to the DICOM data on the server; that is, controlling *who* is supposed to see *what*. Recent security requirements such as HIPAA introduced severe constraints on access to medical data, when most physicians should view only the patients assigned to them. While PS3.18 suggests the use of secure socket protocol (HTTPS, which we all use in online banking and other secure

---

[8]The objectUID would be enough to identify the object, but as you remember, DICOM requires that all higher-level UIDs be provided as well, which is why we still need to provide seriesUID and studyUID.

13.4 DICOM and WWW

web applications), this protocol secures the entire site, but does not solve the problem of limiting user access to certain parts of the data. Add here a practically unavoidable need for user privileges (administrators, read-only, write-only, suspended users) and you end up with a pretty complex user management model that needs to be programmed into any teleradiology system, which is not yet present in DICOM.

A good direction for solving many of these problems on the web – that in my opinion could have been pursued more aggressively – is the adaptation of the eXtensible Markup Language (XML) standard. XML is a more powerful extension of HTTP. PS3.18 briefly mentions XML (see more in DICOM supplement 148), but it does not make much use of it; point of fact, the entire DICOM standard can be rewritten in XML. Sure, rewriting DICOM in XML would be quite an endeavor, but it might be relatively easy if one starts on the web application side, in PS3.18. Reasons for a wider XML adaptation include:

1. XML is supported by many current standards, applications, and systems – from local to web browsers. This includes some healthcare standards, such as the most recent version of HL7 (3.0), the standard for hospital information systems.
2. XML is ideal for complex data structures, such as DICOM objects. It is already used with some of them, such as Structured Reports.
3. XML is text-based, which minimizes the dependency of the computer architecture (like Endian types that DICOM has to deal with). It also makes it far easier to understand and troubleshoot.
4. XML is present in many development environments, and is well-known to many software engineers – unlike DICOM. In the clinical application development area, it would really help to have more people knowing what they are doing.

XML management of data and security, accompanied by more functional client processing, is much closer to what current teleradiology systems do. Meanwhile, PS3.18 sets a very minimal starting point for extending DICOM into web-based, teleradiology applications. Hopefully, PS3.18 will keep growing, offering more functionality and data processing power, which are so critical in radiology – teleradiology included.

Never Fall for Buzzwords

I was recently attending a presentation from a well-known PACS company promoting their teleradiology system. From the first words, the system was labeled as truly web-based, which was emphasized throughout the presentation.

However, when we proceeded to the actual software demo, it became immediately obvious that the software did not run in a web browser (real meaning of web-based), and used the browser only for the install and initial login. The rest of the work was carried out in the large installable client component – nothing different from a standalone PACS workstation. The fact that your PACS workstation connects to a *reeeeally* remote archive does not make it web-based.

As I already pointed out several times, private industry keeps developing – and promoting – its own data exchange standards. DICOM MINT (Medical Imaging Network Transport) is a good example of competing with the standard WADO approach. Using the same HTTP-XML technology, MINT attempts to make some additional enhancements in the DICOM data-exchanging mechanism by adding the following functionality:

- Support for image metadata exchange without exchanging the images. By image metadata MINT understands all nonbinary information about the images, such as various image parameters embedded in DICOM image IODs (image width and bit depth tags, for instance). If only metadata needs to be known, transferring it without the actual images significantly minimizes the network traffic.
- Support for batch image transfers. Except for multiframe IODs, DICOM would transfer any study or series image-by-image. MINT can send all images at once, merged into a single binary buffer. This eliminates DICOM negotiations for each image download, potentially improving the transfer speed (see Fig. 9.21). Nevertheless, let's keep in mind that it is association negotiation that, at the minimal expense of very short-coded messages, makes DICOM particularly robust.
- Support for private and non-DICOM data types. Example: MINT can transfer manufacturer-specific volume data or documents. In essence, MINT treats any data as metadata (nonbinary attributes), accompanied by a list of binary objects. The latter can be used to support various data formats, private included.
- Support for tracking and synchronizing data changes (using the MINT changelog mechanism) when the same study gets modified or deleted on different servers. This cannot be done without developing new tools for a DICOM study comparison, and this is what MINT employs.

At the time this book was written, the MINT project was still under development. If you are curious about the project, you can find MINT specifications and updates at http://code.google.com/p/medical-imaging-network-transport. The site also provides a brief technical overview. In the end, only time will tell whether MINT finds it place next to DICOM and WADO.

13.5 DICOM Email

Recently, especially in teleradiology applications, DICOM email has made an interesting comeback. No, we are not talking about JPEGs stuck into email messages – that was a dead end. With more recent developments in DICOM Media Storage,[9] it has become possible to look at email from a very different and fresh perspective.

Here is the main idea: if it's easy and common to write DICOM files onto flash drives, CDs, and DVDs, what prevents us from considering an email message as another sort of file media? Nothing really. So, we can define the same types of file sets, services (FSC, FSR, FSU), and media applications as we discussed in Chap. 10,

---

[9] See Chap. 10 of this book and PS3.10–3.12 of the DICOM standard.

13.5 DICOM Email

but now for working with email messages. This is exactly what was done in PS3.12 Annex K and a couple of DICOM supplements: extending DICOM applications to support email as DICOM media exchange protocol.

Why do we keep coming back to email though? Isn't it enough to have PACS? Ideally, yes, because email was never meant to support the same scale of volume and robustness required for hospital-level digital imaging. Consequently, email has never been meant to compete with DICOM networks. But the reality is that many imaging facilities – and most individual practitioners (radiologists, experts) – do not have PACS and might not have it anytime soon. In applications such as teleradiology, connecting all these people becomes the most essential task; and if no PACS are available, we can use CDs, DVDs, and yes, even email.

Without going into the nitty gritty (much of which are still either unsupported, or *work in progress* in DICOM working groups[10]), DICOM email can be viewed as the exchange of DICOM data over email protocol. That is, instead of standard DICOM networking built on top of the TCP/IP protocol, we build DICOM email on top of SMTP (Simple Mail Transfer Protocol) networking.[11] This involves several steps.

First of all, DICOM files must be converted into text because only text is genuinely supported by all email programs. As we know, DICOM files are binary; they are written as sequences of binary bytes, not text characters. However, there is a standard that does this conversion: MIME (Multipurpose Internet Mail Extensions[12]). MIME is already routinely used in email: all files attached to email messages become MIME-encoded before they are sent to their destinations. So, just like with any other data encoding, DICOM reserves Transfer Syntax to represent MIME encapsulation: 1.2.840.10008.1.2.6.1 (see DICOM Supplement 54).

There also should be a mechanism for dealing with large data sizes, so typical for medical images. Have you noticed that your email program might not let you attach more than 10 MB to a single message? Remember, email was originally designed for letters, not for CT studies. Fortunately, DICOM email can deal with large data in a reliable way. First of all, MIME can take care of the file size limit issue. When a DICOM file becomes too large it can be broken into several pieces, each of them being within the predefined limits. Second, it is not unreasonable to send one image per email. As experiments indicate, this "interleaved" transport provides the same time and performance compared to emailing image batches (Weisser et al. 2007). Third, ZIP comes in handy as a nearly universal (and lossless) data compression and packaging tool available in many applications (see Annex L in DICOM PS3.11). DICOM email software can zip your DICOM file set into a single file, apply optional encryption, and feed it into the MIME encoder (potentially breaking it into smaller chunks); the rest will follow. This completes the entire DICOM email chain, as shown in Fig. 13.5. And, thanks to encryption, even public email servers can be used without any risk to compromise confidential patient records.

---

[10] For example, it is still unclear whether DICOMDIR should be used in DICOM MIME emails.

[11] And SMTP, in turn, is based on TCP/TP.

[12] For an excellent MIME overview, see Wikipedia, http://en.wikipedia.org/wiki/MIME.

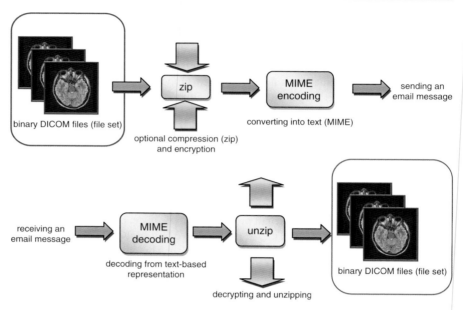

Fig. 13.5 DICOM over email: protocol view

If you attach DICOM files to email messages manually, you will attain pretty much the same results. So why bother with DICOM FSR/FSC standardization? Because DICOM MIME support opens the door for *automated email processing* that can be integrated into your PACS and teleradiology workflow (Fig. 13.6). If your DICOM application can act as a DICOM MIME FSC or FSR (see Sect. 10.3.2) – that is, if it can create emails from DICOM files, or read DICOM files from emails – you get another valuable channel for exchanging DICOM data. Email starts working for you just like any other media type – CD or DVD for example. The beauty is that with email the files will be sent to their destination nearly instantaneously, as opposed to other hard copy media.

In short, the combination of diagnostic DICOM quality and email ubiquitousness creates an attractive mix, capable of running teleradiology projects. In Germany, DICOM email was used to connect dozens of regional hospitals, with more than a million emails shared over 3 years (Weisser et al. 2007). All you need is to add a DICOM email software plug-in to your PACS workstations (some companies provide DICOM email brokers). Another obvious benefit of the DICOM email solution is that it is implemented over a functioning email channel: no networks to setup, no AEs to configure, no firewalls to open.

But before we get too excited, bear in mind that, despite its apparent simplicity, DICOM MIME email protocol was never meant to be the primary distribution channel for your image exchange projects. Rather, it should be considered the most minimal workaround when absolutely nothing else is available. DICOM email inherits many of the problems of the present DICOM media storage protocols discussed

13.5 DICOM Email

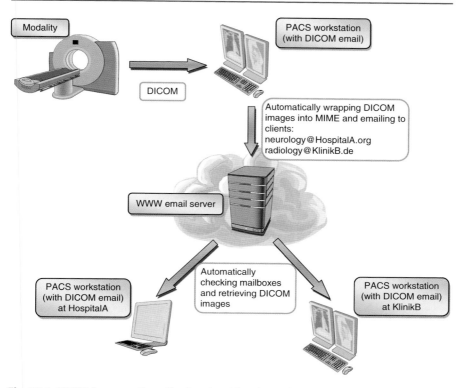

Fig. 13.6 DICOM over email: application view. Note that multiple email servers and destinations can easily be supported for fail-over cases (Weisser et al. 2007)

earlier (see Sect. 10.4). For example, it cannot query and it cannot negotiate image types or compression formats (it cannot negotiate anything, in fact). It is asynchronous; you cannot use it for real-time applications (when several radiologists should share and manipulate the same data at the same time). It can work only in the very basic, least-efficient, and most-supervised form, which makes its wide implementation rather impractical. Establishing a solid DICOM network will always provide you with much richer and more robust functionality, and this should be your ultimate goal even for low-volume teleradiology projects.

Email Limitations
Whatever transfer method you choose to use for DICOM data, you will inherit all the problems of the method. In the case of DICOM email, large DICOM data loads may easily overflow mailbox quotas; direct connection to an email server from a remote DICOM application may be rejected for security reasons; complex architecture and proprietary protocols of certain email applications

might not fit well into direct data transfer. Never assume that working through a more "popular" data exchange method will be easier compared to using the original DICOM networking.

And, as I mentioned, DICOM email implementation does need special broker software. If you see "Send as email" in your PACS interface, this almost never implies compliance with DICOM MIME FSR/FSC media storage. As always, the presence of a DICOM MIME support declaration in your application's DICOM Conformance Statement is the only means to verify that the application indeed does DICOM-compliant email transfers.

"Ubiquitous and Inexpensive Fax Machine"

Just in case you find automatic DICOM emails a bit too exotic, consider integrating your PACS with a ... fax machine. The framework and its successful use are explained in (Rothpearl et al. 2010). Certainly, we are not talking about faxing diagnostic images; but for the reports, physician notes, and patient charts automatic "DICOM faxing" can be a valuable time saver. A special software plug-in can automatically register incoming DICOM studies, and receive faxes, related to them – converting them into DICOM images, and storing them in the PACS to accompany the original image data from the modalities. If you add the simplicity of the fax machine (compared even to a flatbed scanner), that even the most computer-adverse hospital staff can handle, you would certainly appreciate the efficiency of fax-to-PACS interface.

I can't wait for DICOM Twitter ☺

13.6 Vox Populi – Vox Dei

Looking back, I remember the times when computer literacy was viewed as an advanced knowledge. Some 10 years ago, I had to train one brilliant radiologist how to double-click: the professor was 70ish years old, never used computers, and just could not get the second click timing right. For better or worse, the times have changed and many of today's kids start tapping keyboard buttons well before they learned to write. Besides, writing without a keyboard? How medieval!

In short, our patients are getting increasingly computer-proficient and even DICOM-proficient in some cases. This profoundly changes the role of the patient in the DICOM workflow, and in teleradiology in particular. Increasingly more patients want to be involved with their digital imaging. Only a few years ago, we used to give them plain films, then CDs. Now they often want to view their images online. Have you noticed "Patient login" buttons on newer clinical websites? Do you have one on yours (Fig. 13.7)?

13.6 Vox Populi – Vox Dei

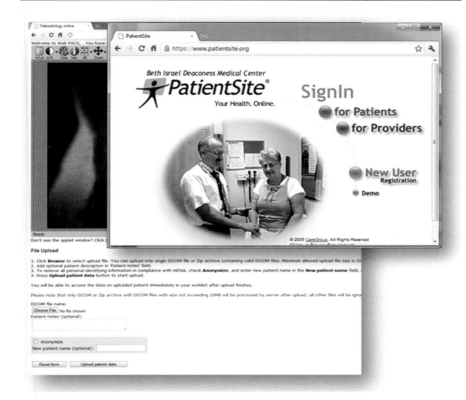

Fig. 13.7 Patients getting in charge of their medical data. "File upload" section in teleradiology website, to allow patients upload their DICOM images. "For Patients" link into a hospital EPR system, to view records, labs, appointments, and payment history online

There are several reasons for patients to be more integrated into the imaging workflow:

- As I just mentioned, medical imaging gets more and more accessible with off-the-shelf PCs, tablets, and smartphones. You do not need special overpriced hardware to look at your chest X-ray. In addition, the web is filled with free DICOM viewers; major software and OS vendors consider making DICOM one of their natively supported formats. DICOM has become quite public.
- Films, CDs, and other "material" media take time to carry and export. For patients living a few time zones away from the expert physicians they want to consult, even mailing these media sounds archaic and sluggish. Moreover, many patients now shop for doctors just like they shop for new shoes – getting in touch with many online and all over the world. Burning CDs for all of them? Hopping on a world-cruise to visit? Certainly not: if we can Google our physicians, if we can Skype them, we should be able to "DICOM" them as well!
- There are increasingly more regional and even national Electronic Patient Record (EPR) initiatives promoting unified patient records. If planned wisely, they all include providing the patients with access to their medical images and reports (Fig. 13.8).

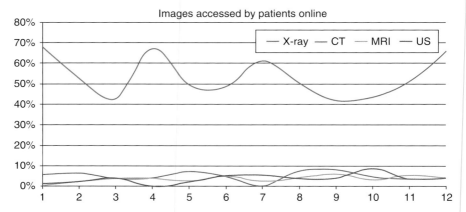

Fig. 13.8 Percent of images viewed by patients monthly in online teleradiology system in 2010; East Tallinn Central Hospital, Estonia (Ross et al. 2011). There were 3750 (11 per day) patients accessing their images from outside the hospital

- Many countries already implement electronic ID cards, which can be used to easily verify patient identity online. Many large organizations also provide their employees with IDs they can use in affiliated hospitals – including accessing their information online. This solves the perpetual problem of online confidentiality.
- With tons of medical and technical expertise available online, more patients are becoming proficient at interpreting their medical records. Well, they do not read their images *yet*; but they do want to see and understand them, especially when serious consequences are in play. Their appetite for personal health management is fueled by a multitude of online applications from Google Health and online DNA profiles to countless PDA apps. In short, "online healthcare" is getting progressively more like online banking applications where clients want to be informed and in control.
- We are all becoming increasingly mobile: changing places, hospitals, and computers. We want our clinical data to be visible to us anywhere at any time. Online patient access to hospitals and teleradiology has become inevitable.

All these factors contribute to increasing patient involvement in medical imaging projects. If you are in charge of starting one, keep them in mind. And if you want to create a vanguard implementation, consider supporting DICOM file uploading to you teleradiology system. Patients holding medical data CDs would prefer to upload their images to your company online, especially if they are contemplating some treatment at your facility. At this point, it may get quite complex: the patients will have to be able to locate DICOM files/folders on their CDs, zip them,[13] and upload them via some intuitive user interface that your system should provide. It still sounds a bit too much even for some physicians, but we live in the age of Picasa and YouTube, so many more patients are becoming comfortable with this job. Make sure your hospital is.

---

[13]Important step not only to compress, but also to upload dozens of DICOM files at once in a single package.

13.7 From PACS to PDAs?

13.7.1 "Pocket Radiology"

Netbooks, iPhones, iPods, iPads, Androids, tablets – what's next on your shopping list? The landscape of portable computing devices has changed dramatically over the past few years, creating channels for a flood of new applications. What used to be available only on desktops now easily fits into our pockets, which makes the notion of "pocket radiology" an alluring prospect as well. And do not forget the human aspect: the "Pod-Pad-Tablet" revolution has electrified the radiological community, which is more than willing to integrate new gadgets into their otherwise monotonous routines.

Well, the technology has really delivered this time: pixel pitch, brightness, and contrast of the mobile gadgets have met the American College of Radiology (ACR) requirements for medical monitors. What's more, gadget monitor resolution can easily accommodate several CT or MR images at their original size. As a result, multiple reports have demonstrated that the quality of diagnostic image interpretations even on iPhones and the like was essentially the same as on usual PACS workstations[14] – in fact, sometimes it was even *better*. Radiologists were so afraid to miss something on tablets that they looked far more carefully and found more compared to usual workstation viewing. After some debate, the U.S. Food and Drug Administration (FDA) cleared the first mobile application (www.mimsoftware.com) to be used on iPhones and iPads for diagnostic purposes (Fig. 13.9).

> **Busy Workstation? Use Your iPad!**
> The FDA cautiously suggested that the first mobile app should be used diagnostically only when "the physician does not have access to a workstation." This filled many comments with humor: there is no way to enforce this rule, or even to specify what "does not have access" implies. In essence, the gate has been opened, and little "ifs" attached to it will make no difference.

Another less expected turn was the appearance of the first truly mobile modalities. Certainly, mobile MRI trucks have been running around for years; small X-ray scanners dropped by parachute from military planes, and portable ultrasound boxes carried in cases. But in early 2011 MobiUS (mobisante.com), a smartphone-based ultrasound system, received its FDA and European clearances (Fig. 13.9). Undoubtedly, more will follow. And they should: my new smartphone gives me more disk space than my 5-year-old laptop, and offers a plethora of imaging, security, and health- and data-management apps that most PACS managers can only dream about.

---

[14] http://www.auntminnie.com/mobile.aspx?Sec=mobile&Sub=1&ItemID=93897

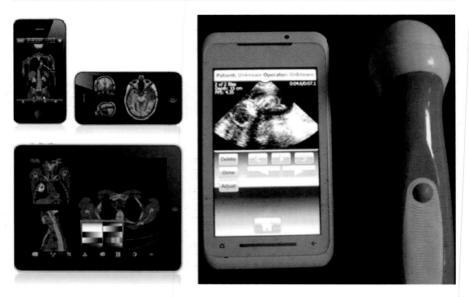

Fig. 13.9 MIM mobile diagnostic software (*left*) and MobiUS smartphone-based ultrasound machine (*right*)

What can we conclude from all of this? Because all three layers of traditional PACS architecture (Fig. 1.1) have been partially or fully implemented with mobile devices, carrying the entire PACS in your pockets no longer sounds like a joke.

But we are not there yet. Pocket CT scanners can still make a couple of Sci-Fi movies; PDAs and tablets still take significantly longer to display and to process images the right way, contributing to considerable fatigue and lack of serious image processing. Yet as I am writing this book, the rivaling gadget manufacturers are announcing their new models; and the curious public never tires from overnight lines at the computer stores. By the time you read these lines, "gadget radiology" will be advancing full speed.

What can it offer?

- *Disk space* – Not a problem. With an average DICOM study taking some 50–500 MB of disk space, an off-the-shelf computer these days can hold months of data for a small imaging center or even a midsize hospital. In addition, pocket-sized USB drives are commonplace; many people use them for offline or project-based storage. Smaller devices including cell phones can easily store several GBs of DICOM data on their SD cards, but they do not have to. Instead, they can store and display a great many medical images in compressed multimedia formats (JPEG for still images, MP3 and AVI for videos).
- *Reliability* – Because conventional computers and handhelds are primarily used as thin clients (that is, for display purposes only) the issue of reliable data storage is bypassed; all major storage and processing is done on the servers.

13.7 From PACS to PDAs?

- *Security* – Encryption is built into all contemporary networking protocols (wireless included), and various software is available to protect personal computers and storage – including remote device tracking and locking. Also, because personal devices (unlike PACS workstations) are rarely shared, they are less prone to security leaks.
- *Image viewing quality* – Current advances in conventional monitors and graphics cards (resolution and color depth) made them extremely competitive and increased their use in PACS setups. As an example, consider supporting more than eight bits (256 shades) per color channel. Previously, you would have needed a special radiological card to support 10-bit or 12-bit grayscale. Now, many high-end consumer-level graphics cards support rich color display and become more frequently used in digital medicine. PDA and tablet monitors, although 8-bit, also provide excellent contrast and brightness, sufficient for diagnostic viewing.
- *Convenience* – This aspect is commonly overlooked by technical analysis, but in many cases it is the dominant consideration. Many radiologists – like the rest of us – use conventional monitors, computers, and handhelds for most of their day-to-day tasks (checking emails, writing presentations, doing teleradiology); so they would tend to use them for medical imaging as well. People are always more productive and comfortable with something they are used to; switching between different systems or even interfaces is always awkward.
- *Role in healthcare* – Light devices such as PDAs and dictaphones are already routinely used in the other healthcare applications for electronic health records, patient registration, tracking, reporting, and dictation. Therefore, adding image data to mobile devices comes naturally and is immediately appreciated by physicians.
- *Processing power* – With little doubt, large systems can offer more processing power and more memory, making many computational tasks real time. However, beefed-up hardware is often used to compensate for inefficient software implementations. Easily 90% of contemporary digital imaging tasks (including 3D reconstructions, perfusion/diffusion/tensor analysis, volume visualizations, and other processor-intensive tasks) can be successfully executed on plain laptops, in real-time. The remaining 10% are typically immature and poorly designed technology, and will have execution problems anyway.
- *Power* – The main problem with all mobile devices is their battery life. However, technology improvements in this area are increasing battery life and making them lighter in the bargain.

In short, there is no technically unsurpassable limit that would exclude small and portable computers from radiology. On the contrary, the blend of mobility and increasing processing power can make them welcome in many parts of the medical workflow. The same should apply to application design and development: the time for mobile, decentralized DICOM software has really arrived. I hope that "pocket radiology" will make this happen, improving both DICOM and its implementations. iPhones and Droids use their own versions of programming languages, which means that you cannot take your 20-year-old PACS memorabilia code and make it run on your PDA. You will have to rewrite it. And if it gets rewritten, then (in addition to the inevitable bugs) more efficient design and processing can be implemented as well. Most current DICOM vendors have been dragging their DICOM implementations for ages, barely sweetening them with new GUI eye candies, but never taking the risk to actually look under the hood. A few hospitals I am working with still run antiquated DOS-era systems, overpaying the few remaining programmers (well into their retirement ages) as the only people who still remember how the damn things work. But I hope that some "fresh blood" will finally allow the venerable gurus to spend more time fishing, as their golden-aged DICOM applications are put out to pasture, replaced by the new breed. The "pocket radiology" revolution just might be the ticket.

Similar long-deserved updates can happen to DICOM media, which we discussed in detail in the Chap. 10. It seems that CDs, DVDs, and even flash drives are quickly becoming things of the past, giving the way to networked-based data exchange. The entire data-sharing paradigm is going into a mobile, "get it from anywhere" direction where old physical media simply cannot venture. Easy and straightforward approaches to data exchange such as DropBox (www.dropbox.com) can even now offer more to DICOM file sharing than all DVD bundles, gathering dust at the bottom of convenience store shelves.

In the end, PDAs should unchain radiologists from their static workstations, which means that new work patterns will dictate DICOM and PACS changes. DICOM has to become more mobile-friendly; teleradiology should cease to be viewed as opposite to PACS. Undoubtedly, many laughed at the first cell phones, favoring state-of-the-art phone booths. Where are these booths now, I wonder?

> **Just Think About It!**
> "Just think about it!" said a sales rep advertizing to me his smartphone image viewer at a major medical trade show, "You can check your patient's images while playing golf!"
> Just think about it…

13.7.2 Multimedia Expansion

Despite the fact that local-area PACS with their horrifyingly huge servers and bulky workstations are still considered state-of-the-art innovations in most hospitals, their 20-year-old structure is beginning to look more and more archaic – if not annoying. In the new era of increasingly lighter, mobile computers consumers expect the same level of mobility from digital medicine. Wouldn't it be nice to do diagnostic imaging with the ease of SMS or instant messaging?

Part of this search for simplicity has already manifested itself in teleradiology, as we discussed earlier. Freeing radiologists from their static hospital offices and allowing them to read images anywhere was meant not only to maximize productivity but to minimize the boring, user-unfriendly routine. Expanding the freedom of image-reading tools becomes the next natural step.

13.7 From PACS to PDAs?

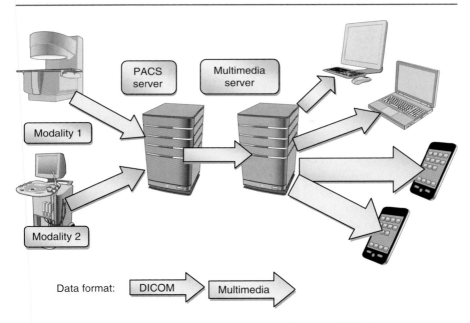

Fig. 13.10 Typical setup for multimedia PACS gateway: PACS server (DICOM) sends image data to its multimedia server (gateway), where the images are converted from DICOM to more common multimedia formats, and distributed to various mobile devices

Just like in the case of telemedicine, physicians started experimenting with more convenient image-viewing strategies several years ago. This led to different multimedia extensions to DICOM servers, actively employed by current telemedicine. When used as add-ons to a robust, fully functional PACS (taking care of all mainstream diagnostics) mobile, multimedia extensions become increasingly popular, opening secluded hospital reading rooms around the world (Fig. 13.10).

Certainly, it would be sheer folly to advocate replacing robust PACS workstations with multimedia PDAs; in spite of their proliferation, PDAs cannot pragmatically scale to the large and even routine tasks of digital image processing. But when you shop for any radiology system, pay particular attention to its multimedia capabilities, openness, and mobility. Avoid isolated installations in which each task can be done only on a dedicated machine under well-defined, idealized conditions. Apart from being just plain annoying, isolated solutions are simply inflexible – they leave you no options when something goes wrong. Explore laptops, tablet computers, PDAs, smartphones, MP3 players, and anything else that holds promise. Explore DICOM routers; a new breed of devices that convert DICOM into various multimedia formats and provide built-in support for many popular mobile gadgets. If they solve part of your problems today, they will help you even more tomorrow (Meehan et al. 2005; Raman et al. 2004). Citing Paul J. Chang, a prominent radiologist and explorer of new technologies: *"If technology got us into this mess, maybe technology can get us out of it."*

Cool vs. Practical

More hands-on advice: learn the hidden limitations of each technology. "Cool" and "practical" may have opposite meanings. Sometimes small portable devices can create problems that you've never experienced on a regular "large" device. For example, how do you work on a smartphone? Using a stylus is not particularly convenient – they get lost all the time. And with a stylus in one hand and a smartphone in the other, you cannot do or hold anything else. A touch-screen is much better and has become a trend in most popular phone models.

This seemed like an improvement before I noticed that many people, advocating their use at radiology conferences, were carrying towels in their pockets. Why? Fingerprints. If you are concerned about image quality, you will have to keep wiping touch-screen monitors all the time, to have the images as clear as possible. As an alternative, I have seen surgeons slip their touch-screen gadgets into plastic bags so they could use the screens while working in gloves in potentially messy environments. Well, the plastic bags were protecting the gadgets, but looking at the images through wrinkled plastic wasn't much fun.

This is the point when you realize that each device is designed for a particular use, and forcing it into the other areas may not look as exciting as it sounds. Ergonomic handles, spill- and drop-resistant casing, easy-to-clean monitors are the bare bone requirements for mobile clinical gadgets. Add integrated barcode and RFID scanners (to scan patient tags, for example), smart card readers (for those clinics implementing smart card IDs), convenient device interfaces (USB, swappable batteries, charging cradles), full control over system settings, software, and upgrades – whew! Now you are getting close to what practical clinical applications require. Can you do all this with your PDA?

13.7.3 Thin and Thick DICOM

Of the most important concepts you need to grasp in teleradiology is that of thin and thick clients. It's pretty simple: client "thickness" translates into its ability to understand and process data. A thick client, just like your standalone PC or workstation, is capable of storing, parsing, and processing the data on its own. A thin client cannot do all this; it depends on another computer (a server) to do all the computing tasks and it only shows the results.

Both client types are quite popular in medical imaging for their own reasons. Let's consider thick clients first. They are independent so they can work on dedicated tasks. As far as DICOM is concerned, thick clients have enough processing power to understand and manipulate DICOM data and to perform DICOM networking tasks. In short, they are self-sufficient and usually DICOM-compliant; most PACS companies sell them as "advanced workstations." The flip side of this full functionality is its cost: having everything in one package is expensive, and managing multiple independent thick clients takes considerable resources as well (Fig. 13.11).

13.7 From PACS to PDAs?

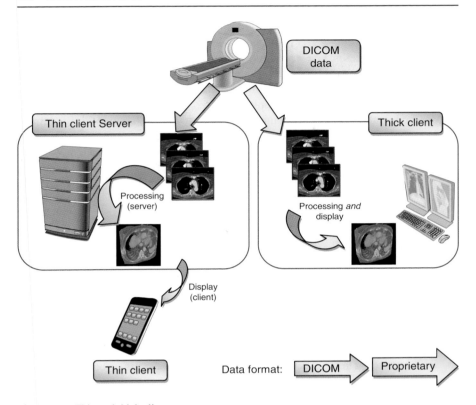

Fig. 13.11 Thin and thick clients

Thin client is what happens when you move all the expensive and resource-hungry processing to a server and give the users a way to view the data remotely. When you do 3D CT reconstructions on your Droid smartphone, you should realize that no current smartphone has enough processing power to run 3D imaging algorithms in real time. Instead, everything gets done on a server that your smartphone (thin client) is connected to. In other words, thin clients take user input, send it to the server (where it is processed), and display the results. Therefore, it is assumed that you are always connected to the server; otherwise, your thin client would be totally useless.

What does it mean in DICOM terms? DICOM is a complex standard, so thin clients usually do not mess with it; instead, relaying all DICOM tasks to their servers. Take our 3D rendering example: the server will do all DICOM networking to fetch the original images from another DICOM node (AE), it will parse DICOM files, it will render 3D images. Then, because the thin client is DICOMless, the server will convert the 3D image into JPEG screenshot and send it to the thin client for display. If you want to look at this 3D image from a slightly different angle, or with different window/level, your request will be sent to the server again, the 3D image will be re-rendered, and the updated JPEG screenshot will be re-sent to you for viewing on your thin client monitor.

Current networks (WiFi included) are already capable of providing sufficient bandwidth to make these frequent client–server communications seamlessly fast (although in some cases, you would notice that your thin client might freeze between two consecutive screenshots). This brings us to the main advantage of thin client architecture: it is less expensive and more manageable because everything important is done on a server and then simply presented to all thin client users.

Many clinical practices moved into thin clients under this assumption, and many of them were right. However, just for completeness, let's mention some thin client problems as well. The first – all thin clients depend on a server – is already known to us. So for example, if the network connection to the server is not available or goes down, thin clients become completely useless. The second problem is the single server bottleneck; if something takes the server down, it will render all thin clients useless as well. This "something" does not have to be a major disaster. Several thin clients may request complex 3D renderings at the same time, exhausting the server's computing power. Thin clients are just like shared phone lines: great when used sparsely, painful otherwise.

This partially dilutes the great "low cost" thin client assumption. Let's say you have six radiologists and you want to buy a thin client system. How powerful should it be? The vendor will charge you proportionally for the number of clients supported. You may think that only three of your radiologists will use the system at once, and buy the three-client version. But then if four or more radiologists try to use it, it won't work. On the other hand, if you try to minimize the risks and pay for six concurrent clients, it would cost you close to the same as buying six independent thick client licenses, even though most of the time only three of them will be used.

Note that the thin client-to-server interaction (as described above) is not DICOM, so it uses some proprietary protocol. In some cases, hospitals fall for this because it relieves them from doing any DICOM work. Say, you want to provide teleradiology readings to a remote facility, and they happen to have a thin client system already. Instead of working on a DICOM connection to load their images into your workstations, you just get an account to run their thin clients and the images are available to you right away, a la carte. Yes, it works sometimes, and when it does it's great. But now think about providing teleradiology services to another hospital that also happens to have *its own* thin client solution. Very soon, your radiologists will end up working with different thin clients – different functionality, different interfaces – which will certainly drive them crazy.

You might be surprised, but most PACS workstations from major PACS vendors often work like thin clients – in particular, with no understanding of DICOM. The main processing is done on the PACS servers, the images are sent to the workstations in a proprietary format, and only the most primitive tasks such as window/level are run on the workstations. Personally, I never liked this arrangement: once again, it creates a single-server bottleneck, which immediately invites too many problems (more discussion in Chap. 15). If vendors implement DICOM and PACS functionality anyway to make their systems work, why limit the implementation to a single server?

13.7.4 New Gadgets, Old Technology?

As Ecclesiastes wisely observed a while ago, "What has been will be again, what has been done will be done again; there is nothing new under the sun." This cannot be more true for a technical revolution. The recent explosion of mobile technology mimicked the triumph of personal computers some 20 years ago when each manufacturer wanted to be the one and the only – and the least compatible with all the others.

Mobile gadgets came out with various platforms, systems, and technology. If any company attempted to support them all, it would be a Herculean task. They would have to rewrite DICOM software in several different languages and, what's worse, keep developing and maintaining it this way. This is highly unpractical and costly, so the companies chose the path of the least resistance: implementing DICOM with the most universal – that is, the most primitive – tools that all gadgets can understand. In terms of image display, it means one thing: converting DICOM images to JPEG to display them in web browsers.[15]

This really kicks us back to the old problems discussed in the beginning of the teleradiology chapter. No surprise; doing DICOM on smartphones *is* teleradiology anyway.

When JPEG+HTML comes to medical imaging, you can say goodbye to any image processing. The only way to process images then will be to do it on a DICOM-capable server, sending JPEG screenshots to the smartphone. This applies even to the most primitive tasks such as window/level.

For DICOM, nearly all current PACS applications on PDAs work as thin clients.[16] In other words, what appears to you as a nice app running on your little smartphone or tablet often comes with a huge server attached, complete with proportionally huge upfront and maintenance costs. In some cases it is great, fitting into contemporary cloud and Software as a Service (SaaS) models. In other cases, when you really want to do things locally, you would be out of luck. And the outlook doesn't get any better when the entire software distribution channel becomes the property of the smartphone vendor; and everything in it – from your data to that powerful server some 1000 miles away – runs in proprietary, vendor-specific, and totally-unknown-to-you format. We have been there too many times before.

The same thing happens when new buzzwords are used to paint over old workflows. Consider for a moment "cloud computing." First, let's set the record straight, cloud computing does not equate to storing your data remotely: "Company X provided us with a great cloud computing solution, and they run our data center from now on!" This is not cloud computing, but a simple server outsourcing as you might get it from many hosting providers. And to make it even worse, it takes the old single-vendor problem discussed in Sect. 12.3 to the cloud level: "Can my cloud

---

[15] At the time this book was written, Apple declined to support Java on its mobile devices.
[16] This will change soon as more DICOM developers turn to PDAs, and PDA memory/networking reach PACS-sufficient levels.

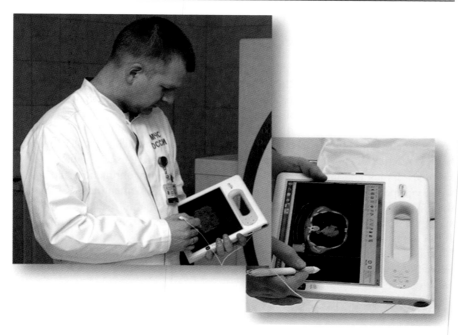

Fig. 13.12 Physician with tablet PC, designed for hospital applications (http://arcerm.ru/en/). The tablet runs standalone PACS workstation software (thick client), and has enough processing power even for real-time 3D imaging. Images are transmitted via hospital WiFi

talk to your cloud, and whose cloud is to blame?" We've had quite enough of this prattle with PACS, let's learn from our mistakes this time around. True cloud computing implies a convenient, easily shareable pool of computing resources that can be rapidly allocated to different tasks, at minimal setup or management cost. By definition, this cannot be vendor-specific or proprietary. On the contrary (just as we tried to describe in Sect. 15.2.4), it should rely on standards and diverse interfaces to provide maximum freedom and flexibility.

A similar approach should be taken in portable radiology. "Mobile" was never meant to stand for "deficient." Many mobile devices can go beyond joyriding the web and gaming. Some have scalable processing power, durable design, and useful interfaces (such as card readers, imperative for many hospital practices). When released from the bondage of particular vendors and web stores, they can provide physicians and medical IT with better functionality and more flexibility for their practical work applications (Fig. 13.12).

I can only hope that after the smoke clears from the initial gadget explosion and we've seen enough ultrasound loops posted on YouTube that the true medical technology will catch up; just like it did after JPEGs in email attachments. On the other hand, this is a natural process: every trendy thing will somehow affect radiologists, who after all are humans, just like the rest of us. Let's experiment with mobile processing and sharing, let's make medical imaging part of the popular social networks.

These days, we can do much more online than we can waiting in a hospital line. So as long as image quality remains a priority, sharing images with new gadgets should benefit all of us.

13.8 Starting Your Teleradiology Project

Okay, you're a trained radiologist and you were just invited to join a teleradiology project; or better still, you have to run one. What DICOM-related aspects will be of particular importance to you?

By far, the most important question would be whether the project images will be acquired in a DICOM-compliant manner. We have already spent the bulk of this chapter explaining the reasons for DICOM-based teleradiology, yet one cannot underestimate the importance of this issue. In short, the images must be acquired, stored, transmitted, and presented to you in their original DICOM format.[17] For that reason, the image acquisition site should employ a DICOM server through which all images will be routed from the modalities and stored for further retrieval and interpretation.

The next step will be accessing these images remotely and, just as we discussed in Sect. 6.2.4, you will most likely be presented with the bandwidth vs. compression dilemma (speed vs. quality). Make sure their PACS server provides sufficient compression options and study them visually to evaluate possible effects on the image quality. Retrieve the same study remotely with different compression methods and measure the time it takes. Then select the fastest of those, providing most adequate image quality.

What should your viewing workstation be? This is simply a question of monitor selection and it's been flogged to death over the past few years. If you refer to the teleradiology guidelines,[18] both American and European, you will see that the choice of viewing equipment is really up to you. It makes sense; no official recommendation can replace the sense of comfort and optimal viewing that you should create for yourself. Despite the PACS vendors lobby, often forcing purchases of the most expensive and least flexible viewing solutions you can ever waste your money on, general experience shows that a decent 24-inch, off-the-shelf LCD monitor with 400 cd/m² luminance and 1000:1 contrast would satisfy most radiologists' needs – even for high-resolution plain film readings (Hayes). Moreover, some studies indicate that higher monitor luminance (600 cd/m²) might even hinder radiology performance (Ridley 2006) (see Sect. 6.3.3). Color (RGB) monitors, due to their design, inevitably produce more blurred and less bright images than pure grayscale monitors simply because some of the backlight energy and some of the monitor

---

[17] If some images are not in DICOM format, make your best effort to convert them into DICOM format with DICOM-importing software and to acquire them with the best possible digital resolution.

[18] I recommend you check out (TeleradUSA), (TeleradEurope).

resolution is spent on coloring the pixels. However, color monitors are more universal: you will need color display for many image types, and limiting yourself to grayscale becomes increasingly more restrictive.

Figure out how the images should flow to you: whether you will be pulling them, or they will be pushed to you, or you will be viewing them in a web-enabled viewer (essentially, synonymous to pulling). Pulling takes time; you will have to pick a study and wait until it downloads to your computer. However, from all points of view pulling is also the simplest way of accessing images; and if your study load is not overwhelming, pulling will suffice.

If you have to read large amounts of images for a remote site – especially if you are working in a group of radiologists located at the same place and limited by strict turnaround time – I would recommend setting a more solid pushing workflow in which the images will be pushed to you right after they are acquired. You will have to set up a server at your site so that the remote imaging center or hospital can configure their DICOM server to relay all new studies to yours. In this event, by the time you need to look at the images, they will be preloaded to your local server – you and your group members won't have to wait for the images to download. It also eliminates downloading duplicates, when several teleradiology group members are loading the same study from a remote location (for whatever reason), stressing the network with unnecessary overload. Reading preloaded images is a much more pleasant experience.

The need for having a local teleradiology server brings up another important point: if you plan to provide teleradiology services from your facility, do not use your hospital PACS server. Instead, set up a new dedicated teleradiology server and use it to store all external images that you will be receiving for viewing. Mixing your local patients with teleradiology "strangers" in a single PACS archive would be a disaster – different names, different protocols, different storage and archiving policies will make it a total mess. If you have a good DICOM-compliant PACS (which I have been advocating on every single page of this book), you will be able to add your teleradiology server to your PACS workstation configurations so that your radiologists would be able to view all images, local or not, on the same workstations. Convenience matters; but do not mix the archives, keep them task-specific.

Apart from getting all your equipment together, I suggest you think about few other key aspects that are imperative for your success. They are particularly important if you are considering starting a teleradiology business.

1. You cannot run any teleradiology practice without IT support. Networking, computer, application, and software problems can kill your business well before the first image download, so you need a trained IT professional standing by. Find one ahead of time and share with him the layout of your entire data flow. This will enable him to come up with the most adequate and cost-efficient solution. Some of the elements in this solution may be hard to modify later, so plan ahead carefully and always leave some cushion for expansion.

13.8 Starting Your Teleradiology Project

2. Do not forget to temper your expectations and the expectations of your fellow radiologists. Most importantly, remote images will never load to your workstations as flawlessly as the images from your PACS server next door. Remote access will require more time. Moreover, your remote image provider might have different rules on organizing patient data, and on presenting the information to you. Review them before the project starts, but be flexible if you cannot change something. Remember that your remote site might have no interest in revolutionizing their workflow just to match yours. (And consider this: What if your contract with them ends tomorrow?)
3. If you are planning on expanding your business, never borrow solutions from others – the sites you serve in particular. You will end up with a dozen systems to run. Review what is available and what is best on the market, and start building your own practice with your own software and hardware setup – tailored to *your* needs. Running an independent system is one of the main requirements for your project scalability.
4. Emphasize the simplicity of access to your teleradiology images. They should be available to you and your colleagues virtually anywhere: on hospital workstations, on home PCs, even on smartphones when needed (urgent cases). You might need to sort out all these options based on their display quality and accessibility, but you *must* have them.

While many still consider teleradiology an inferior attachment to standard PACS, the reality could not be further from the truth. The time has come when teleradiology nets stretch over multiple time zones, countries, and even continents; and nothing in current technology will prevent teleradiology networks from expanding further still. Scalability becomes one of the main problems in these ever-growing networks: one of the most common misconceptions in building wide-area PACS is the idea that everything should have *direct* connection to everything. A workstation in a chest X-ray reading room in hospital A is expected to talk directly to a CR scanner in hospital B *and* print images on a DICOM printer in hospital C.

Sound familiar? Sure! This is another mental attempt to create a point-to-point DICOM network – a beast that has already caused so many problems even on a small, local PACS level. If cell phone networks and internet provider companies stayed with the same approach, we would never have cell phones or the internet. So let's abandon this idea once and forever.

As experience shows, the projects consisting of independent, self-sufficient components are the most scalable ones. We will explore this concept more in Chap. 15, but for now, if you are trying to build a system that can grow, ask yourself a few very simple questions: "Would my project still work if the reading room in hospital A needs to move because of a water pipe leak?" "What if the CR scanner in hospital B changes its IP address?" "What if the DICOM printer in hospital C runs out of film?" Most importantly, these questions are not about any fail-over or backup policies you might have, and certainly should implement; they are about ensuring that the components of your expanding workflow are truly independent and functional.

> **Predators or Allies?**
> There is one important item in any teleradiology project that has absolutely nothing to do with DICOM: personal relationships. Many hospitals tend to view expanding teleradiology practices as predators, threatening their business, jobs, and quality standards. Moreover, when patients and referring physicians learn that their images will be read *somewhere else*, they may get concerned as well. Therefore, the pros and cons of any teleradiology project should be weighed ahead of time, with very clear boundaries of responsibilities defined for the local and remote radiology groups. If anything is questionable, prioritize the quality, and the quantity will follow.

13.9 Conclusion

Summarizing the technical and DICOM-related aspects of teleradiology, we can (at least initially) focus our attention on the three most important characteristics: image transmission speed, network reliability, and image quality. They are directly related. The only way to increase image transmission speed is to improve the networks and to increase the use of lossy image compression (see 6.2.2), which may, however, lead to degraded image quality.

To avoid overuse of lossy compression and to make image downloading over networks more manageable, teleradiology adopted several popular solutions:

- *Thumbnails* – Smaller copies of images (usually also one image per series) are presented to the remote radiologist. The radiologist decides what he wants to download by clicking on specific thumbnails.
- *Filtering key images* – Done by trained technologists who might remove the least important or least informative images, excluding them from transmission. Only selected images are then sent for remote reading.
- *Image postprocessing and reconstructions* – Performed by trained technologists and imaging labs to replace large image volumes with a more compact, postprocessed representation. A reduced set of postprocessed images are then sent for remote reading.

Reliable teleradiology networking requires dynamic, self-adjustable, and self-healing networks. This part can be strengthened only with appropriate changes in the current static DICOM design.

Imagine one of the simplest tasks in a dynamic network environment: enumerating currently active DICOM nodes to see which ones are working and can be used. The most natural way would be to C-Echo all network nodes and count those that replied. But many static DICOM nodes will not accept C-Echo from unknown AEs; they will respond only to a few privileged applications from their *white lists*. As a result, if we want to write an application that finds the optimal DICOM path on a complex DICOM network, we won't be able to do this with the current DICOM.

13.9 Conclusion

The same thing is true for network-wide C-Find (searching for data on a network, not on an archive). The same is true in general for all DIMSE relaying, for recovering interrupted C-Stores, and for so much more. All this needs to change to make DICOM networks really scalable, which merits a new extension in the DICOM standard enabling them to work in peer-to-peer mode. In other words, teleradiology networks should be allowed to connect with any and all participants and workstations wherever they might be.

Think about Skype, social networking, instant messaging, and the myriad of similar applications – this is what teleradiology needs to embrace. Otherwise, even the most advanced teleradiology networks will lag behind contemporary communication paradigms. Think about more exotic technology – mobile plug-and-play modality blocks,[19] hospital trains and ships,[20] portable modalities – that, when properly equipped with DICOM interfaces, represent another dimension on teleradiology projects. With little doubt, teleradiology should and will become an integral part of PACS, finding a more elaborate technical representation in standards such as DICOM. Learning and standardizing new processes is really the most efficient way to ensure their correctness. I might repeat myself, but there is no conceptual boundary between conventional *local* PACS and *wide-area* PACS, or teleradiology. Hopefully, soon enough, local PACS will be well forgotten and digital imaging without distance constraints will become a true radiology standard.

---

[19] http://www.x-ions.ch/index-uk.php
[20] http://en.wikipedia.org/wiki/Hospital_ship, http://en.wikipedia.org/wiki/Hospital_train

Standards and System Integration in Digital Medicine

14

> *I go checking out the reports – digging up the dirt*
> *You get to meet all sorts in this line of work*
> *Treachery and treason – there's always an excuse for it*
> *And when I find the reason I still can't get used to it*
>
> – Dire Straits, "Private Investigations"

If you are interested in PACS workflow organization and management, I suggest you read an excellent book by Dreyer et al. (2005). In this chapter, we will glance only at the DICOM-related standards that are supposed to make everything fit together.

Why, even within DICOM, has product integration become such a big hassle? Let me answer this with a simple question: If two DICOM products conform to the same parts (SOPs) of the DICOM standard, do they conform to each other? Do not rush to say "Yes," as it would be a mistake. Sure, theoretically "Yes" is the right answer. Practically though, any DICOM product leaves plenty of room for mistakes and incorrect assumptions.

Although DICOM is called a *standard*, it is really a guideline, a big fat 16-volume *suggestion* on how things should be done if you and your vendors are nice enough to take the 16 volumes into consideration. If a DICOM vendor makes a mistake in its DICOM implementation – or falsely claims conformance, or "understands something differently," or just does not care to follow DICOM at all – there will be no penalty handed down and no blame assigned. In fact, when caught in these situations, most DICOM vendors would usually say something like "DICOM is too complex, its DICOM's fault." What DICOM really needs, in addition to less complexity, is a nice set of teeth to transform itself from scapegoat to industry authority. Before this happens, you as a customer will be responsible for making sense of standard implementation and integration – so read carefully. And by the way, there are *other* standards, too.

14.1 HL7: HIS and RIS

By far, PACS is the main imaging tool in the modern radiological workflow; to many radiologists, PACS *equals* radiology. However, PACS do not solve (and, in fact, were never meant to solve) the other abundant data-processing tasks that are imperative for current clinical enterprises. Patient scheduling, billing, financials, reports, worklists, labs, and many other items that record the complete patient path through a healthcare system are commonly managed by another important tool: the Hospital Information System, or *HIS* (often accompanied by the Radiology Information System, or *RIS*).

HIS and RIS take care of processing *anything but images*. HIS works as the central repository for all patient-related information, and RIS does the same job at the radiology department level (in many cases, you can view RIS as a radiology-specific part of HIS). Consequently, HIS and RIS are text-based systems, recording textual data about different states and conditions of the clinical workflow. The concept of this workflow can be structured in many ways, but almost always it begins with an *admittance event* when a new patient arrives at the hospital. This event binds the patient with the facility and its staff. The patient demographics are recorded (linking the patients to their previous visits, if any), insurance is verified, and appropriate examinations and clinicians are allocated and scheduled (Fig. 14.1).

Both HIS and RIS use a different data standard, HL7,[1] to represent data and associated events. HL7 is not meant to deal with images or any other nontextual data – it is meant to eliminate an archaic paper-based workflow. You might get a small taste of HL7 by looking at the following sample:

```
MSH|^~\&|ADT|N|ADT|MEDSC|200601081527||ADT^A08|RE|P|3.2|||||ASCII|
EVN|A08|200601080823||||||PID|1||3175875|1127278|SAMPLE^JOE^^^^||19
901334|M|||5400 Lake Villa Dr^^Metairie^LA^70001-1230||(405)555-
2920|||SINGLE|||||||||||||N|
MSH|^~\&|ADT|N|ADT|MEDSC|200601081527||ADT^A08|RE|P|3.2|||||ASCII|
EVN|A08|200601080812||||||PID|1||1487999|677931|TEST^BARBARA^F^^^||
19560216|F|||132 Austin Rd^^Someville^LA^70132-6582||(555)132-
7890|||MARRIED|||987-11-1324|||||||||||N|
MSH|^~\&|ADT|N|ADT|MEDSC|200601081511||ADT^A08|RE|P|3.2|||||ASCII|
EVN|A08|200601080832||||||PID|1||3057088|1051999|INCOGNITO^MONICA^A
NN^^^||19780117|F|||PO Box 1324^^Jefferson^LA^83625-3184||(555)423-
1423|||OTHER|||512-11-1425|||||||||||N|
```

Unlike binary DICOM abracadabra (remember Fig. 11.1?), you can almost read the entire HL7 message without knowing anything about the HL7 format: patient names, addresses, dates, phone numbers, marital statuses are very simple to spot. You might even figure out HL7 syntax. This particular example illustrates patient demographics fed from an HIS. The prefix MSH (**MeS**sage **H**eader) opens each new

---

[1] Health Level 7. Visit www.hl7.org for more information.

14.1 HL7: HIS and RIS

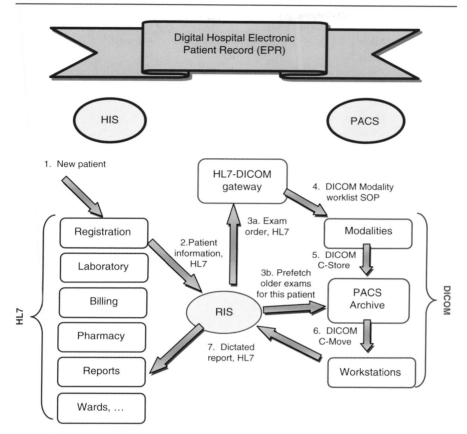

Fig. 14.1 HIS, PACS, RIS (Radiology Information System), and a typical path of a scheduled radiology exam

HL7 message, and a new line terminates it. Each message is a sequence of *segments*, where each segment has a three-character *segment name* followed by segment data *fields*, separated by field-delimiting *pipe* (|) characters. For example, the PID segment contains patient data fields, the EVN (event) segment contains fields with code and time of the related event (such as admittance to the hospital), and so on. If any field is empty, it is left blank between its pipes.

Look at EVN segment specifications in Table 14.1 – you might notice many similarities with the way DICOM defines its data elements.

As you can see from the table, EVN supports seven fields: the first two are present in our HL7 sample message above, the others are left blank (making a sequence of pipes with nothing in between). Similar to using VR types in DICOM, each field has its own HL7 data type: ID stands for ID string, TS for time string, and so on. Fields can be required and can have default values.

The most popular versions of HL7 (2.3, 2.4, 2.5) have been around for a long time; and while the encoding flexibility of HL7 2.X was overgrowing the original

Table 14.1 EVN (event) segment format

Field #	Name	Data type	Required	Default
1	Event Type Code	ID	No	–
2	Recorded Date/time	TS	Yes	–
3	Date/time Planned Event	TS	No	–
4	Event Reason Code	IS	No	–
5	Operator ID	XCN	No	–
6	Event Occurred	TS	No	–
7	Event Facility	HD	No	–

solid structure, its information structure was lagging behind increasingly complex workflows. In 2001, a completely new HL7 version 3.0 was released, changing both the format and the underlying organization of HL7 data. Just like DICOM 3.0, HL7 3.0 adopted object-oriented design (see Sect. 5.7.5) to represent the entire information flow as an interaction between data objects. This paradigm shift led to the alteration in the HL7 format: the clumsy pipes were abandoned and the much more appropriate and powerful XML (eXtensible Markup Language) was used:

```
<ns0:ADT_A04_22_GLO_DEF
xmlns:ns0="http://microsoft.com/HealthCare/HL7/2X">
<EVN_EventType>
    <EVN.1_EventTypeCode>A08</EVN.1_EventTypeCode>
    <EVN.2_DateTimeOfEvent>200601080823</EVN.2_DateTimeOfE
    vent>
    <EVN.3_DateTimePlannedEvent>200601080823</EVN.3_DateTi
    mePlannedEvent>
    <EVN.4_EventReasonCode>01</EVN.4_EventReasonCode>
</EVN_EventType>
<PID_PatientIdentification>
    <PID.1_SetIdPatientId>3175875</PID.1_SetIdPatientId>
    <PID.2_PatientIdExternalId>
        <PID.5_PatientName>
            <PN.0_FamiliyName>Sample</PN.0_FamiliyName>
            <PN.1_GivenName>Joe</PN.1_GivenName>
        </PID.5_PatientName>
    </PID.2_PatientIdExternalId>
</PID_PatientIdentification>
    ….
```

Albeit long-awaited, HL7 3.0 was perceived as a dramatic change from the previous HL7 versions, which is why the majority of clinical practices and large, hard-to-evolve

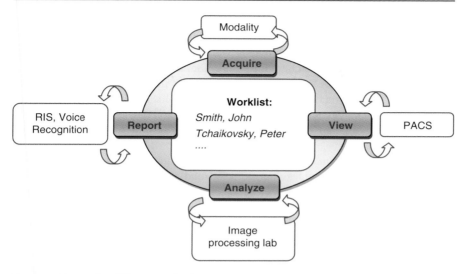

Fig. 14.2 Integrating different applications into a single worklist-driven interface. "View" button will launch PACS interface, "Analyze" will schedule the study for advanced image lab processing, "Acquire" will add it to Modality Worklist, "Report" will run voice recognition system

14.3 IHE: Integration Profiles

So, my dear radiology professional, are you still interested in the *ideal* integration scenario? You are not alone, and somebody started working on making your life easier a decade ago. By 1998, it was finally understood that standards alone do not guarantee efficiently integrated workflow, and something else needed to be done to cross the standards borders. This understanding launched the *Integrating the Healthcare Enterprise* (IHE) initiative.[4]

The main point of IHE is to promote the *coordinated* use of established healthcare standards (mainly DICOM and HL7) for better, effective, and easier-to-implement computer system integration. This is achieved through a collaborative effort from healthcare providers and the industry. The main result of IHE is the definition of *integration profiles* designed to solve identified integration problems.

Here is the list of some profiles (see (IHEProfiles) for the most updated profile listing):

- *Scheduled Workflow (SWF)* integrates ordering, scheduling, imaging acquisition, storage, and viewing for Radiology exams.
- *Patient Information Reconciliation (PIR)* coordinates reconciliation of the patient record when images are acquired for unidentified (for example, trauma), or misidentified patients.

---

[4] Visit http://www.ihe.net for more information.

- *Postprocessing Workflow (PWF)* provides worklists, status and result tracking for postacquisition tasks, such as Computer-Aided Detection or Image Processing.
- *Reporting Workflow (RWF)* provides worklists, status and result tracking for reporting tasks, such as dictation, transcription, and verification.
- *Import Reconciliation Workflow (IRWF)* manages importing images from CDs, hardcopy, etc. and reconciling identifiers to match local values.
- *Portable Data for Imaging (PDI)* provides reliable interchange of image data and diagnostic reports on CDs for importing, printing, or optionally, displaying in a browser.
- *Nuclear Medicine Image (NM)* specifies how Nuclear Medicine images and result screens are created, exchanged, used, and displayed.
- *Mammography Image (MAMMO)* specifies how Mammography images and evidence objects are created, exchanged, used, and displayed.
- *Evidence Documents (ED)* specifies how data objects such as digital measurements are created, exchanged, and used.
- *Simple Image and Numeric Report (SINR)* specifies how Diagnostic Radiology Reports (including images and numeric data) are created, exchanged, and used.
- *Key Image Note (KIN)* lets users flag images as significant (for example, for referring, for surgery, etc.) and add notes.
- *Consistent Presentation of Images (CPI)* maintains consistent intensity and image transformations between different hardcopy and softcopy devices.
- *Presentation of Grouped Procedures (PGP)* facilitates viewing and reporting on images for individual requested procedures (for example, head, chest, abdomen) that an operator has grouped into a single scan.
- *Image Fusion (FUS)* specifies how systems creating and registering image sets and systems displaying fused images create, exchange, and use the image, registration and blended presentation objects.
- *Cross Enterprise Document Sharing (XDS)* registers and shares electronic health record documents between healthcare enterprises, ranging from physician offices to clinics to acute care in-patient facilities.
- *Cross-enterprise Document Sharing for Imaging (XDS-I)* extends XDS to share images, diagnostic reports, and related information across a group of care sites.
- *Teaching File and Clinical Trial Export (TCE)* lets users flag images and related information for automatic routing to teaching file authoring or clinical trials management systems.
- *Access to Radiology Information (ARI)* shares images, diagnostic reports, and related information inside a single network.
- *Audit Trail and Node Authentication (ATNA)* Radiology Option defines Radiology-specific audit trail messages.
- *Charge Posting (CHG)* provides timely procedure details from modalities to billing systems.
- *Consistent Time (CT)* ensures system clocks and time stamps of computers in a network are well synchronized (median error less than 1 s).

Each IHE profile essentially defines the information-exchanging steps (*IHE transactions*), standards, and formats that each *IHE actor* (information system or

14.3 IHE: Integration Profiles

application) needs to follow to understand the other actors. In other words, each IHE profile gives you the best possible integration sequence for its project, assuring that it will comply with the existing standards (HL7, DICOM) on each device, and will work correctly where the standards meet each other. For example, the HIS-RIS-PACS integration problems, outlined earlier in this chapter, are addressed with the Scheduled Workflow profile particularly concerned with making HIS-RIS-PACS work in sync. Scheduled Workflow profile (our *ideal* integration solution, shown with arrows on our diagram in Sect. 14.1) paves the most correct information path through HIS, RIS, and PACS borders to register, scan, and report a patient's study. Portable Data for Imaging (PDI) profile[5] helps with some of the DICOM media problems discussed in Sect. 10.4.

A more detailed description of profiles can be found in (IHEkey); but IHE is not only a collection of integration recipes, it has developed itself into an industry etiquette that more and more vendors are starting to pay attention to (IHEvendors). Vendors follow IHE etiquette similarly to establishing DICOM compliance – by claiming compliance to certain IHE profiles. To confirm these claims, many vendors participate in the IHE-run *connectathons* (http://www.ihe.net/Connectathon/) – hands-on interoperability tests, verifying IHE profile compliance.

Recent developments in IHE have greatly influenced DICOM, which had to introduce new SOPs for better intersystem integration. On the flip side, DICOM and HL7 have become the main driving force behind most IHE projects. IHE documents and profiles are written in a very practical and easy-to-follow manner. I recommend that you visit the IHE website (www.ihe.net) before you embark on your first large integration project. Do not forget to ask your vendors which IHE profiles they support, and what benefits this can bring to your practice.

---

[5]http://wiki.ihe.net/index.php?title=Portable_Data_for_Imaging

Disaster PACS Planning and Management

15

In memory of Bart Ponze.

In late August and early September of 2005, two massive hurricanes – Katrina and Rita – hit the gulfshore states of the USA, devastating the region and creating havoc for every person, business, institution, and industry.

At that time, I happened to be working in Louisiana with two large state-wide clinical organizations. Both had their headquarters in New Orleans – the epicenter of the hurricane devastation.

Needless to say, the majority of local radiologists and clinicians found themselves displaced and disconnected, unable to come to their usual workplaces (if they even still existed). The hospital system binding the entire workflow went to pieces. Ironically, the need for such binding structure had never been higher. The fallout of medical treatment needs for the afflicted people of the area rose at an alarming rate. Everything depended on how soon the pieces could be repaired and patched back together. Establishing some kind of teleradiology network had become the only means of reconnecting the broken healthcare workflow.

My colleagues and I were responsible for solving the PACS part of the Katrina puzzle, and we had to make many unusual decisions to find viable solution. We had to build a distributed PACS network system from scratch, DICOM-connecting hospital tents, mobile modality units, and telecommuting radiologists into a single functional network (Fig. 15.1). This experience is summarized below.

Before we proceed with this analysis, I would like to express my deepest respect to all those who worked in the affected areas. Only your exceptional professionalism and dedication saved so very many lives, and made so many good things possible during such a very difficult and trying time.

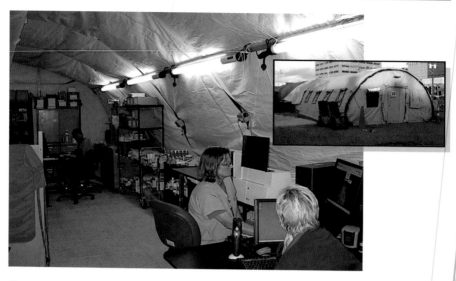

Fig. 15.1 New Orleans, USA, late 2005 – running our teleradiology system from a tent

15.1 What It Takes to Kill a PACS

Building a Godzilla-proof PACS has been a favorite subject of countless books, papers, and presentations. I remember quite a few of them. One suggested a triple PACS server; if anyone of the three identical components goes down, the remaining two would suffice for redundant, error-correcting functionality.[1] Another advertised itself with an *axe* concept: if we let a blindfolded maniac wielding an axe into the PACS room and let him smash his axe once into any PACS component, the PACS should still work.

> Lizzie Borden took an axe
> And gave her mother forty whacks,
> When she saw what she had done,
> She gave her father forty-one.

The image of Lizzie Borden axing PACS servers in a network closet does indeed appear quite thrilling except for one little caveat: somehow it is assumed that *the room itself* stays intact. But the wrath of Mother Nature knows no bounds and can go much further than the zeal of our blindfolded villain. The pre-Katrina PACS system, provided by a major PACS manufacturer, was located on the seventh floor of a solid concrete building. It had backup servers, power generators, tapes, and many other safety features located in the same area. It was naturally assumed that if

---

[1] Similar to mirroring hard drives in RAID.

anything takes down a solid concrete building, we would have much bigger problems than worrying about the PACS. This assumption was wrong.

Here is a brief list of mortal wounds that our imaging network suffered during the hurricane:

1. *Severe power loss in the hurricane-affected area.* The power was out for weeks. When it returned it was not stable. Meanwhile, the power was still reliably available in neighboring cities as close as 50–70 miles away.
2. *Severe connectivity loss.* While our PACS servers survived the hit, they lost network connectivity. One obvious reason for this was the same loss of power, but it was not the only reason. For example, one local telecommunication provider had located all its backup power generators on the first floor. They were quickly submerged during the flood, taking down the entire wide area network. Our servers were on the seventh floor; they remained totally intact, but lost connectivity as well because they were dependent on the same sunken provider – the quintessential weakest link scenario.
3. *Loss of technical support and onsite personnel.* Almost everybody evacuated to safer areas as the storm approached. Many systems quit simply because there was no one there to push the *Restart* button.
4. *Complete collapse of the public utility infrastructure.* In the immediate aftermath there was no water, gas, power, telecommunications, and all but a very few roads were flooded to a depth of several feet. The city was under strict martial law. This went on for several weeks. So although the PACS hardware was undamaged, there was no practical way to get to the data. As a consequence, patients fled the city without their medical records.
5. *Multiple technical problems.* For example, routers sporadically changing their IP addresses, servers running in overheated rooms (the servers restarted, but the cooling did not), physical damage, and so much more.

> **Know Your Weakest Link!**
> It's saddening to see more technological disasters happening because of some unexpected "secondary" failures. Look at the recent earthquake tragedy in Japan. While the Fukushima nuclear plant itself withstood the enormous quake, its cooling system and low-lying power generators did not,[2] leading to subsequent plant overheating, explosions, and radiation leaks. This issue is very similar to the low-lying power generators and cooling problems which contributed to the infrastructure collapse during Katrina. Your entire operation – as high-tech as it might be – is as stable as its weakest piece, and you have to know this piece before it's too late.

6. *Multiple logistical, administrative, personal problems and unstable, chaotic work environment.* When the centralized chain of command failed and fell to

---

[2] http://en.wikipedia.org/wiki/Fukushima_I_nuclear_accidents

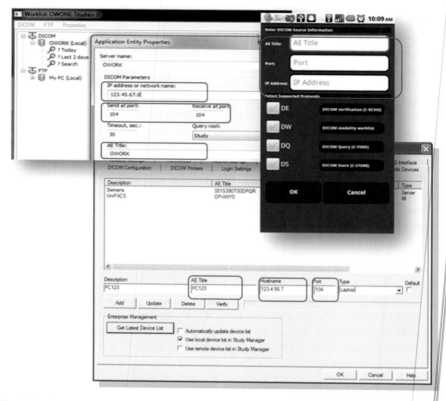

Fig. 15.2 Setting DICOM connectivity in different PACS software (from standalone to PDA). Different views, but same basic connectivity properties: IP address, DICOM (AE) title, and port

pieces, and when personal issues overwhelmed everyone, even the smallest problems turned into major obstacles.

Now, if we return to the beginning of this chapter, axing PACS servers looks more like child's play compared to New Orleans in September 2005 (Fig. 15.2). You might ask the question: "If a disaster of this scale happens in our area, why should we worry about the PACS? Shouldn't we concentrate more on lifesaving issues?"

But is not the main goal of PACS to be a lifesaving system?

Should it not be most available at the time when it is most needed?

Since when have we assumed that PACS is nothing but a complex, whimsical, and expensive monster that needs to be constantly baby-sat; one that we have to buy and maintain at exorbitant costs, considering ourselves lucky when it runs even under the normal conditions?

Unfortunately, most current PACS would easily freeze for hours because of a minor computer virus, incorrect patient ID, wrong mouse click, or a failing hard drive – incurring an average of $150/employee/h losses (Langer 2005). Most contemporary PACS are rigid, bulky, centralized systems having very little to do with

DICOM Applications: Usual and Not 16

Sure enough, DICOM is all about digital imaging in medicine, and PACS is all about DICOM. But in addition to PACS, there is a whole world of DICOM-driven applications out there, and it is definitely worth looking at. I randomly picked a few for this chapter, just to give you an idea of their variety.

16.1 Temporal Image Analysis

Temporal imaging is a perfect example of most complex patient data analysis driven by a single DICOM element: the image time stamp. There are several clinical applications (such as perfusion) that study how different organs and tissues respond to temporal factors (Fig. 16.1). Imagine that a patient was injected with a contrasting agent; a special substance that appears bright on CT images. As blood flow transports the contrast agent through various organs and tissues, temporal CT images are made at specific locations, say every second or so. Tissues with contrast appear brighter (proportionally to their pharmokinetic properties), and tumors – invisible otherwise – become more apparent on the benign tissue background.

In essence, we add time as another imaging dimension (hence the "4D" label used for temporal imaging).

To quantify this process, one needs to know the exact time stamp for each image. Where does the stamp come from? From the DICOM tags called Acquisition Time (0008,0032) and Content Time (0008,0033). The time stamps are set there in TM VR format (HHMMSS.FFFFFF) – precise to one millionth of a second.[1] Moreover, they are set by the imaging device (such as CT scanner) immediately when the images are acquired, so you do not need to worry about any other "time-setting" arrangements.

Time, measured precisely and instantaneously, becomes a gold mine for clinical image analysis, and another pitfall for PACS vendors. I have seen software from a

---

[1] Temporal image analysis is probably the main reason to have time measurements set to such an outstanding precision.

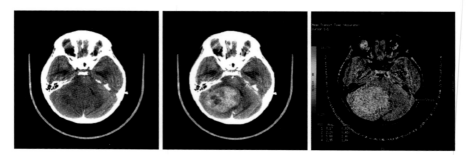

Fig. 16.1 CT brain perfusion: two of the 45 original CT images (taken with one-second delay, note brighter contrast areas on the second image), and mean transit time map (result of temporal image analysis) clearly showing damaged brain area

very reputable PACS vendor that was able to process time stamps done only on its own CT scanners. You should probably be able to guess why; the time stamps were stored in private tags instead of the standard (0008,0032) or (0008,0033) tags. The reason? None whatsoever, really.

16.2 DICOM Localization

Raise your hands, my dear hospital project managers if you have started receiving phone calls *from other countries* with the "I cannot understand your data" message? I will bet some of you might be getting quite accustomed to this already; and the more time flies, the merrier it will become.

Radiology is going global, and so do patient names, reports, and all related information, seasoned with local formats, dialects, and culture. Our fellow radiologists and physicians would definitely prefer to do business in their native languages; and typing Chinese or Hebrew names in Latin is not a practical option.

So how do we integrate foreign languages into DICOM with its default Latin character set, and one byte per character convention, inherited from the good old days? Specific Character Set (0008,0005) attribute comes to the rescue[2] – well, sort of. This attribute defines the selection of language (characters) used in DICOM textual data such as patient names (Table 16.1). Specific Character Set (0008,0005) is applied to the attributes with Value Representation of SH, LO, ST, PN, LT, or UT – the attributes containing text strings. If (0008,0005) is not provided, we revert to the Latin default (Table 16.2).

When (0008,0005) is provided, then DICOM application should do its best to support the correct characters, at least in the user interface to display text strings in the specified language. From a programming point of view, this is not a rocket science – all it takes is to grab the data bytes from textual DICOM elements, such as Patient

---

[2] Section 6.1 in DICOM PS3.5.

16.2 DICOM Localization

Table 16.1 Character repertoires defined in DICOM

Character set description	Defined term
Default repertoire (ISO-IR 6)	None
Latin alphabet No. 1	ISO_IR 100
Latin alphabet No. 2	ISO_IR 101
Latin alphabet No. 3	ISO_IR 109
Latin alphabet No. 4	ISO_IR 110
Cyrillic	ISO_IR 144
Arabic	ISO_IR 127
Greek	ISO_IR 126
Hebrew	ISO_IR 138
Latin alphabet No. 5	ISO_IR 148
Japanese	ISO_IR 13
Thai	ISO_IR 166
Unicode	ISO_IR 192
Chinese	GB18030

Table 16.2 DICOM default character repertoire (not shown are control characters ESC, LF, FF, CR)

SP	0	@	P	`	p
!	1	A	Q	a	q
"	2	B	R	b	r
#	3	C	S	c	s
$	4	D	T	d	t
%	5	E	U	e	u
&	6	F	V	f	v
'	7	G	W	g	w
(	8	H	X	h	x
)	9	I	Y	i	y
*	:	J	Z	j	z
+	;	K	[	k	{
,	<	L	\	l	|
-	=	M	]	m	}
.	>	N	^	n	~
/	?	O	_	o	

Name (0010,0010), and run them through a language-conversion routine – readily available on any computing platform. However, even this step becomes a challenge for most DICOM application developers, as can be seen in Fig. 16.2.

But this little task of proper language display only scratches the surface of the far deeper internationalization issues.

First of all, what is the origin of the correct (0008,0005) value? When radiologists or receptionists type a patient name in a Greek hospital, they do not really click

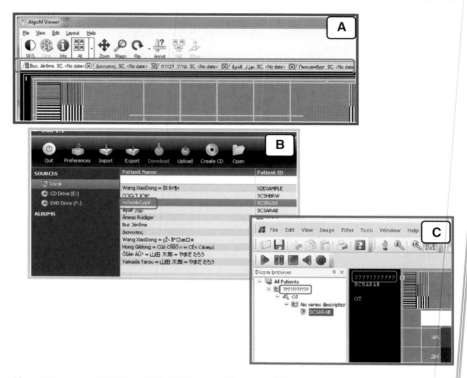

Fig. 16.2 Testing DICOM (0008,0005) with different DICOM software. Application A displayed all patient names correctly, using their respective character sets. Application B stumbled on some languages; application C was not prepared to handle foreign characters at all, replacing them with question marks

on some "use Greek encoding" button to apply the proper character repertoire. The language value most likely comes from two principal sources:
- Language settings in the program interface (when programs come in *localized*, language-specific versions)
- Language settings on the computer (such as "Region and Language" in Windows)

You would expect them to be perfectly right and in sync, and you are certainly right – in theory. In reality, the more a hospital grows, the more it is exposed to a mixture of various regional and language settings. Our imaginary Greek hospital can buy a modality unit from a US manufacturer, and innocently forget to change its default Latin repertoire. The same hospital can buy a plain PC from a French company, and again forget to set regional settings to Greece. The very same hospital can expand its operations to an international affiliate in China, and import a few Chinese-encoded DICOM files from there… And in each of these cases, before it gets noticed the hospital PACS will be inundated with incorrectly localized patient data, virtually impossible to fix. As radiology goes global, so do the devices and data that radiologists mix in their practices; and their localization capabilities quite often are not equal to the task.

16.3 Radiation Dose Monitoring

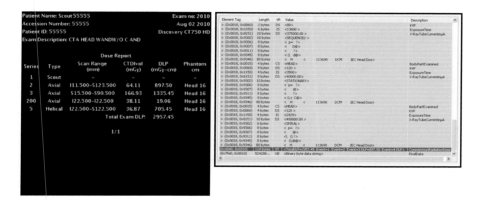

Fig. 16.3 (*Left*) Example of dose report image from GE Discovery CT750HD scanner. For each scanned series, Weighted Volume CT Dose Index ($CTDI_{vol}$) and Dose-Length Product (DLP) are shown, along with the total exam DLP. (*Right*) DICOM tags for the same image, displayed with nonproprietary software. You can see the mixture of standard and unreadable values, but the total report does show in the highlighted (0040,0310) tag

radiation report image to the original CT scan sequence (Fig. 16.3). The image would show total radiation doses used for each scanned series, based on some phantom calibration used for the scanner.

Well, the report image was better than nothing, but what could one do with this image in a busy hospital? All dose numbers need to be stored in a database, instead of being presented in a screenshot. Grabbing them from the image pixels would require OCR (Optical Character Recognition), which is complex and inefficient in the clinical context.

Instead of the screenshot reports dead-end, more efforts were expected from DICOM to standardize dose reporting in a legible, easy-to-automate format. Steps in this direction have become more apparent in the recent DICOM editions. Part 3.3 of the DICOM standard introduces the Radiation Dose module (see Table C.4-16 in DICOM PS3.9), shown here in Table 16.3. Note that (0040,0310) attribute was used to report radiation dose for the CT scan from Fig. 16.3 (selected line in the right image).

Storing dose data in the standardized DICOM tags was already better than screenshots, and many were able to take advantage of it. Nonetheless, image-based data reporting suffered from several problems. First, DICOM defined most of these tags as optional, which resulted in different tag support at different vendors. Second, storing study-specific information in individual SOP instances is not robust by definition. Some images can be removed, manipulated, or replaced; others can be sent to the PACS server before the study is finished (therefore containing incomplete dose data).

Table 16.3 Radiation dose module

Attribute name	Tag	Attribute description
Anatomic Structure, Space, or Region Sequence	(0008,2229)	Anatomic structure, space, or region that has been exposed to ionizing radiation. The sequence may have zero or one Items
>Include 'Code Sequence Macro' Table 8.8-1		No Baseline Context ID is defined
Total Time of Fluoroscopy	(0040,0300)	Total duration of X-Ray exposure during fluoroscopy in seconds (pedal time) during this Performed Procedure Step
Total Number of Exposures	(0040,0301)	Total number of exposures made during this Performed Procedure Step. The number includes nondigital and digital exposures
Distance Source to Detector	(0018,1110)	Distance in mm from the source to detector center. Note: This value is traditionally referred to as Source Image Receptor Distance (SID)
Distance Source to Entrance	(0040,0306)	Distance in mm from the source to the surface of the patient closest to the source during this Performed Procedure Step. Note: This may be an estimated value based on assumptions about the patient's body size and habitus
Entrance Dose	(0040,0302)	Average entrance dose value measured in dGy at the surface of the patient during this Performed Procedure Step. Note: This may be an estimated value based on assumptions about the patient's body size and habitus
Entrance Dose in mGy	(0040,8302)	Average entrance dose value measured in mGy at the surface of the patient during this Performed Procedure Step. Note: This may be an estimated value based on assumptions about the patient's body size and habitus
Exposed Area	(0040,0303)	Typical dimension of the exposed area at the detector plane. If Rectangular: row dimension followed by column; if Round: diameter. Measured in mm. Notes: 1. This may be an estimated value based on assumptions about the patient's body size and habitus. 2. This attribute is used in the X-Ray Acquisition Dose Module with units in cm (see Section C 8.7.8 Table C.8-33)
Image and Fluoroscopy Area Dose Product	(0018,115E)	Total area-dose-product to which the patient was exposed, accumulated over the complete Performed Procedure Step and measured in dGy*cm*cm, including fluoroscopy. Notes: 1. The sum of the area dose product of all images of a Series or a Study may not result in the total area dose product to which the patient was exposed. 2. This may be an estimated value based on assumptions about the patient's body size and habitus
Comments on Radiation Dose	(0040,0310)	User-defined comments on any special conditions related to radiation dose encountered during this Performed Procedure Step
Exposure Dose Sequence	(0040,030E)	Exposure Dose Sequence will contain Total Number of Exposures (0040,0301) items plus an item for each fluoroscopy episode not already counted as an exposure

Table 16.3 (continued)

Attribute name	Tag	Attribute description
>Radiation Mode	(0018,115A)	Specifies X-Ray radiation mode. Enumerated Values: CONTINUOUS PULSED
>KVp	(0018,0060)	Peak kilo voltage output of the x-ray generator used. An average in the case of fluoroscopy (continuous radiation mode).
>X-Ray Tube Current in μA	(0018,8151)	X-Ray Tube Current in μA. An average in the case of fluoroscopy (continuous radiation mode)
>Exposure Time	(0018,1150)	Time of X-Ray exposure or fluoroscopy in ms
>Filter Type	(0018,1160)	Type of filter(s) inserted into the X-Ray beam (for example, wedges). See C.8.7.10 and C.8.15.3.9 (for enhanced CT) for Defined Terms
>Filter Material	(0018,7050)	The X-Ray absorbing material used in the filter. May be multivalued. See Sects. C.8.7.10 and C.8.15.3.9 (for enhanced CT) for Defined Terms
>Comments on Radiation Dose	(0040,0310)	User-defined comments on any special conditions related to radiation dose encountered during the episode described by this Exposure Dose Sequence Item

Therefore, in the few past years, a more comprehensive radiation dose reporting started making its way into the DICOM: Radiation Dose Structured Reports (RDSR), detailed in PS3.16, and DICOM Supplements 127 and 150 (Fig. 16.4). The use of RDSR makes more sense than sprinkling study-wide dosage data over the individual DICOM images. Fortunately, it seems that the concept of RDSRs is getting gradually popular with modality vendors, and will hopefully provide a unified dose reporting mechanism in the future. At the same time, anything about structured reporting is still news to the PACS vendors, and most current PACS lack sufficient (if any) SR support. This adds another layer of implementation complexity, so if you want to go with RDSRs, get in touch with your modality and PACS manufacturers to make sure they are up-to-date with your expectations.

Finally, all DICOM can offer is a radiation report (dose) for the study in question. If you need to track older patient irradiation events, you inevitably need another software application in which DICOM reports from each scan will be stored to compute cumulative patient doses. But then, you must consider the problems of patients travelling between various hospitals (where their irradiation events were not recorded or were recorded differently), retrospective scans, unreported scans, and so on. One way to solve this problem could be mobile patient records: patients carrying their medical information on smart cards or other portable media. The most critical patient data, radiation dose included, can be stored there cumulatively and backed up to a safe location at each hospital visit. This is still very much a "dream technology," but the recent advances in mobile and cloud processing can make it a reality. In short, radiation dose tracking needs work – within DICOM and outside – to provide standardized data and interfaces for reliable dose records.

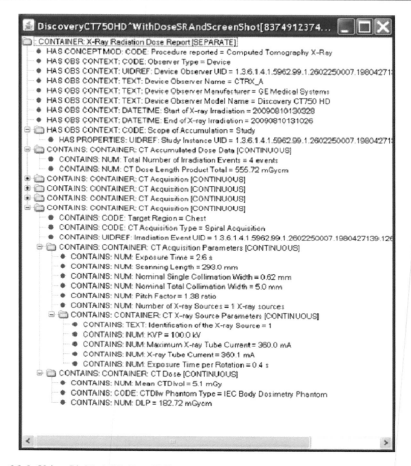

Fig. 16.4 Using PixMed SR DoseUtility tool to display the contents of Radiation Dose SR; http://www.dclunie.com/pixelmed/software/webstart/DoseUtilityUsage.html

And now? If you are concerned about robust radiation dose tracking (as you should be), keep pressure on your CT and X-ray vendors; ask for DICOM dose reporting. At least this will help all of us move in the right direction.

> **Next Time...**
> A couple of years ago my colleagues and I were charged with setting an automated dose reporting system in which radiation dose values would be read directly from scanned DICOM images. We went to several CT scanner manufacturers and waded through many layers of their engineering and technical

support just to find out that none of them provided any standard dose reporting. Adding a dose report image to a CT scan was considered state-of-the-art then, but the mere idea of running OCR against a PACS archive sent shivers down our spines. So we asked where the numbers came from and were told some vague stories about the raw data reports nested deeply into proprietary scanner architecture. Were these numbers accurate? Who knows! And when we asked about using DICOM for making radiation data available, the answer was the same as for any other nonexisting functions: "We do not have it right now, but we will have it in our next revolutionary model."

With a little luck, this situation will soon change and robust radiation dose tracking with DICOM will become commonplace on all irradiating devices. Keep in mind that without standardized dose reporting, one cannot even tell that the radiation numbers in some proprietary formats are accurate.

16.4 DICOS

It is interesting to see how DICOM finds unusual applications in seemingly remote areas such as airport security (having nothing to do with the security we just discussed). Digital Imaging and COmmunications in Security (DICOS) provides an example of DICOM expanding well beyond the original medical realm. As much as we are already accustomed to the use of X-rays for security checks, new elaborate security threats call for more elaborate detection tools, which can be borrowed from digital medicine. DICOS makes an attempt to adjust the DICOM object model and attributes to the needs of security checks (Fig. 16.5).

For its own needs, DICOS changes the DICOM information model to the hierarchy of Owner (highest level), Object of Inspection (OOI), Scan, and Series of objects. When John Smith walks with his suitcases through an airport security gate, he, his suitcases, and his laptop bag become the OOIs. Note that John may or may not be the Owner of some of these items, which makes him different from a DICOM Patient who definitely owns all his body parts. For the rest, DICOS scan corresponds to DICOM Study, and Series (data obtained on a particular scanning device) to DICOM modality-specific Series. Modality (scanning device) can vary from traditional X-ray or CT to less usual devices such as security trace detectors or even manual inspection. TDR, or Threat Detection Report (for Series, Scan, OOI or Owner), including information regarding the properties, locations, and probabilities of suspicious objects, becomes the ultimate outcome of the DICOS data analysis.

It is interesting to note that DICOS stresses the use of intelligent computer algorithms to detect and evaluate threats. Initial threat detection (image regions, ROI, containing potential threats), threat classification (such as assignment of threat probabilities to each detected ROI), and final threat aggregation (collecting all threats to make an overall assessment of the security risk) can hardly be done "by

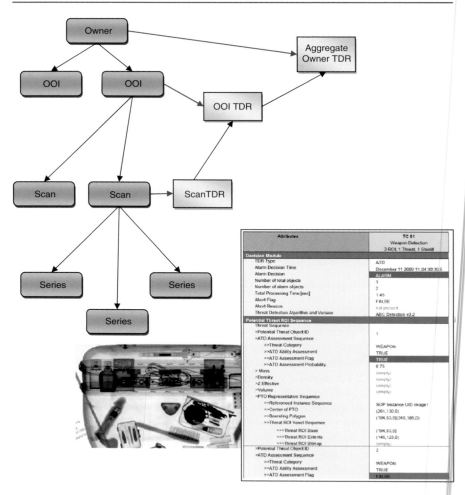

Fig. 16.5 DICOS information model

hand" without extensive use of computerized data analysis. This puts DICOS very close to clinical CAD (Computer-Aided Diagnosis): both rely on intelligent number crunching to estimate and measure the importance of certain image details.

DICOS inherits another important DICOM functionality: data transmission. The same SOP model (see Sect. 7.2) is used to transmit and store DICOS data, whether it is CT images or Threat Detection Reports. On the other hand, some DICOM functions such as information encryption and protection still have to make their way to DICOS. The introduction of "see-through" devices in airports has already raised understandable concern about passenger privacy. Verbal assurances that the security images will be deleted and will not be distributed illegally certainly do not work in the age of digital permissiveness; and if patient confidentiality is not protected by the standard, it will not be protected at all. In general, if you think about DICOM, the only "medical" part of it is its Data Dictionary, which translates clinical attributes into otherwise purely abstract objects. In other words, scanning for guns and explosives can be implemented with the same DICOM tools used for scanning tumors and plaques. When we see DICOS using DICOM for security, we can easily imagine that one day some DICOS tools (trace detectors and image-processing algorithms perhaps) may as well find some other clinical use. All rivers run into the sea...

16.5 Coloring DICOM Images: Science and Art

Grayscale images, films, and monitors has ruled medical imaging for ages; and I can remember that even just 10 years ago many of my radiologist friends would consider any color as sheer distraction. This was somewhat expected: most of the core DICOM modalities – CT, MR, ultrasound, and X-ray – were meant to image one-dimensional data, such as tissue density; there was nothing to color. Slowly but surely the dull grayscale landscape of medical imaging has started to change, and DICOM has had to catch up.

If the color is not in the original DICOM data, where might it come from? From any kind of postprocessing, increasing the original data dimensionality. Volumetric imaging is a perfect (and quite old) example of enhancing monochrome DICOM images with color. Think about complex 3D or even 4D (3D plus time) renderings, when multiple anatomic structures and organs overlap in a single image. Doing them with grayscale would hide most structures behind the others, barely conveying any information. Color is another story: even the three basic color channels (Red, Green, and Blue) provide you with an infinite number of mixtures, sufficient to differentiate between the most subtle shades. Adding a fourth palette channel – Alpha transparency – allow us to make objects semitransparent, providing another layer of visual complexity.

Coloring called for *palettes:* tables, mapping original imaging data (such as grayscale densities) into different colors. Consistently with two-byte/pixel DICOM grayscale, DICOM palettes are also two-byte per color channel, meaning that palette color data may range from (0,0,0) minimum to (65535,65535,65535) maximum (R,G,B). Compare this to (0,0,0) to (255,255,255) in bitmap/JPEG images and conventional monitors (Fig. 16.6).

Complex image postprocessing was only one of the many ways to introduce color. As another example, consider new dual-energy CT: the images are obtained simultaneously at two different energy levels, yet they are often presented in a single picture. Adding another energy dimension changes the old CT density display (Hounsfield units, HUs); different materials with the same HUs look different in dual-energy visualization: so color naturally shows the mixtures of different "basis" materials (such as iodine and water). Think about functional imaging, when certain processes (blood flow, tumor growth, brain impulses) have to be visualized on top

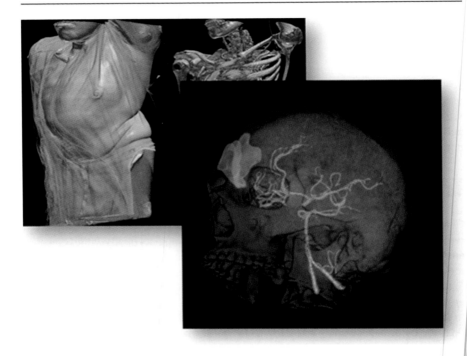

Fig. 16.6 Color in CT volume rendering helps visualize different structures, otherwise overlapping in grayscale or hidden behind the other anatomy. Images by Anders Persson (NewScientist) and Maryellen O'Rourke (BIDMC Advanced Imaging Lab)

of the usual imagery – color becomes the only meaningful way to make it possible. Consider hybrid imaging, when images from different modalities – PET and MR, PET and CT, MR and CT, and so on – are *fused* together; one needs color to differentiate between the image types.

I think you get the idea: whether the color is present in the original data or not, it may be essential for informative image display. Therefore, during the past 2 years DICOM has made several steps to enrich its color portfolio. Standard color palettes (Hot metal, Hot iron, PET, and such) finally made their debut in the DICOM Data Dictionary (Fig. 16.7). It was a good move: before palette standardization, each vendor implemented coloring on its own, often making the results incompatible with the others. Moreover, in 2009 DICOM added color palettes to its Information Model (PS3.3), treating them as separate entities meant to colorize otherwise monochrome data. Consequently, the Color Palette IOD was introduced (section A58 in PS3.3) to handle the palette lookup table – the table that maps the original grayscale values into RGB colors.

To manage palettes, DICOM now offers Color Palette Storage and Query/Retrieve SOPs (Table 16.4, see DICOM PS3.4, Annex W and X) so that DICOM applications can search and send palettes to each other, just like they search and send the images.

16.5 Coloring DICOM Images: Science and Art

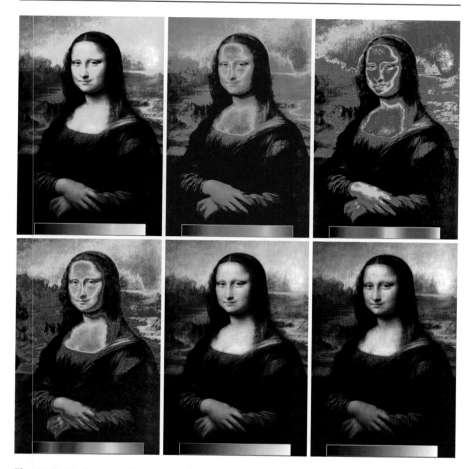

Fig. 16.7 Playing with Gioconda and popular PACS palettes. Hot iron, Hot, French, Spectral, Thermal, Grayscale

Table 16.4 Service classes to manage color palettes in DICOM

SOP class name	SOP class UID
Color Palette Information Model – STORE	1.2.840.10008.5.1.4.39.1
Color Palette Information Model – FIND	1.2.840.10008.5.1.4.39.2
Color Palette Information Model – FIND	1.2.840.10008.5.1.4.39.3
Color Palette Information Model – FIND	1.2.840.10008.5.1.4.39.4

Technically, Color Palette Storage and Query/Retrieve SOPs work just like image-exchanging SOPs: we simply extend C-Find, C-Get, C-Move, and C-Store to palette IODs. Consider palette storage: the interacting AEs (SCP and SCU with

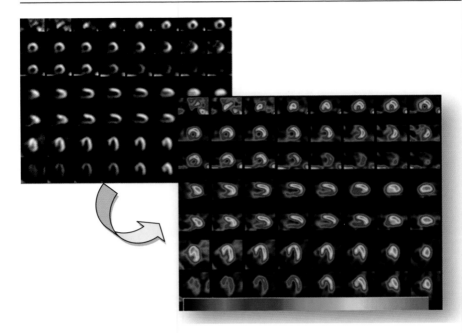

Fig. 16.8 Coloring original grayscale image with spectral palette. Note better segmentation of different tissue intensities

respect to palette storage SOP) start with the usual association negotiation and follow the usual C-Store protocol (see Sect. 7.3); but instead of image IODs, palette IODs are attached to C-Store DIMSE messages. DICOM does not define (yet), what Color Palette Storage SCU is supposed to do after it receives the palette; it is left to the application developers (DICOM Conformance Statement). You may add this palette to your application interface, apply it to current images, or do something else altogether (Fig. 16.8).

La vie en rose
Color often comes from various image-processing options provided in DICOM software. This has one important implication: if you see a colorful image in your DICOM software, it does not mean that the original image data has color as well. Quite often, the original might be in plain grayscale. I have seen many cases when radiologists were puzzled, sending colorful images from one workstation to another just to discover that the second workstation shows them in grayscale. "Where did all my colors go?" The answer is simple: grayscale data remained grayscale, and even if it was displayed in color by some software, opening it on another workstation will still produce a grayscale view.

16.5 Coloring DICOM Images: Science and Art

These tricks are particularly frequent in nuclear and functional imaging, where applications add default colors to the original data to highlight certain processes. Your best bet in preserving this coloring would be taking image screenshots (DICOM SC images, see Sect. 8.2), recording the images just as they appear on the screen.

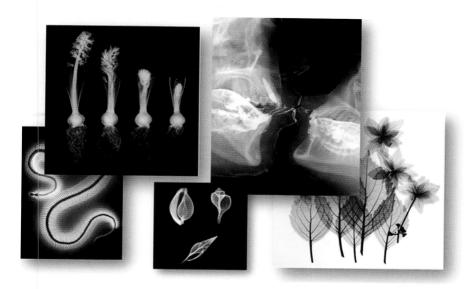

Fig. 16.9 X-ray art – X-ray flowers by Hugh Turvey, X-ray Genus Python by LUßO, X-ray kiss, X-ray seashells by Bert Myers, X-ray leaves by Albert Koetsier (XRayArt)

Speaking of color, I would be remiss if I did not mention the most fascinating application of medical imaging: X-ray art and photography. What started as a pure entertainment for artistically inclined MDs has taken on a life of its own, becoming the preferred tool for many professional artists. I cannot wait for DICOM to be taught in art colleges (Fig. 16.9).

19.2 Naïve Questions That MDs Like to Ask and Salesmen Like to Brag About

19.2.1 Do I Get the Original Image Resolution If I Buy Your PACS?

Sorry, but this question is naïve and meaningless at the same time. As long as the PACS is DICOM-compliant (which is always the case) it will not in any way attempt to change the image resolution. If your CT image was acquired as a 512×512 pixel matrix with two bytes/pixel grayscale it will always stay that way. This is one of the reasons we have DICOM, in fact.

The only thing that can affect the image resolution is lossy image compression (see Sect. 6.2.2). No, it will not change the number of pixels either, but it can introduce compression artifacts, sometimes making the images look less sharp (reducing your perceptual resolution, if you will). But in DICOM-compliant systems, the default image transfer format is always uncompressed; that is, you will get *exactly* the same image as it was acquired on the modality. Compression will be enabled only if you want to do so.

Moreover, your potential PACS vendor has already obtained their 510K premarket approval from the FDA, thus committing to maintaining the original image quality. According to the FDA requirements, images that undergo any quality-degrading modifications (such as lossy compression) should be clearly labeled as such when they appear on the screen.

Variations of this question might include "Can you show color images?" or "Can you show large X-rays?" and so on. They *must* show them because of DICOM, and not because of their *groundbreaking technology*.

19.2.2 Is Your System Web-based?

Do not ask it this way. Ask instead whether the system can run in a web browser. This is the true meaning of *web-based*. If they reply "yes," ask for a demo. You should see their entire system running as a plug-in within a web-browser window (not next to it, and not in another window; see Fig. 19.1).

19.2.3 Can You Connect to My CT Scanner (MR, US, PET, and So On)?

Yes, they sure can, as long as your scanner and their PACS are:
1. DICOM-compliant
2. Both support the same Image Storage SOP class, corresponding to your image type (such as CT Image Storage SOP – scanner as SCU, PACS as SCP, see Sect. 7.11). This should be clearly stated in the PACS' DICOM Conformance Statement.

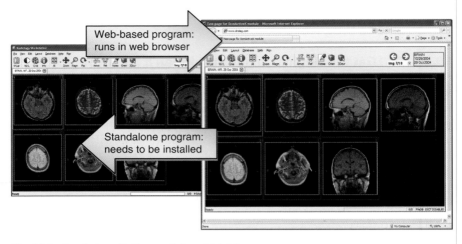

Fig. 19.1 Stand-alone (*left*) vs. web-based (*right*)

Once again, DICOM connectivity is not a *great favor* from your PACS company for which you should be eternally grateful. PACS companies that cannot get their DICOM straight should consider doing anything else but medical imaging.

19.2.4 Do You Have 3D Imaging (Perfusion, Diffusion, Volume Measurements, and So On)?

Never be satisfied with a verbal "yes" for any advanced image processing. Always ask for a demonstration. You might be surprised by what some companies call "3D" or "perfusion imaging." If they demonstrate this to you, check not only the quality, but the speed of the image processing (ask them to use a large data set as well, a few thousand images). I have seen *state-of-the-art commercial* programs run for half an hour doing perfusion maps that other *freeware* programs can do in a few seconds. Most basic features such as zoom or window/level are very much the same with any PACS company, but advanced processing can sometimes be replaced by low-quality or inefficient substitutes.

They might also answer "No, but our developers are working on this, and it will be available in the next version, very soon." Just *walk away*. This is their nice way of saying "Half a year from now (if not later) you will get a beta-system, clinically untested, and full of bugs." Besides, software companies work on their own version development cycles; they will not rush one bit to keep you happy.

19.2.5 Does Your System Support Multitasking (Multithreading, 64-Bit Processors, and So On, and So On)?

It is okay to play computer guru with them only if you really know what you are asking. But the answer will be "yes" anyway, because these features (multitasking,

multithreading, 64-bit math, and so on) are not the features of the PACS software – they are the features of the operating systems and processors that the PACS is running on. I have seen a PACS demo that started with "We have developed a 64-bit PACS." To my liking, this was a horrible start, because:
- They simply ran their PACS on a 64-bit computer (processor), they did not invent it.
- They used an engineering term that will not mean anything to most MDs. Advertising PACS from a technical viewpoint is always a mistake.
- It just made it sound like a shampoo commercial: "And your hair volume is three times larger!"

Besides, I have my own collection of insane engineering claims that I have heard at various PACS shows. "Multitasking means several processors," and "All monitors can show eight bits at most," and so many more. It just does not get you anywhere, whether the answer is correct or completely wrong.

19.2.6 Can I Use Your System for Teleradiology?

Yes, you can ask this question and if you happen to speak with an honest guy, you might even get a reasonable answer. However, please check Chap. 13 on teleradiology. Your main questions should really be:
1. Do they have a web-based (see above) or thin client solution? Thin client means a *lighter* application version, such as image viewing software that can run on virtually any computer and can load images from the central PACS server. If they ask you to install their entire PACS workstation on each computer that needs to view the images remotely this will likely be a very expensive and inefficient way of implementing your teleradiology project.
2. What kind of lossless and lossy image compression do you support (see Sect. 6.2)?
3. Can they do preloading and how? In particular, can their server do scheduled preloading from the remote facilities – for example, preload from there all of today's MR studies by 8 AM tomorrow morning?
4. Their licensing terms: do they license every viewing workstation, or can they give you a better server-based license – preferably based on concurrent users? The latter means that you will be paying licensing fees only for the *currently active users*, and not for their total number. You could have 100 teleradiology clients attached to your PACS server, but only 10 at most will be active at any time. With concurrent licensing, you pay for only 10 licenses.
5. Their references from teleradiology practices that use their system.

It also does not hurt to ask your questions in a more defined form, such as "Can I use your product in Israel to read the images from a US-based hospital?"

19.2.7 How Fast Can You Transfer the Images?

"Very fast, certainly!" Just kidding.

Once again, there is only one way that your PACS company can influence DICOM image transfer rates and that's by using image compression. So please look at Sect. 6.2 and ask them instead what compression types (Transfer Syntaxes) they use, and what compression ratios they achieve.

The rest depends on the speed of your network – or to be more precise, on the slowest link within your network. For example, uncompressed CT images take:

$$512 \times 512 \times 2 \text{ bytes} = 521 \times 512 \times 16 \text{ bits}.$$

If you have a T1 line, it transfers at 1.5 Mbit/s speed, and it will take:

$$(512 \times 512 \times 16)/(1.5 \text{ Mbit/s}) = 3 \text{ seconds}$$

per CT image to transmit. Apart from reducing the image size with compression, there is nothing else your PACS company can do with this formula.

19.2.8 How Much Data Can I Store In Your PACS?

This is another question that has nothing to do with the PACS. You will always store as much data as your hardware can handle; that is, as much as the size of your hard drive(s).

If you run out of hard drive space, you will need to consider:
1. Deleting or compressing unused files – older studies, for example. This always makes sense because it minimizes your hardware/storage expenses.
2. Increasing storage capacity:
   - Upgrading your existing hard drives to larger capacity models.
   - Attaching additional storage (disk arrays, tape libraries, optical jukeboxes) to your PACS.

Number two must be done by your PACS vendor. So ask them ahead of time whether they have a strategy for increasing their storage volume and how much it will cost you (it will not be cheap). Also, ask them about the largest current site they have – this will help you know at least how much data they have been able to handle so far.

You can easily run into PACS providers who advertise that they do not have any offline storage and will keep all your data online forever. This is nonsense. First of all, it means that they have no strategy to deal with large data volumes when diversified offline solutions become very cost-efficient (slower, less expensive storage types for less frequently used images). Second, sooner or later (especially in a large project/practice) you *will* fill your current online storage, and you *will* run out of server and rack space – what then?

19.2.9 Is Your DICOM Software Secure?

I think we are getting to the main point here: avoid "yes-no" questions because the answer will always be "yes." It would be better to ask: "*What* makes your system secure (if anything)?" Is it using DICOM PS3.15? Does it have audit? What HIPAA requirements does it implement? What encryption types does it use, if any? See Chap. 11.

19.2.10 Do You Have Full-Fidelity DICOM?

Sometimes vendors come to you with "full-fidelity DICOM" proposals, and you might wonder, what they are talking about. In fact, I am wondering as well: either we have a standard or we do not. Many things, obvious in DICOM, are frequently exaggerated for sales purposes: you shouldn't be excited over "multimodality worklists" (C-Find works with any modality), "full-fidelity images" or "unlimited connectivity." Never treat DICOM as a luxury – it is your most essential survival tool.

19.2.11 Do You Have Free DICOM?

A friend of mine who runs the online marketing for a private PACS company told me that "free DICOM" is one of the most frequently used keywords users type to look for PACS products. Well, I hope that at the end of this book we have a very clear idea of what DICOM is. It is a standard, a set of rules, and therefore it is completely free. You can always download it from DICOM home page, http://medical.nema.org.

What is *not* free are DICOM products and services – software, hardware, and consulting. In fact, the simplest of them can be free – such as the variety of DICOM file viewers available online – but they will never suffice to implement a serious clinical project. Prepare to pay.

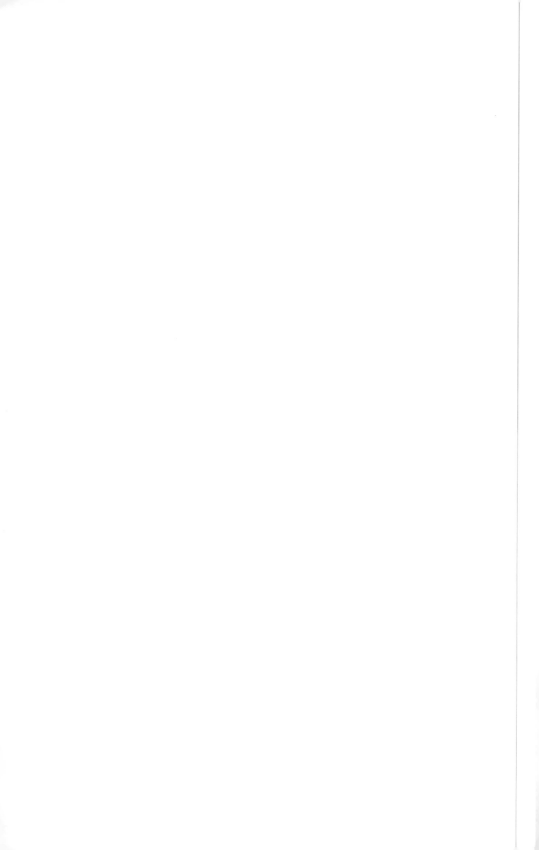

Appendix

DICOM Command Dictionary

Table A.1 DICOM command dictionary

Message field	Keyword	Tag	VR	VM	Description of field
Command Group Length	CommandGroupLength	(0000,0000)	UL	1	The even number of bytes from the end of the value field to the beginning of the next group
Affected SOP Class UID	AffectedSOPClassUID	(0000,0002)	UI	1	The affected SOP Class UID associated with the operation
Requested SOP Class UID	RequestedSOPClassUID	(0000,0003)	UI	1	The requested SOP Class UID associated with the operation
Command Field	CommandField	(0000,0100)	US	1	This field distinguishes the DIMSE operation conveyed by this Message. This field shall be set to one of the following values: 0001H C-STORE-RQ 8001H C-STORE-RSP 0010H C-GET-RQ 8010H C-GET-RSP 0020H C-FIND-RQ 8020H C-FIND-RSP 0021H C-MOVE-RQ 8021H C-MOVE-RSP 0030H C-ECHO-RQ 8030H C-ECHO-RSP 0100H N-EVENT-REPORT-RQ 8100H N-EVENT-REPORT-RSP 0110H N-GET-RQ 8110H N-GET-RSP 0120H N-SET-RQ 8120H N-SET-RSP 0130H N-ACTION-RQ 8130H N-ACTION-RSP 0140H N-CREATE-RQ 8140H N-CREATE-RSP 0150H N-DELETE-RQ 8150H N-DELETE-RSP 0FFFH C-CANCEL-RQ

Table A.1 (continued)

Message field	Keyword	Tag	VR	VM	Description of field
Message ID	MessageID	(0000,0110)	US	1	Implementation-specific value that distinguishes this Message from other Messages
Message ID Being Responded To	MessageID Being RespondedTo	(0000,0120)	US	1	Shall be set to the value of the Message ID (0000,0110) field used in associated request Message
Move Destination	Move Destination	(0000,0600)	AE	1	Shall be set to the DICOM AE Title of the destination DICOM AE to which the C-STORE sub-operations are being performed
Priority	Priority	(0000,0700)	US	1	The priority shall be set to one of the following values: LOW = 0002H MEDIUM = 0000H HIGH = 0001H
Data Set Type	Command DataSet Type	(0000,0800)	US	1	This field indicates if a Data Set is present in the Message. This field shall be set to the value of 0101H if no Data Set is present; any other value indicates a Data Set is included in the Message
Status	Status	(0000,0900)	US	1	Confirmation status of the operation. See Annex C
Offending Element	Offending Element	(0000,0901)	AT	1-n	If status is Cxxx, then this field contains a list of the elements in which the error was detected
Error Comment	ErrorComment	(0000,0902)	LO	1	This field contains an application-specific text description of the error detected
Error ID	ErrorID	(0000,0903)	US	1	This field shall optionally contain an application-specific error code
Affected SOP Instance UID	AffectedSOPInstanceUID	(0000,1000)	UI	1	Contains the UID of the SOP Instance for which this operation occurred
Requested SOP Instance UID	RequestedSOPInstanceUID	(0000,1001)	UI	1	Contains the UID of the SOP Instance for which this operation occurred
Event Type ID	EventTypeID	(0000,1002)	US	1	Values for this field are application-specific
Attribute Identifier List	Attribute Identifier List	(0000,1005)	AT	1-n	This field contains an Attribute Tag for each of the n Attributes applicable

Table A.1 (continued)

Message field	Keyword	Tag	VR	VM	Description of field
Action Type ID	ActionTypeID	(0000,1008)	US	1	Values for this field are application-specific
Number of Remaining Sub-operations	NumberOfRemainingSuboperations	(0000,1020)	US	1	The number of remaining C-STORE sub-operations to be invoked for the operation
Number of Completed Sub-operations	NumberOfCompletedSuboperations	(0000,1021)	US	1	The number of C-STORE sub-operations associated with this operation that have completed successfully
Number of Failed Sub-operations	NumberOfFailedSuboperations	(0000,1022)	US	1	The number of C-STORE sub-operations associated with this operation that have failed
Number of Warning Sub-operations	NumberOfWarningSuboperations	(0000,1023)	US	1	The number of C-STORE sub-operations associated with this operation that generated warning responses
Move Originator Application Entity Title	MoveOriginatorApplicationEntityTitle	(0000,1030)	AE	1	Contains the DICOM AE Title of the DICOM AE that invoked the C-MOVE operation from which this C-STORE sub-operation is being performed
Move Originator Message ID	MoveOriginatorMessageID	(0000,1031)	US	1	Contains the Message ID (0000,0110) of the C-MOVE-RQ Message from which this C-STORE sub-operation is being performed

DICOM Transfer Syntaxes

Table A.2 provides a list of DICOM Transfer Syntaxes, available in 2009 version of the standard.

Table A.2 DICOM transfer syntaxes

Transfer syntax UID	Transfer syntax name
1.2.840.10008.1.2	Implicit VR Little Endian: Default Transfer Syntax for DICOM
1.2.840.10008.1.2.1	Explicit VR Little Endian
1.2.840.10008.1.2.1.99	Deflated Explicit VR Little Endian
1.2.840.10008.1.2.2	Explicit VR Big Endian
1.2.840.10008.1.2.4.100	MPEG2 Main Profile @ Main Level
1.2.840.10008.1.2.4.50	JPEG Baseline (Process 1): Default Transfer Syntax for Lossy JPEG 8 Bit Image Compression
1.2.840.10008.1.2.4.51	JPEG Extended (Process 2 & 4): Default Transfer Syntax for Lossy JPEG 12 Bit Image Compression (Process 4 only)

(continued)

Table A.2 (continued)

Transfer syntax UID	Transfer syntax name
1.2.840.10008.1.2.4.52	JPEG Extended (Process 3 & 5) (Retired)
1.2.840.10008.1.2.4.53	JPEG Spectral Selection, Non-Hierarchical (Process 6 & 8) (Retired)
1.2.840.10008.1.2.4.54	JPEG Spectral Selection, Non-Hierarchical (Process 7 & 9) (Retired)
1.2.840.10008.1.2.4.55	JPEG Full Progression, Non-Hierarchical (Process 10 & 12) (Retired)
1.2.840.10008.1.2.4.56	JPEG Full Progression, Non-Hierarchical (Process 11 & 13) (Retired)
1.2.840.10008.1.2.4.57	JPEG Lossless, Non-Hierarchical (Process 14)
1.2.840.10008.1.2.4.58	JPEG Lossless, Non-Hierarchical (Process 15) (Retired)
1.2.840.10008.1.2.4.59	JPEG Extended, Hierarchical (Process 16 & 18) (Retired)
1.2.840.10008.1.2.4.60	JPEG Extended, Hierarchical (Process 17 & 19) (Retired)
1.2.840.10008.1.2.4.61	JPEG Spectral Selection, Hierarchical (Process 20 & 22) (Retired)
1.2.840.10008.1.2.4.62	JPEG Spectral Selection, Hierarchical (Process 21 & 23) (Retired)
1.2.840.10008.1.2.4.63	JPEG Full Progression, Hierarchical (Process 24 & 26) (Retired)
1.2.840.10008.1.2.4.64	JPEG Full Progression, Hierarchical (Process 25 & 27) (Retired)
1.2.840.10008.1.2.4.65	JPEG Lossless, Hierarchical (Process 28) (Retired)
1.2.840.10008.1.2.4.66	JPEG Lossless, Hierarchical (Process 29) (Retired)
1.2.840.10008.1.2.4.70	JPEG Lossless, Non-Hierarchical, First-Order Prediction (Process 14 [Selection Value 1]): Default Transfer Syntax for Lossless JPEG Image Compression
1.2.840.10008.1.2.4.80	JPEG-LS Lossless Image Compression
1.2.840.10008.1.2.4.81	JPEG-LS Lossy (Near-Lossless) Image Compression
1.2.840.10008.1.2.4.90	JPEG 2000 Image Compression (Lossless Only)
1.2.840.10008.1.2.4.91	JPEG 2000 Image Compression
1.2.840.10008.1.2.4.92	JPEG 2000 Part 2 Multi-component Image Compression (Lossless Only)
1.2.840.10008.1.2.4.93	JPEG 2000 Part 2 Multi-component Image Compression
1.2.840.10008.1.2.4.94	JPIP Referenced
1.2.840.10008.1.2.4.95	JPIP Referenced Deflate
1.2.840.10008.1.2.5	RLE Lossless
1.2.840.10008.1.2.6.1	RFC 2557 MIME encapsulation

DICOM SOPs

Table A.3 provides a list of DICOM SOP classes, available in 2009 version of the standard.

Table A.3 DICOM service-object pairs (SOPs)

UID value	UID name
1.2.840.10008.1.1	Verification SOP Class
1.2.840.10008.1.3.10	Media Storage Directory Storage
1.2.840.10008.1.9	*Basic Study Content Notification SOP Class (Retired)*
1.2.840.10008.1.20.1	Storage Commitment Push Model SOP Class
1.2.840.10008.1.20.2	*Storage Commitment Pull Model SOP Class (Retired)*
1.2.840.10008.1.40	Procedural Event Logging SOP Class
1.2.840.10008.1.42	Substance Administration Logging SOP Class
1.2.840.10008.3.1.2.1.1	*Detached Patient Management SOP Class (Retired)*
1.2.840.10008.3.1.2.1.4	*Detached Patient Management Meta SOP Class (Retired)*
1.2.840.10008.3.1.2.2.1	*Detached Visit Management SOP Class (Retired)*
1.2.840.10008.3.1.2.3.1	*Detached Study Management SOP Class (Retired)*
1.2.840.10008.3.1.2.3.2	*Study Component Management SOP Class (Retired)*
1.2.840.10008.3.1.2.3.3	Modality Performed Procedure Step SOP Class
1.2.840.10008.3.1.2.3.4	Modality Performed Procedure Step Retrieve SOP Class
1.2.840.10008.3.1.2.3.5	Modality Performed Procedure Step Notification SOP Class
1.2.840.10008.3.1.2.5.1	*Detached Results Management SOP Class (Retired)*
1.2.840.10008.3.1.2.5.4	*Detached Results Management Meta SOP Class (Retired)*
1.2.840.10008.3.1.2.5.5	*Detached Study Management Meta SOP Class (Retired)*
1.2.840.10008.3.1.2.6.1	*Detached Interpretation Management SOP Class (Retired)*
1.2.840.10008.4.2	Storage Service Class
1.2.840.10008.5.1.1.1	Basic Film Session SOP Class
1.2.840.10008.5.1.1.2	Basic Film Box SOP Class
1.2.840.10008.5.1.1.4	Basic Grayscale Image Box SOP Class
1.2.840.10008.5.1.1.4.1	Basic Color Image Box SOP Class
1.2.840.10008.5.1.1.4.2	*Referenced Image Box SOP Class (Retired)*
1.2.840.10008.5.1.1.9	Basic Grayscale Print Management Meta SOP Class
1.2.840.10008.5.1.1.9.1	*Referenced Grayscale Print Management Meta SOP Class (Retired)*
1.2.840.10008.5.1.1.14	Print Job SOP Class
1.2.840.10008.5.1.1.15	Basic Annotation Box SOP Class
1.2.840.10008.5.1.1.16	Printer SOP Class
1.2.840.10008.5.1.1.16.376	Printer Configuration Retrieval SOP Class
1.2.840.10008.5.1.1.18	Basic Color Print Management Meta SOP Class
1.2.840.10008.5.1.1.18.1	*Referenced Color Print Management Meta SOP Class (Retired)*
1.2.840.10008.5.1.1.22	VOI LUT Box SOP Class
1.2.840.10008.5.1.1.23	Presentation LUT SOP Class
1.2.840.10008.5.1.1.24	*Image Overlay Box SOP Class (Retired)*
1.2.840.10008.5.1.1.24.1	*Basic Print Image Overlay Box SOP Class (Retired)*

(continued)

Table A.3 (continued)

UID value	UID name
1.2.840.10008.5.1.1.26	*Print Queue Management SOP Class (Retired)*
1.2.840.10008.5.1.1.27	*Stored Print Storage SOP Class (Retired)*
1.2.840.10008.5.1.1.29	*Hardcopy Grayscale Image Storage SOP Class (Retired)*
1.2.840.10008.5.1.1.30	*Hardcopy Color Image Storage SOP Class (Retired)*
1.2.840.10008.5.1.1.31	*Pull Print Request SOP Class (Retired)*
1.2.840.10008.5.1.1.32	*Pull Stored Print Management Meta SOP Class (Retired)*
1.2.840.10008.5.1.1.33	Media Creation Management SOP Class UID
1.2.840.10008.5.1.4.1.1.1	Computed Radiography Image Storage
1.2.840.10008.5.1.4.1.1.1.1	Digital X-Ray Image Storage – For Presentation
1.2.840.10008.5.1.4.1.1.1.1.1	Digital X-Ray Image Storage – For Processing
1.2.840.10008.5.1.4.1.1.1.2	Digital Mammography X-Ray Image Storage – For Presentation
1.2.840.10008.5.1.4.1.1.1.2.1	Digital Mammography X-Ray Image Storage – For Processing
1.2.840.10008.5.1.4.1.1.1.3	Digital Intra-oral X-Ray Image Storage – For Presentation
1.2.840.10008.5.1.4.1.1.1.3.1	Digital Intra-oral X-Ray Image Storage – For Processing
1.2.840.10008.5.1.4.1.1.2	CT Image Storage
1.2.840.10008.5.1.4.1.1.2.1	Enhanced CT Image Storage
1.2.840.10008.5.1.4.1.1.3	*Ultrasound Multi-frame Image Storage (Retired)*
1.2.840.10008.5.1.4.1.1.3.1	Ultrasound Multi-frame Image Storage
1.2.840.10008.5.1.4.1.1.4	MR Image Storage
1.2.840.10008.5.1.4.1.1.4.1	Enhanced MR Image Storage
1.2.840.10008.5.1.4.1.1.4.2	MR Spectroscopy Storage
1.2.840.10008.5.1.4.1.1.4.3	Enhanced MR Color Image Storage
1.2.840.10008.5.1.4.1.1.5	*Nuclear Medicine Image Storage (Retired)*
1.2.840.10008.5.1.4.1.1.6	*Ultrasound Image Storage (Retired)*
1.2.840.10008.5.1.4.1.1.6.1	Ultrasound Image Storage
1.2.840.10008.5.1.4.1.1.6.2	Enhanced US Volume Storage
1.2.840.10008.5.1.4.1.1.7	Secondary Capture Image Storage
1.2.840.10008.5.1.4.1.1.7.1	Multi-frame Single Bit Secondary Capture Image Storage
1.2.840.10008.5.1.4.1.1.7.2	Multi-frame Grayscale Byte Secondary Capture Image Storage
1.2.840.10008.5.1.4.1.1.7.3	Multi-frame Grayscale Word Secondary Capture Image Storage
1.2.840.10008.5.1.4.1.1.7.4	Multi-frame True Color Secondary Capture Image Storage
1.2.840.10008.5.1.4.1.1.8	*Standalone Overlay Storage (Retired)*
1.2.840.10008.5.1.4.1.1.9	*Standalone Curve Storage (Retired)*
1.2.840.10008.5.1.4.1.1.9.1	*Waveform Storage – Trial (Retired)*
1.2.840.10008.5.1.4.1.1.9.1.1	12-lead ECG Waveform Storage
1.2.840.10008.5.1.4.1.1.9.1.2	General ECG Waveform Storage
1.2.840.10008.5.1.4.1.1.9.1.3	Ambulatory ECG Waveform Storage
1.2.840.10008.5.1.4.1.1.9.2.1	Hemodynamic Waveform Storage
1.2.840.10008.5.1.4.1.1.9.3.1	Cardiac Electrophysiology Waveform Storage
1.2.840.10008.5.1.4.1.1.9.4.1	Basic Voice Audio Waveform Storage
1.2.840.10008.5.1.4.1.1.9.4.2	General Audio Waveform Storage

Table A.3 (continued)

UID value	UID name
1.2.840.10008.5.1.4.1.1.9.5.1	Arterial Pulse Waveform Storage
1.2.840.10008.5.1.4.1.1.9.6.1	Respiratory Waveform Storage
1.2.840.10008.5.1.4.1.1.10	*Standalone Modality LUT Storage (Retired)*
1.2.840.10008.5.1.4.1.1.11	*Standalone VOI LUT Storage (Retired)*
1.2.840.10008.5.1.4.1.1.11.1	Grayscale Softcopy Presentation State Storage SOP Class
1.2.840.10008.5.1.4.1.1.11.2	Color Softcopy Presentation State Storage SOP Class
1.2.840.10008.5.1.4.1.1.11.3	Pseudo-Color Softcopy Presentation State Storage SOP Class
1.2.840.10008.5.1.4.1.1.11.4	Blending Softcopy Presentation State Storage SOP Class
1.2.840.10008.5.1.4.1.1.11.5	XA/XRF Grayscale Softcopy Presentation State Storage
1.2.840.10008.5.1.4.1.1.12.1	X-Ray Angiographic Image Storage
1.2.840.10008.5.1.4.1.1.12.1.1	Enhanced XA Image Storage
1.2.840.10008.5.1.4.1.1.12.2	X-Ray Radiofluoroscopic Image Storage
1.2.840.10008.5.1.4.1.1.12.2.1	Enhanced XRF Image Storage
1.2.840.10008.5.1.4.1.1.13.1.1	X-Ray 3D Angiographic Image Storage
1.2.840.10008.5.1.4.1.1.13.1.2	X-Ray 3D Craniofacial Image Storage
1.2.840.10008.5.1.4.1.1.13.1.3	Breast Tomosynthesis Image Storage
1.2.840.10008.5.1.4.1.1.12.3	*X-Ray Angiographic Bi-Plane Image Storage (Retired)*
1.2.840.10008.5.1.4.1.1.20	Nuclear Medicine Image Storage
1.2.840.10008.5.1.4.1.1.66	Raw Data Storage
1.2.840.10008.5.1.4.1.1.66.1	Spatial Registration Storage
1.2.840.10008.5.1.4.1.1.66.2	Spatial Fiducials Storage
1.2.840.10008.5.1.4.1.1.66.3	Deformable Spatial Registration Storage
1.2.840.10008.5.1.4.1.1.66.4	Segmentation Storage
1.2.840.10008.5.1.4.1.1.66.5	Surface Segmentation Storage
1.2.840.10008.5.1.4.1.1.67	Real World Value Mapping Storage
1.2.840.10008.5.1.4.1.1.77.1	*VL Image Storage – Trial (Retired)*
1.2.840.10008.5.1.4.1.1.77.2	*VL Multi-frame Image Storage – Trial (Retired)*
1.2.840.10008.5.1.4.1.1.77.1.1	VL Endoscopic Image Storage
1.2.840.10008.5.1.4.1.1.77.1.1.1	Video Endoscopic Image Storage
1.2.840.10008.5.1.4.1.1.77.1.2	VL Microscopic Image Storage
1.2.840.10008.5.1.4.1.1.77.1.2.1	Video Microscopic Image Storage
1.2.840.10008.5.1.4.1.1.77.1.3	VL Slide-Coordinates Microscopic Image Storage
1.2.840.10008.5.1.4.1.1.77.1.4	VL Photographic Image Storage
1.2.840.10008.5.1.4.1.1.77.1.4.1	Video Photographic Image Storage
1.2.840.10008.5.1.4.1.1.77.1.5.1	Ophthalmic Photography 8 Bit Image Storage
1.2.840.10008.5.1.4.1.1.77.1.5.2	Ophthalmic Photography 16 Bit Image Storage
1.2.840.10008.5.1.4.1.1.77.1.5.3	Stereometric Relationship Storage
1.2.840.10008.5.1.4.1.1.77.1.5.4	Ophthalmic Tomography Image Storage
1.2.840.10008.5.1.4.1.1.78.1	Lensometry Measurements Storage
1.2.840.10008.5.1.4.1.1.78.2	Autorefraction Measurements Storage
1.2.840.10008.5.1.4.1.1.78.3	Keratometry Measurements Storage
1.2.840.10008.5.1.4.1.1.78.4	Subjective Refraction Measurements Storage
1.2.840.10008.5.1.4.1.1.78.5	Visual Acuity Measurements
1.2.840.10008.5.1.4.1.1.78.6	Spectacle Prescription Reports Storage

(continued)

Table A.3 (continued)

UID value	UID name
1.2.840.10008.5.1.4.1.1.79.1	Macular Grid Thickness and Volume Report Storage
1.2.840.10008.5.1.4.1.1.88.1	*Text SR Storage – Trial (Retired)*
1.2.840.10008.5.1.4.1.1.88.2	*Audio SR Storage – Trial (Retired)*
1.2.840.10008.5.1.4.1.1.88.3	*Detail SR Storage – Trial (Retired)*
1.2.840.10008.5.1.4.1.1.88.4	*Comprehensive SR Storage – Trial (Retired)*
1.2.840.10008.5.1.4.1.1.88.11	Basic Text SR Storage
1.2.840.10008.5.1.4.1.1.88.22	Enhanced SR Storage
1.2.840.10008.5.1.4.1.1.88.33	Comprehensive SR Storage
1.2.840.10008.5.1.4.1.1.88.40	Procedure Log Storage
1.2.840.10008.5.1.4.1.1.88.50	Mammography CAD SR Storage
1.2.840.10008.5.1.4.1.1.88.59	Key Object Selection Document Storage
1.2.840.10008.5.1.4.1.1.88.65	Chest CAD SR Storage
1.2.840.10008.5.1.4.1.1.88.67	X-Ray Radiation Dose SR Storage
1.2.840.10008.5.1.4.1.1.88.69	Colon CAD SR Storage
1.2.840.10008.5.1.4.1.1.104.1	Encapsulated PDF Storage
1.2.840.10008.5.1.4.1.1.104.2	Encapsulated CDA Storage
1.2.840.10008.5.1.4.1.1.128	Positron Emission Tomography Image Storage
1.2.840.10008.5.1.4.1.1.129	*Standalone PET Curve Storage (Retired)*
1.2.840.10008.5.1.4.1.1.130	Enhanced PET Image Storage
1.2.840.10008.5.1.4.1.1.131	Basic Structured Display Storage
1.2.840.10008.5.1.4.1.1.481.1	RT Image Storage
1.2.840.10008.5.1.4.1.1.481.2	RT Dose Storage
1.2.840.10008.5.1.4.1.1.481.3	RT Structure Set Storage
1.2.840.10008.5.1.4.1.1.481.4	RT Beams Treatment Record Storage
1.2.840.10008.5.1.4.1.1.481.5	RT Plan Storage
1.2.840.10008.5.1.4.1.1.481.6	RT Brachy Treatment Record Storage
1.2.840.10008.5.1.4.1.1.481.7	RT Treatment Summary Record Storage
1.2.840.10008.5.1.4.1.1.481.8	RT Ion Plan Storage
1.2.840.10008.5.1.4.1.1.481.9	RT Ion Beams Treatment Record Storage
1.2.840.10008.5.1.4.1.2.1.1	Patient Root Query/Retrieve Information Model – FIND
1.2.840.10008.5.1.4.1.2.1.2	Patient Root Query/Retrieve Information Model – MOVE
1.2.840.10008.5.1.4.1.2.1.3	Patient Root Query/Retrieve Information Model – GET
1.2.840.10008.5.1.4.1.2.2.1	Study Root Query/Retrieve Information Model – FIND
1.2.840.10008.5.1.4.1.2.2.2	Study Root Query/Retrieve Information Model – MOVE
1.2.840.10008.5.1.4.1.2.2.3	Study Root Query/Retrieve Information Model – GET
1.2.840.10008.5.1.4.1.2.3.1	*Patient/Study Only Query/Retrieve Information Model – FIND (Retired)*
1.2.840.10008.5.1.4.1.2.3.2	*Patient/Study Only Query/Retrieve Information Model – MOVE (Retired)*
1.2.840.10008.5.1.4.1.2.3.3	*Patient/Study Only Query/Retrieve Information Model – GET (Retired)*
1.2.840.10008.5.1.4.1.2.4.2	Composite Instance Root Retrieve – MOVE
1.2.840.10008.5.1.4.1.2.4.3	Composite Instance Root Retrieve – GET
1.2.840.10008.5.1.4.1.2.5.3	Composite Instance Retrieve Without Bulk Data – GET
1.2.840.10008.5.1.4.31	Modality Worklist Information Model – FIND

Table A.3 (continued)

UID value	UID name
1.2.840.10008.5.1.4.32.1	General Purpose Worklist Information Model – FIND
1.2.840.10008.5.1.4.32.2	General Purpose Scheduled Procedure Step SOP Class
1.2.840.10008.5.1.4.32.3	General Purpose Performed Procedure Step SOP Class
1.2.840.10008.5.1.4.32	General Purpose Worklist Management Meta SOP Class
1.2.840.10008.5.1.4.33	Instance Availability Notification SOP Class
1.2.840.10008.5.1.4.34.1	RT Beams Delivery Instruction Storage (Supplement 74 Frozen Draft)
1.2.840.10008.5.1.4.34.2	RT Conventional Machine Verification (Supplement 74 Frozen Draft)
1.2.840.10008.5.1.4.34.3	RT Ion Machine Verification (Supplement 74 Frozen Draft)
1.2.840.10008.5.1.4.34.4	Unified Worklist and Procedure Step Service Class
1.2.840.10008.5.1.4.34.4.1	Unified Procedure Step – Push SOP Class
1.2.840.10008.5.1.4.34.4.2	Unified Procedure Step – Watch SOP Class
1.2.840.10008.5.1.4.34.4.3	Unified Procedure Step – Pull SOP Class
1.2.840.10008.5.1.4.34.4.4	Unified Procedure Step – Event SOP Class
1.2.840.10008.5.1.4.37.1	General Relevant Patient Information Query
1.2.840.10008.5.1.4.37.2	Breast Imaging Relevant Patient Information Query
1.2.840.10008.5.1.4.37.3	Cardiac Relevant Patient Information Query
1.2.840.10008.5.1.4.38.1	Hanging Protocol Storage
1.2.840.10008.5.1.4.38.2	Hanging Protocol Information Model – FIND
1.2.840.10008.5.1.4.38.3	Hanging Protocol Information Model – MOVE
1.2.840.10008.5.1.4.38.4	Hanging Protocol Information Model – GET
1.2.840.10008.5.1.4.41	Product Characteristics Query SOP Class
1.2.840.10008.5.1.4.42	Substance Approval Query SOP Class

Example of Matching Attributes from Different DICOM Providers

Table A.4 shows DICOM attributes supported for study queries with different vendors and products. The products were chosen randomly, and their versions change all the time; but as you can see, even the same vendor may use very different attribute sets in different applications. Moreover (this is not shown in the table), the degrees of attribute matching (required, unique, optional) may vary greatly as well.

Table A.4 DICOM attributes supported for Study queries in different vendor products: GE Centricity (GE1), GE PACS-IW (GE2), Siemens Leonardo (Sim1), Siemens Syndo Plaza (Sim2), Toshiba CT scanner (T), Vital Vitrea (V)

Tag	Description	GE1	GE2	Sim1	Sim2	T	V
(0008,0020)	Study Date	*	*	*	*	*	*
(0008,0030)	Study Time	*	*	*	*	*	*
(0008,0050)	Accession Number	*	*	*	*	*	*
(0008,0061)	Modalities In Study	*	*	*		*	
(0008,0090)	Referring Physician's Name	*	*	*	*		

(continued)

Table A.4 (continued)

Tag	Description	GE1	GE2	Sim1	Sim2	T	V
(0008,1030)	Study Description	*	*	*	*	*	*
(0008,1032)	Procedure Code Sequence	*					
(0010,0010)	Patient's Name	*	*	*		*	*
(0010,0020)	Patient ID	*	*	*		*	*
(0010,0021)	Issuer of Patient ID	*					
(0010,0030)	Patient's Birth Date	*	*				
(0010,0040)	Patient's Sex	*	*			*	
(0010,1000)	Other Patient IDs	*					
(0010,2160)	Ethnic Group	*					
(0020,000D)	Study Instance UID	*	*	*	*	*	*
(0020,0010)	Study ID	*	*	*	*	*	*
(0020,1206)	Number of Study Related Series	*	*	*	*		
(0020,1208)	Number of Study Related Instances	*	*	*	*	*	*
(0008,1060)	Name of Physician Reading Study			*	*	*	
(0008,0054)	Retrieve AE Title			*			
(0032,000a)	Study Status ID						
(0010,0032)	Patient's Birth Time		*				
(0010,4000)	Patient Comments						
(0010,1010)	Patient's Age		*			*	
(0010,1020)	Patient's Size		*				
(0010,1030)	Patient's Weight		*				
(0018,0015)	Body Part				*		
(0038,0300)	Patient Location				*		
(0008,0080)	Institution Name				*		

C-Find Bytes

If you are developing DICOM applications – or in any other way dealing with DICOM on the very fine level – it is definitely worth looking at the DICOM bytes, just as we did earlier with C-Echo. C-Find is easy enough to follow, and at the same time, it is more complex and considerably longer. However, reviewing this nicely formatted sample on paper will prepare you for looking through kilobytes of ugly error log dumps, if you ever have to. So let us see in the finest detail how DICOM will encode and send a C-Find message.

C-Find-Rq includes, as we just learned, two DICOM objects: command (DIMSE) and data (IOD, describing search criteria). The command object will be written in DICOM as shown in Table A.5.

It will be immediately followed by the data object, and Table A.6 gives an example of C-Find-Rq IOD. In our case, we decided to search for all studies for patients, whose names start with PIAN, performed after April 1, 2007 (see fields in bold).

Table A.5 C-Find-Rq DIMSE example

Byte #	1	2	3	4	5	6	7	8	9	10	11	12	13	14	15	16
Decimal	0	0	0	0	4	0	0	0	76	0	0	0	0	0	2	0
Binary	00	00	00	00	04	00	00	00	4C	00	00	00	00	00	02	00

g = 0000, e = 0000, VR length = 4, VR value = 76 = 0x4C, g = 0000, e = 0002

Byte #	17	18	19	20	21	22	23	24	25	26	27	28	29	30	31	32
Decimal	28	0	0	0	20	'.'	'2'	'.'	'8'	'4'	'0'	'.'	'1'	'0'	'0'	'0'
Binary	1C	00	00	00	31	2E	32	2E	38	34	30	2E	31	30	30	30

VR length = 28, VR value = "1.2.840.10008.5.1.4.1.2.2.1" (27 characters and trailing 0), corresponds to *Study root* C-Find

Byte #	33	34	35	36	37	38	39	40	41	42	43	44	45	46	47	48
Decimal	'8'	'.'	'5'	'.'	'1'	'.'	'4'	'.'	'1'	'.'	'2'	'.'	'2'	'.'	'1'	0
Binary	38	2E	35	2E	31	2E	34	2E	31	2E	32	2E	32	2E	31	00

Byte #	49	50	51	52	53	54	55	56	57	58	59	60	61	62	63	64
Decimal	0	0	0	1	2	0	0	0	32	0	0	0	16	1	2	0
Binary	00	00	00	01	02	00	00	00	20	00	00	00	10	01	02	00

g = 0000, e = 0100, VR length = 2, Val = 0x0020, g = 0000, e = 0110, VR length = 2

Byte #	65	66	67	68	69	70	71	72	73	74	75	76	77	78	79	80
Decimal	0	0	4	0	0	0	0	7	2	0	0	0	0	0	0	0
Binary	00	00	04	00	00	00	00	07	02	00	00	00	00	00	00	00

Val = 0x0102, g = 0000, e = 0700, VR length = 2, Val = 0

Byte #	81	82	83	84	85	86	87	88
Decimal	0	8	2	0	0	0	2	1
Binary	00	08	02	00	00	00	02	01

e = 0800, VR length = 2, Val = 0x0102

Total DICOM object length: 88 bytes = 12 bytes + 76 bytes, where:
(0000,0000) "group length" element length: 12 bytes
Length after (0000,0000) element: 76 bytes
(equals to (0000,0000) element value)

Table A.6 C-Find-Rq IOD example

Byte #	1	2	3	4	5	6	7	8	9	10	11	12	13	14	15	16
Decimal	8	0	0	0	4	0	0	0	88	0	0	0	8	0	32	0
Binary	8	0	0	0	4	0	0	0	58	0	0	0	8	0	20	0
	g = 0008			e = 0000				VR length = 4				VR value = 88 = 0x58			e = 0020	

Byte #	17	18	19	20	21	22	23	24	25	26	27	28	29	30	31	32
Decimal	10	0	0	0	'2'	'0'	'0'	'7'	'0'	'4'	'0'	'T'	'-'	32	8	0
Binary	0A	0	0	0	32	30	30	37	30	34	30	31	2D	20	8	0
	VR length = 10				VR value = 20070401- (date: April 1, 2007 or after)										g = 0008	

Byte #	33	34	35	36	37	38	39	40	41	42	43	44	45	46	47	48
Decimal	48	0	0	0	0	0	8	0	80	0	0	0	0	0	8	0
Binary	30	0	0	0	0	0	8	0	50	0	0	0	0	0	8	0
	e = 0030				VR length = 0				g = 0008				e = 0050			

Byte #	49	50	51	52	53	54	55	56	57	58	59	60	61	62	63	64
Decimal	80	0	6	0	0	0	'S'	'T'	'U'	'D'	'Y'	32	8	0	84	0
Binary	52	0	6	0	0	0	53	54	55	44	59	20	8	0	54	0
	e = 0052				VR length = 6			VR value = STUDY (with blank at the end)							e = 0054	

Byte #	65	66	67	68	69	70	71	72	73	74	75	76	77	78	79	80
Decimal	0	0	0	0	8	0	97	0	0	0	0	0	8	0	144	0
Binary	0	0	0	0	8	0	61	0	0	0	0	0	8	0	90	0
	VR length = 0				g = 0008		e = 0061				VR length = 0		g = 0008		e = 0090	

Byte #	81	82	83	84	85	86	87	88	89	90	91	92	93	94	95	96
Decimal	0	0	0	0	8	0	48	16	0	0	0	0	8	0	96	16
Binary	0	0	0	0	8	0	30	10	0	0	0	0	8	0	60	10
	VR length = 0				g = 0008		e = 1030		VR length = 0				g = 0008		e = 1060	

C-Find Bytes

Byte #	97	98	99	100	101	102	103	104	105	106	107	108	109	110	111	112
Decimal	0	0	0	0	16	0	0	0	4	0	0	0	62	0	0	0
Binary	0	0	0	0	10	0	0	0	4	0	0	0	3E	0	0	0
		VR length = 0			g = 0010				VR length = 4				VR value = 62			

Byte #	113	114	115	116	117	118	119	120	121	122	123	124	125	126	127	128
Decimal	16	0	0	0	6	0	0	0	'P'	'I'	'A'	'N'	'*'	32	16	0
Binary	10	0	0	0	6	0	0	0	50	49	41	4E	2A	20	10	0
	g = 0010		e = 0000		VR length = 6				VR value = PIAN*						g = 0010	

Byte #	129	130	131	132	133	134	135	136	137	138	139	140	141	142	143	144
Decimal	32	0	0	0	0	0	16	0	48	0	0	0	0	0	16	0
Binary	20	0	0	0	0	0	10	0	30	0	0	0	0	0	10	0
	e = 0020			VR length = 0			g = 0010		e = 0030		VR length = 0				g = 0010	

Byte #	145	146	147	148	149	150	151	152	153	154	155	156	157	158	159	160
Decimal	50	0	0	0	0	0	16	0	64	0	0	0	0	0	16	0
Binary	32	0	0	0	0	0	10	0	40	0	0	0	0	0	10	0
	e = 0032		VR length = 0				g = 0010		e = 0040		VR length = 0				g = 0010	

Byte #	161	162	163	164	165	166	167	168	169	170	171	172	173	174	175	176
Decimal	0	16	0	0	0	0	16	0	0	64	0	0	0	0	17	0
Binary	0	10	0	0	0	0	10	0	0	40	0	0	0	0	11	0
	e = 1000		VR length = 0				g = 0010		e = 4000		VR length = 0				g = 0011	

Byte #	177	178	179	180	181	182	183	184	185	186	187	188	189	190	191	192
Decimal	0	0	4	0	0	0	8	0	0	0	17	0	21	0	0	0
Binary	0	0	4	0	0	0	8	0	0	0	11	0	15	0	0	0
	e = 0000		VR length = 4				VR length = 8				g = 0011		e = 0015		VR length =	

(continued)

Table A.6 (continued)

Byte #	193	194	195	196	197	198	199	200	201	202	203	204	205	206	207	208
Decimal	0	0	32	0	0	0	4	0	0	0	24	0	0	0	32	0
Binary	0	0	20	0	0	0	4	0	0	0	18	0	0	0	20	0
	=0		g = 0020		e = 0000		VR length = 4								g = 0020	
Byte #	209	210	211	212	213	214	215	216	217	218	219	220	221	222	223	224
Decimal	13	0	0	0	0	0	32	0	16	0	0	0	0	0	32	0
Binary	0D	0	0	0	0	0	20	0	10	0	0	0	0	0	20	0
	e = 000D								e = 0010		VR length = 0				g = 0020	
Byte #	225	226	227	228	229	230	231	232	233	234	235	236	237	238	239	240
Decimal	8	18	0	0	0	0	50	0	0	0	4	0	0	0	8	0
Binary	8	12	0	0	0	0	32	0	0	0	4	0	0	0	8	0
	e = 1208		VR length = 0				g = 0032		e = 0000		VR length = 4				VR value =	
Byte #	241	242	243	244	245	246	247	248	249	250	251	252	253	254	255	256
Decimal	0	0	50	0	10	0	0	0	0	0	136	0	0	0	4	0
Binary	0	0	32	0	0a	0	0	0	0	0	88	0	0	0	4	0
	= 8		g = 0032		e = 000a		VR length = 0				g = 0088		e = 0000		VR length =	
Byte #	257	258	259	260	261	262	263	264	265	266	267	268	269	270		
Decimal	0	0	8	0	0	0	136	0	48	1	0	0	0	0		
Binary	0	0	8	0	0	0	88	0	30	1	0	0	0	0		
	= 0		VR length = 8				g = 0088		e = 0030		VR length = 0					

As you can see, the supplied data object contains search criteria for the studies to be found – in our case, all studies for the PIAN* patient (the first letters of the patient name are PIAN) .When C-Find SCP receives this DIMSE + IOD object pair, it will try to match the search keys from the C-Find-Rsp in its database and will reply with all the matches found. So, the replying C-Find-Rsp will be issued for each match, containing two parts: DIMSE to encode the C-Find response command, and data IOD to return any matches. The C-Find-Rsp DIMSE is shown in Table A.7.

And an example of a matched object that will be attached to the DIMSE is here, as C-Find-Rsp IOD is shown in Table A.8. Bold fields show matches for the original search parameters provided in C-Find-Rq IOD, and a few more attributes (such as study time) are returned in the other fields.

Table A.7 C-Find-Rsp DIMSE example

Byte #	1	2	3	4	5	6	7	8	9	10	11	12	13	14	15	16
Decimal	0	0	0	0	4	0	0	0	86	0	0	0	0	0	2	0
Binary	00	00	00	00	04	00	00	00	56	00	00	00	00	00	02	00
	g = 0000		e = 0000		VR length = 4				VR value = 86 = 0x56				g = 0000		e = 0002	
Byte #	17	18	19	20	21	22	23	24	25	26	27	28	29	30	31	32
Decimal	28	0	0	0	'1'	'.'	'2'	'.'	'8'	'4'	'0'	'.'	'1'	'0'	'0'	'0'
Binary	1C	00	00	00	31	2E	32	2E	38	34	30	2E	31	30	30	30
	VR value = 28				VR value = "1.2.840.10008.5.1.4.1.2.2.1" (27 characters and trailing 0), corresponds											
Byte #	33	34	35	36	37	38	39	40	41	42	43	44	45	46	47	48
Decimal	'8'	'.'	'5'	'.'	'1'	'.'	'4'	'.'	'1'	'.'	'2'	'.'	'2'	'.'	'1'	0
Binary	38	2E	35	2E	31	2E	34	2E	31	2E	32'	2E	32	2E	31	00
	to *Study root* C-Find															
Byte #	49	50	51	52	53	54	55	56	57	58	59	60	61	62	63	64
Decimal	0	0	0	1	2	0	0	0	32	128	0	0	32	1	2	0
Binary	00	00	00	01	02	00	00	00	20	80	00	00	20	01	02	00
	g = 0000		e = 0100		VR length = 2				Val = 0x8020		g = 0000		e = 0120		VR length =	
Byte #	65	66	67	68	69	70	71	72	73	74	75	76	77	78	79	80
Decimal	0	0	4	0	0	0	0	7	2	0	0	0	0	0	0	0
Binary	00	00	04	00	00	00	00	07	02	00	00	00	00	00	00	00
	= 2		Val = 4		g = 0000		e = 0700		VR length = 2				Val = 0		g = 0000	
Byte #	81	82	83	84	85	86	87	88	89	90	91	92	93	94	95	96
Decimal	0	8	2	0	0	2	1	0	0	0	0	9	2	0	0	0
Binary	00	08	02	00	00	00	02	01	00	00	00	09	02	00	00	00
	e = 0800		VR length = 2				Val = 0x0102		g = 0000		e = 0900		VR length = 2			
Byte #	97	98	Total DICOM object length: 98 bytes = 12 bytes + 86 bytes, where: (0000,0000) "group length" element length: 12 bytes Length after (0000,0000) element: 86 bytes (equals to (0000,0000) element value)													
Decimal	0	255														
Binary	00	ff														
	Val = 0x00FF															

Table A.8 C-Find-Rsp IOD example

Byte #	1	2	3	4	5	6	7	8	9	10	11	12	13	14	15	16
Decimal	8	0	0	0	4	0	0	0	148	0	0	0	8	0	32	0
Binary	8	0	0	0	4	0	0	0	94	0	0	0	8	0	20	0
	g = 0008				VR length = 4				VR value = 148				g = 0008		e = 0020	
Byte #	17	18	19	20	21	22	23	24	25	26	27	28	29	30	31	32
Decimal	8	0	0	0	'2'	'0'	'0'	'7'	'0'	'4'	'2'	'6'	8	0	48	0
Binary	8	0	0	0	32	30	30	37	30	34	32	36	8	0	30	0
	VR length = 8				VR value = 20070426 (April 26, 2007) (matched study date)								g = 0008		e = 0030	
Byte #	33	34	35	36	37	38	39	40	41	42	43	44	45	46	47	48
Decimal	6	0	0	0	'1'	'5'	'5'	'5'	'5'	'9'	8	0	80	0	8	0
Binary	6	0	0	0	31	35	35	35	35	39	8	0	50	0	8	0
	VR length = 6				VR value = 155559 (15:55:59 time)						g = 0008		e = 0050		VR length =
Byte #	49	50	51	52	53	54	55	56	57	58	59	60	61	62	63	64
Decimal	0	0	'4'	'3'	'3'	'6'	'2'	'3'	'8'	32	8	0	82	0	6	0
Binary	0	0	34	33	33	36	32	33	38	20	8	0	52	0	6	0
= 8			VR value = 4336238								g = 0008		e = 0052		VR length =
Byte #	65	66	67	68	69	70	71	72	73	74	75	76	77	78	79	80
Decimal	'S'	'T'	'S'	'T'	'U'	'D'	'Y'	32	8	0	84	0	10	0	0	0
Binary	0	0	53	54	55	44	59	20	8	8	54	0	0a	0	0	0
= 6			VR value = STUDY (with blank at the end)								g = 0008		e = 0054		VR length = 10
Byte #	81	82	83	84	85	86	87	88	89	90	91	92	93	94	95	96
Decimal	'L'	'I'	'B'	'Z'	'5'	'3'	'7'	'E'	'C'	'A'	8	0	86	0	6	0
Binary	4C	31	42	5A	35	33	37	45	43	41	8	0	56	0	6	0
	VR value = L1BZ537ECA										g = 0008		e = 0056		VR length =

Byte #	97	98	99	100	101	102	103	104	105	106	107	108	109	110	111	112
Decimal	0	0	'O'	'N'	'L'	'I'	'N'	'E'	8	0	97	0	2	0	0	0
Binary	0	0	4F	4E	4C	49	4E	45	8	0	61	0	2	0	0	0

VR value = DX | VR value = ONLINE | g = 0008 | e = 0061 | VR length = 2

Byte #	113	114	115	116	117	118	119	120	121	122	123	124	125	126	127	128
Decimal	'D'	'X'	8	0	144	0	12	0	0	0	'B'	'O'	'D'	'I'	'O'	94
Binary	44	58	8	0	90	0	0C	0	0	0	42'	4F	44	49	4F	5E

g = 0008 | e = 0090 | VR length = 12 | VR value =

Byte #	129	130	131	132	133	134	135	136	137	138	139	140	141	142	143	144
Decimal	'K'	'E'	'L'	'L'	'Y'	32	8	0	48	16	18	0	0	0	'C'	'H'
Binary	4B	45	4C	4C	59	20	8	0	30	10	12	0	0	0	43	48'

= BODIO KELLY | g = 0008 | g = 1030 | VR length = 18 | VR value =

Byte #	145	146	147	148	149	150	151	152	153	154	155	156	157	158	159	160
Decimal	'E'	'S'	'T'	32	'('	'P'	'A'	32	'A'	'N'	'D'	32	'L'	'A'	'T'	')'
Binary	45'E'	53	54	20	28	50	41	20	41	4E	44	20	4C	41	54	29

= CHEST (PA AND LAT)

Byte #	161	162	163	164	165	166	167	168	169	170	171	172	173	174	175	176
Decimal	16	0	0	0	4	0	0	0	62	0	0	0	16	0	16	0
Binary	10	0	0	0	4	0	0	0	3E	0	0	0	10	0	10	0

g = 0010 | e = 0000 | VR length = 4 | VR value = 62 | g = 0010 | e = 0016

Byte #	177	178	179	180	181	182	183	184	185	186	187	188	189	190	191	192
Decimal	12	0	0	0	'P'	'I'	'A'	'N'	'Y'	'K'	'H'	'^'	'O'	'L'	'E'	'G'
Binary	0C	0	0	0	50	49	41	4E	59	4B	48	5E	4F	4C	45	47

VR length = 12 | VR value = PIANYKH^OLEG (matched patient name)

(continued)

Table A.8 (continued)

Byte #	193	194	195	196	197	198	199	200	201	202	203	204	205	206	207	208
Decimal	16	0	32	0	8	0	0	0	'2'	'1'	'8'	'5'	'9'	'0'	'8'	32
Binary	10	0	20	0	8	0	0	0	32	31	38	35	39	30	38	20
	g=0010					VR length=8			VR value=2185908 (with trailing blank)							

Byte#	209	210	211	212	213	214	215	216	217	218	219	220	221	222	223	224
Decimal	16	0	48	0	8	0	0	0	'1'	'9'	'6'	'8'	'1'	'1'	'0'	'8'
Binary	10	0	30	0	8	0	0	0	31	39	36	38	31	31	30	38
	g=0010		e=0030		VR length=8				VR value=19681108 (patient birth date, YYYYMMDD)							

Byte#	225	226	227	228	229	230	231	232	233	234	235	236	237	238	239	240
Decimal	16	0	64	0	2	0	0	0	'M'	32	17	0	0	0	4	0
Binary	10	0	40	0	2	0	0	0	4D	20	11	0	0	0	4	0
	g = 0010		e = 0040		VR length = 2				Value = M (sex)		g = 0011		e = 0000		VR length	

Byte #	241	242	243	244	245	246	247	248	249	250	251	252	253	254	255	256
Decimal	0	0	14	0	0	0	17	0	21	0	6	0	0	0	'C'	'H'
Binary	0	0	0E	0	0	0	11	0	15	0	6	0	0	0	43	48
= 4			VR value = 14				g = 0011		e = 0015		VR length = 6				VR value =	

Byte #	257	258	259	260	261	262	263	264	265	266	267	268	269	270	271	272
Decimal	'E'	'S'	'T'	32	32	0	0	0	4	0	0	0	84	0	0	0
Binary	45	53	54	20	20	0	0	0	4	0	0	0	54	0	0	0
CHEST					g = 0020		e = 0000		VR length = 4				VR value = 84			

Byte #	273	274	275	276	277	278	279	280	281	282	283	284	285	286	287	288
Decimal	32	0	13	0	50	0	0	0	'1'	'.'	'2'	'.'	'1'	'2'	'4'	'.'
Binary	20	0	0D	0	32	0	0	0	31	2E	32	2E	31	32	34	2E
	g = 0020		e = 000D		VR length = 50				VR value =							

Byte #	289	290	291	292	293	294	295	296	297	298	299	300	301	302	303	304
Decimal	'1'	'1'	'3'	'5'	'3'	'2'	'.'	'1'	'0'	'.'	'4'	'5'	'.'	'5'	'7'	'.'
Binary	31	31	33	35	33	32	2E	31	30	2E	34	35	2E	35	37	2E

= 1.2.124.113532.10.45.57.434.20070426.154359.4155112

C-Find Bytes

Byte #	305	306	307	308	309	310	311	312	313	314	315	316	317	318	319	320
Decimal	'4'	'3'	'.'	'2'	'0'	'0'	'7'	'0'	'4'	'2'	'6'	'.'	'1'	'5'	'4'	'3'
Binary	34	33	2E	32	30	30	37	30	34	32	36	2E	31	35	34	33
Byte #	321	322	323	324	325	326	327	328	329	330	331	332	333	334	335	336
Decimal	'5'	'9'	'.'	'4'	'1'	'5'	'5'	'1'	'1'	'2'	32	0	16	0	8	0
Binary	35	39	2E	34	31	35	35	31	31	32	20	0	10	0	8	0
				VR value = 4336238				g = 0020				e = 0010		VR length	
Byte #	337	338	339	340	341	342	343	344	345	346	347	348	349	350	351	352
Decimal	0	0	'4'	'3'	'3'	'6'	'2'	'3'	'8'	32"	32	0	8	18	2	0
Binary	0	0	34	33	33	36	32	33	38	20"	20	0	8	12	2	0
	=8			VR value = 4336238								g = 0020			VR length	
Byte #	353	354	355	356	357	358	359	360	361	362	363	364	365	366	367	368
Decimal	0	0	'6'	':'	50	0	0	0	4	0	0	0	16	0	0	0
Binary	0	0	36	20	32	0	0	0	4	0	0	0	10	0	0	0
	= 2		Value = 6		g = 0032		e = 0000		VR length = 4				VR value = 16			
Byte #	369	370	371	372	373	374	375	376	377	378	379	380	381	382	383	384
Decimal	50	0	10	0	8	0	0	0	'S'	'T'	'A'	'R'	'T'	'E'	'D'	32
Binary	32	0	0A	00	8	0	0	0	53	54	41	52	54	45	44	20
	g = 0032		e = 000a		VR length = 8				VR value = STARTED							

References

Batchelor JS (2006) Meeting the challenge of structured reporting. Published online at http://www.auntminnie.com/index.aspx?Sec=sup&Sub=ris&Pag=dis&ItemId=71510

Bender S, Lederle K, Weiß C, Schoenberg SO, Weisser G (2011) 8-bit or 11-bit monochrome displays-which image is preferred by the radiologist? Eur Radiol 21(5):1088–1096

Branstetter BF IV (ed) (2009) Practical imaging informatics: foundations and applications for PACS professionals. Springer, New York

Cesarani F, Martina MC, Grilletto R, Boano R, Donadoni Roveri AM, Capussotto V, Giuliano A, Celia M, Gandini G (2004) Facial reconstruction of a wrapped Egyptian mummy using MDCT. AJR 183:755–758

Clunie D DICOM structured reporting. PixMed Publishing. Also available electronically from http://www.pixelmed.com/srbook.html

Dreyer KJ, Hirschorn DS, Thrall JH, Mehta A (2005) PACS: a guide to the digital revolution. Springer, New York

Hayes JC. Monitor's megapixels do not affect image interpretation. Online at http://www.diagnosticimaging.com/conference-reports/scar2005/article/113619/1198917

Hirschorn DS, Dreyer KJ Two years experience with using consumer displays in PACS. RSNA 2007, SSG15-05

Horill SC, Prior FW, Bidgood WD, Parisot Ch, Claeys G. DICOM: an introduction to the standard

Huang HK (2004) PACS and imaging informatics. Wiley-Liss, Hoboken

Hussein R, Engelmann U, Schroeter A, Meinzer HP (2004a) DICOM structured reporting, part 2: problems and challenges in implementation for PACS workstations. Radiographics 24:897–909

Hussein R, Engelmann U, Schroeter A, Meinzer HP (2004b) DICOM structured reporting. Radiographics 24(3):891–896

IHE key. http://www.ihe.net/About/upload/iheyr3_integration_profiles.pdf

IHE Profiles. http://www.ihe.net/profiles/

IHE vendors. http://www.ihe.net/resources/ihe_integration_statements.cfm

Kimpe T, Tuytschaever T (2007) Increasing the number of gray shades in medical display systems—How much is enough? J Digit Imaging 20(4):422–432

Langer S (2005) Continuous availability PACS and RIS. Presented at RSNA 2005, Chicago, IL, December 2005

Lewis RS, Sunshine JH, Bhargavan M (2009) Radiology practices' use of external off-hours teleradiology services in 2007 and changes since 2003. AJR 193(5):1333–1339

Meehan CP, Cronin CG, Lohan DG, McCarthy P PACS in your pocket? The PDA as imaging tool of the future. ECR 2005 electronic poster, www.ecr.org

New Scientist. http://www.newscientist.com/gallery/dn16281-animals-and-murder-inside-out/2

Oakley J (2003) Digital imaging: a primer for radiographers, radiologists, and health care professionals. Greenwich Medical Media Limited, London

Oracle DICOM. Oracle database 11g DICOM medical image support. An Oracle White Paper, June 2007. Available online at www.oracle.com

Pattynama PMT (2006) The future of teleradiology. Imaging Manag 6(2):18–20

Raman B, Raman R, Raman L, Beaulieu CF (2004) Radiology on handheld devices: image display, manipulation, and PACS integration issues. Radiographics 24(1):299–310

Ridley EL (2006) Higher monitor luminance levels may hinder performance. Available online at http://www.auntminnie.com/index.asp?sec=ser&sub=def&pag=dis&ItemID=69878, 27 Feb 2006

Rorden C. Web page. http://www.cabiatl.com/mricro/dicom/index.html

Ross P, Siinmaa P, Pohjonen HK Extending image sharing to patients using web-based PACS and EPR. ECR 2011 conference

Rothpearl A, Sanguinetti R, Killcommons J (2010) Development of a fax-based system for incorporating nondigital paper-based data into DICOM imaging examinations. J Digit Imaging 23(1):81–86

Tan CK, Ng JC, Xu X, Poh CL, Guan YL, Sheah K (2011) Security protection of DICOM medical images using dual-layer reversible watermarking with tamper detection capability. J Digit Imaging 24(3):528–540, published online: 23 April 2010

Telerad Europe. Teleradiology in the European Union. Available online at http://www.myesr.org/html/img/pool/1_ESR_2006_VII_Telerad_Summary_Web.pdf

Telerad USA. ACR technical standard for teleradiology. American College of Radiology (ACR), effective 1/1/03. Available online at www.acr.org

Vázquez A, Bohn S, Gessat M, Burgert O Evaluation of open source DICOM frameworks. Available online at http://www.dcm4che.org/confluence/download/attachments/271/ossdicom.pdf?version=1

Weisser G, Engelmann U, Ruggiero S, Runa A, Schröter A, Baur S, Walz M (2007) Teleradiology applications with DICOM-e-mail. Eur Radiol 17:1331–1340

XRay Art. http://www.photographymojo.com/2010/10/x-ray-photography-20-incredible-images-of-our-inner-space/

Yu C, Yao Z (2009) XML-based DICOM data format. J Digit Imaging 23(2):192–202

Index

A

A-Abort, 180, 194, 198–199, 201, 204
A-Associate-AC, 180, 181, 190, 191, 194–200, 207
A-Associate-RJ, 180, 184, 194–199
A-Associate-RQ, 180, 181, 190, 191, 194–201, 210
Abstract syntax, 178–185, 188–191, 195, 383
ACR-NEMA, 21–25, 29, 31, 38, 244, 273
AE. *See* Application Entity
AE configuration, 120, 121, 157, 206, 337
AET. *See* Application Entity Title
Anonymization, 236, 245–250, 255–257, 259–262, 293
Application Context, 181, 187–188, 195, 197
Application Entity (AE), 7, 8, 32, 41, 118, 121, 123, 130, 143, 144, 154, 164, 180, 184, 189, 191, 194, 206, 220, 230, 231, 337, 340
Application Entity Title (AET), 118, 135, 220, 393
Application integration, 325–327
A-Release-RP, 194, 199–200
A-Release-RQ, 194, 199–201
Association establishment, 9–10, 113, 177–181, 188, 193, 201, 202, 204–206, 213, 218–220, 231
Audio, 63, 75, 111–113
Audit, 239, 241, 259, 328, 389

B

Big Endian, 30, 36, 184, 189
Bits allocated, 83, 108
Bits stored, 83, 86, 102, 108

C

C-Cancel, 126, 159, 163, 391
C-Echo, 55, 56, 124–133, 135, 137, 146, 161, 164, 183, 201, 210, 316, 370, 374, 378, 391, 400
C-Find, 137, 210, 234, 269, 317, 359, 370, 378, 389
C-Get, 135, 150–165, 209, 212–214, 336, 340, 359, 370, 374, 378, 391
C-Move, 135, 154–165, 209, 210, 213, 234, 321, 336, 359, 370, 374, 378, 391, 393
Color palette, 357–360
Composite, 65, 79, 80, 123, 124, 398
Compression, 24, 62, 81, 173, 184, 219, 250, 284, 337, 364, 375, 381
Connectathon, 329
Contrast ratio, 104, 105
C-Store, 132–137, 143, 144, 146, 150, 151, 154–156, 158–160, 162, 164–166, 202, 210–213, 217, 220, 234, 317, 359, 360, 370, 373, 374, 378, 391–393

D

Data integration, 325–326
Data integrity, 57, 229, 250, 253–254, 325–326
Dcm4che, 369–371
DICM prefix, 218–219
DICOM broker, 146
DICOMDIR, 217–242, 297, 382
DICOM Message Service Elements (DIMSE), 117, 122–130, 132–138, 143–146, 149–150, 154, 158–160, 163, 177, 210, 217, 234, 317, 337, 360, 391, 400, 401, 405

Index

DICOM toolkit (DCMTK), 369, 371
Digital Imaging and Communications in Medicine (DICOM)
   attribute, 7, 39–40, 43, 47, 49, 62, 67, 101, 102, 139, 140, 173, 219, 228–229, 246, 257, 347, 399
   Command Dictionary, 47–48, 163, 391–393
   Command Object, 48, 53, 55, 123, 125, 126, 138, 193, 200
   Conformance Statement, 4, 10, 12, 24, 48, 71, 129, 137, 140, 142–144, 146, 149, 152, 166, 169, 192–193, 206, 232, 257, 268, 269, 300, 337, 360, 373, 385
   converter, 16, 62, 377
   Data Dictionary, 5, 7, 27, 43–49, 52, 53, 63, 66, 69, 71, 81, 84, 85, 125, 164–165, 188, 219, 246–248, 267, 358, 366, 378
   Data Object, 41, 48, 53, 56–57, 87, 100, 123, 129, 132, 138, 152, 193, 200, 211, 217–220, 222, 366
   email, 217, 296–300
   file, 30, 65, 218–234, 364, 381–382
   gateway (*see* DICOM broker)
   information model, 7, 77, 78, 80, 237, 355
   persistent object, 293
   ping, 124, 164, 182
   Print, 4, 9, 12, 119, 122, 175, 182, 315
   pull, 164
   push, 164
   router, 307
   validation, 62, 277–278
Digital Imaging and COmmunications in Security (DICOS), 355–357
Digital signature, 229, 254, 255, 261
DLP. *See* Dose-length product
Dose index, 350, 351
Dose-length product (DLP), 350, 351

E

Electronic Patient Record (EPR), 301, 323–326
Encapsulated PDF, 173–174, 398
Encryption, 172, 228–229, 236, 237, 241, 243, 245, 247, 250–264, 291, 297, 305, 332, 339, 341, 356, 365, 389
EPR. *See* Electronic Patient Record
Error log, 198, 205, 336, 407
Explicit encoding, 51, 52

F

File ID, 221–222, 226, 227, 229–230
File Meta Information, 219, 220, 224
File Set, 224, 229–230, 235
File Set Creator (FSC), 230, 231, 235, 296, 298, 300
File Set Reader (FSR), 230, 231, 235, 296, 298, 300
File Set Updater (FSU), 230, 231, 296
File Transfer Protocol (FTP), 213, 234, 236, 237, 260–261, 292, 383
FSC. *See* File Set Creator
FSR. *See* File Set Reader
FSU. *See* File Set Updater

G

Group length, 53–56, 125, 127, 128, 135, 136, 144, 145, 155, 159, 160, 163, 220, 224, 391, 401, 405

H

Health Insurance Portability and Accountability Act (HIPAA), ix, 246, 248, 249, 257, 262, 294, 389
Hexadecimal, 28–29, 44, 60, 109, 125, 126, 183, 185, 199, 243
Hierarchical, 71, 72, 137, 140–143, 145, 152–154, 158, 165, 171, 192, 394
High bit, 83, 85
HIPAA. *See* Health Insurance Portability and Accountability Act
HIS. *See* Hospital Information System
HL7, ix, 129, 146, 295, 320–327, 371
Hospital Information System (HIS), 16, 261, 273, 294, 295, 320–325, 329
HyperText Markup Language (HTML), 21, 30, 237, 291, 311

I

IE. *See* Information Entity
IHE. *See* Integrating the Healthcare Enterprise
Image
   interpolation, 97–100
   orientation, 85, 101
   position, 77, 85, 100, 101
   reconstructions, 100–102
Implicit encoding, 49, 51
Information Entity (IE), 72, 77, 107
Information Module, 72–77, 79, 80, 173

Index   415

Information Object Definition (IODs), 7, 8, 71–80, 112, 122, 129, 130, 132, 138, 140–146, 148–155, 157–160, 163, 164, 170, 173, 174, 193, 228, 267, 296, 323, 358–360, 364, 367, 371, 400, 402, 405, 406
Integrating the Healthcare Enterprise (IHE), 327–329, 371
IODs. *See* Information Object Definition

J
JND. *See* Just Noticeable Difference
JPEG, 5, 16, 81, 86, 87, 90, 93, 94, 96, 97, 103, 111–114, 179, 185, 186, 189, 190, 237, 242, 273, 282, 284, 285, 290, 291, 293, 294, 296, 304, 309, 311, 312, 357, 367, 368, 370, 393, 394
JPEG2000, 81, 87, 90, 93, 94, 96, 179, 185, 186, 189, 237, 290, 293, 294
JPEG-LS, 81, 87, 93, 94, 185, 189, 190, 237, 290, 394
Just Noticeable Difference (JND), 104, 105

L
List matching, 139, 141, 152, 158
Little Endian, 30, 36, 39, 43, 50, 52, 87, 126, 184, 185, 189, 191, 200, 211, 219, 220, 364, 393
Localization, 37, 344–349
Luminance, 82, 83, 101, 103–105, 313

M
Macro attribute, 72–73
MCH. *See* Message Control Header
M-DELETE, 230, 231
Medical Imaging Network Transport (MINT), 296
Medical Record Number (MRN). *See* Patient ID
Message Control Header (MCH), 200
M-INQUIRE FILE, 230, 234
M-INQUIRE FILE-SET, 230
MINT. *See* Medical Imaging Network Transport
Modality, vii, ix, 3, 38, 46, 62, 68, 70–72, 74, 76, 87, 90, 96, 111, 118, 132, 137, 139, 142, 145–150, 169–171, 173, 174, 180, 182, 186, 220, 225, 228, 270, 277, 317, 326, 327, 331, 337, 346, 347, 353, 355, 370, 371, 373, 374, 377, 378, 381, 385, 389, 395, 397, 398

Modality Worklist, 146–150, 180, 182, 270, 326, 327, 370, 371, 389, 398
MPEG, 75, 112–114, 260, 393
M-READ, 230
Multipurpose Internet Mail Extensions (MIME), 217, 297–300, 394
M-WRITE, 230

N
Normalized, 76, 79, 80, 123

O
Open-source, 253, 273–277, 367, 369–371, 383
Overlay, 69, 76, 79, 83, 108–111, 228, 258, 276, 357, 358, 395, 396

P
Patient ID, 40, 44, 62, 65–71, 73, 74, 76, 133, 139, 141, 142, 149, 152, 153, 158, 227, 238, 246, 247, 250, 256–258, 302, 322, 325, 334, 347, 349, 383, 400
PDA, 283, 302–313, 334
P-Data-TF, 194, 200–201
PDU. *See* Protocol Data Unit
PDV. *See* Protocol Data Value
Perfusion, vii, 101, 170, 305, 339, 343, 344, 378, 386
Picture Archiving and Communication System (PACS), vii, ix, 3, 4, 8, 15, 16, 19–21, 23, 28, 36, 38–41, 47, 48, 68, 69, 87, 90, 96, 97, 99, 103, 105, 106, 109, 111, 114, 117–120, 133, 140, 143, 149, 152–154, 156, 158, 161–164, 166, 170, 173–175, 178, 186–188, 196, 201, 202, 206–212, 217, 218, 228, 229, 233–235, 238–242, 252, 261, 263, 264, 268, 273, 275–278, 281–292, 295, 297, 298, 300, 303–317, 319–321, 323–327, 329, 331–344, 346, 347, 351, 353, 355, 359, 363, 368, 371, 375, 377, 383–389, 399
  cloud, 286, 288, 338, 341
  database, 36, 170, 238–242, 347, 384
PixelMed, 354, 369
Pixel Spacing, 85, 100, 101
Point-to-point, 117, 206–209, 214, 233–234, 258, 281, 292, 315, 336
Preamble, 218–219, 224
Presentation Context, 10, 178, 180, 188–192, 195–197, 200
Presentation Context ID, 191, 200

Private key, 251, 252, 261
Protocol Data Unit (PDU), 193–204, 369
Protocol Data Value (PDV), 200, 201
Pseudonimization, 247
Public key, 251, 252

Q
Query. *See* C-Find

R
Radiation dose, 5, 270, 350–355, 369, 398
Radiology Information System (RIS), 36, 141, 146–149, 261, 285, 320–326, 329, 372, 375, 377
Range matching, 139, 141
Redundancy, 52, 76, 87, 88, 91, 96, 254, 332, 335, 337, 340, 341
Relational, 71, 72, 143, 152, 192, 238, 239, 368
Retrieve. *See* C-Get; C-Move
RIS. *See* Radiology Information System
RLE. *See* Run-Length Encoding
Run-Length Encoding (RLE), 81, 87, 93, 367, 394

S
SC. *See* Secondary Capture
SCP. *See* Service Class Provider
SCU. *See* Service Class User
Secondary Capture (SC), 70–71, 87, 108, 134, 142, 170, 171, 174, 248, 270, 361, 371, 396
Secure DICOM file, 228–229, 261, 262
Sequence matching, 139, 148
Sequencing (SQ), 35, 41–43, 49, 51, 53, 56–62, 73, 75, 108, 139, 148, 223–227, 366
Service Class Provider (SCP), 9, 10, 122, 123, 130, 131, 133, 138, 142–154, 156, 158, 159, 161–163, 165, 166, 175, 179, 183, 184, 189, 192, 206, 231, 237, 269, 326, 340, 359–360, 370, 373, 385, 405
Service Class User (SCU), 9, 10, 122, 123, 130, 133, 138, 144, 145, 150, 152, 154, 156, 159, 165, 166, 183, 189, 192, 231, 237, 269, 340, 359–360, 370, 385
Service-Object Pair (SOP), 8, 42, 48, 66, 67, 70, 73, 79, 125, 129–138, 141, 144–147, 149–152, 155, 157, 159, 160, 164, 166, 169–171, 173, 174, 177, 180, 206, 212, 218–220, 222, 224, 226, 227, 231, 256, 268, 351, 356, 359, 360, 383, 385, 391–397, 399
Single value matching, 140, 152, 158
SOP. *See* Service-Object Pair
Spacing between slices, 85, 101
SQ. *See* Sequencing
SR. *See* Structured Report
Storage Commitment, 169–170, 371, 395
Structured Report (SR), 77, 134, 171–173, 228, 258, 260, 270, 295, 323, 347, 353, 354, 370, 398

T
TCP/IP, 96, 117–119, 124, 164, 177, 185, 201, 206, 208, 217, 232, 282, 285, 297, 369
Teleradiology, 39, 86, 161, 177, 207, 235, 252, 273, 281, 331, 374, 383
Temporal imaging, 101, 343–344
Thick client, 308–310, 312
Thin client, 304, 308–311, 387
Transfer Syntax, 52, 75, 113, 178, 179, 184–191, 195, 196, 200, 211, 212, 218–220, 224, 226, 227, 231, 297, 337, 369, 383, 388, 393–394
Transliteration, 37, 68, 348, 349

U
UID. *See* Unique identifier
Unicode, 28, 345, 348
Unique identifier (UID), 33, 41, 42, 48, 64–67, 70, 71, 73, 125, 129, 130, 132–137, 141, 142, 144–147, 151–153, 155, 157–160, 169, 180, 182, 185, 187, 189, 192, 219, 220, 222, 224–227, 229, 244, 256, 259, 293, 359, 370, 383, 391–400
Universal matching, 139, 140
Upper Layer, 117, 177, 196, 369
User Information Item, 191–193, 200

V
Value Representation (VR), 7, 31, 32, 34–38, 40–52, 54, 55, 57–59, 61, 65, 67, 73, 82, 85, 87, 118, 123, 125–128, 135, 136, 139, 140, 144, 145, 148, 155, 159, 160, 163, 177, 183–185, 189, 196, 211, 218–221, 229, 237, 245, 321, 343, 344, 347, 365–367, 370, 391–393, 401–409
Verification. *See* C-Echo
Video, 16, 63, 74, 76, 85, 99, 111–114, 117, 132, 233, 260, 261, 282–284, 304, 368, 376, 397
VR. *See* Value Representation

W

WADO. *See* Web Access to DICOM Persistent Objects
Waveforms, 77, 107–108, 132, 134, 171, 228, 369, 396, 397
Web Access to DICOM Persistent Objects (WADO), 293, 296, 369, 370
Wildcards, 38, 40, 62, 139–141, 221, 365
Working Group (WG), 22, 24, 297

X

XML, 21, 30, 44, 58, 60, 241, 295, 296, 322, 323, 365, 368–371

Z

ZIP, 81, 87, 93, 203, 211, 236, 237, 246, 284, 297, 302, 383

Printing: Ten Brink, Meppel, The Netherlands
Binding: Stürtz, Würzburg, Germany